A CAREGIVER'S GUIDE TO DEMENTIA

An Unintended Journey

JANET YAGODA SHAGAM

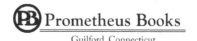
Prometheus Books

Guilford, Connecticut

Prometheus Books

An imprint of Globe Pequot, the trade division of
The Rowman & Littlefield Publishing Group, Inc.
4501 Forbes Blvd., Ste. 200
Lanham, MD 20706
PrometheusBooks.com

Distributed by NATIONAL BOOK NETWORK

British Library Cataloguing in Publication Information Available

Library of Congress Cataloging-in-Publication Data

Names: Shagam, Janet Yagoda, author.
Title: A caregiver's guide to dementia : an unintended journey / Janet
   Yagoda Shagam.
Description: Lanham, MD : Prometheus, [2021] | Includes bibliographical
   references and index. | Summary: "This book is designed to address the
   needs and challenges faced by adult children and other family members
   who are scrambling to make sense of what is happening to themselves and
   the loved ones with dementia in their care. It covers the basics of
   dementia as a brain disorder, its accompanying behaviors, the procedures
   used to diagnose and stage the disease, and the legal aspects of
   providing care for an adult who is no longer competent. Other topics
   covered include family dynamics, caregiver burnout, elder abuse,
   incontinence, finances and paying for care, the challenges same-sex
   families face, and coping with the eventuality of death and estate
   management"—Provided by publisher.
Identifiers: LCCN 2021007322 (print) | LCCN 2021007323 (ebook) | ISBN
   9781633886940 (paperback) | ISBN 9781633886957 (epub)
Subjects: LCSH: Dementia—Patients—Care. | Dementia—Patients—Family
   relationships. | Caregivers.
Classification: LCC RC521 .S53 2021 (print) | LCC RC521 (ebook) | DDC
   616.8/31—dc23
LC record available at https://lccn.loc.gov/2021007322
LC ebook record available at https://lccn.loc.gov/2021007323

CONTENTS

FOREWORD

When the author's mother began to show signs of dementia, Janet Yagoda Shagam had no idea where that journey was going to take her. It was a path unrealized and not one she could have ever imagined.

Many of us find ourselves in that same position. We stumble along caring for our loved one without the time or energy to learn how and what to do.

The author provides us with a comprehensive and easy-to-read book that begins with the first inklings that dementia may have entered your day. Other chapters contain the information caregivers need to understand and manage the behaviors associated with the various kinds of dementia. She also offers tips on communicating with health care providers, suggestions on how to find suitable caregiving arrangements and financial resources, and, perhaps most important, ideas on ways to prevent family conflict. Basically, the author takes readers from diagnosis to settling the estate.

The beauty of *A Caregiver's Guide to Dementia: An Unintended Journey* is that it helps family caregivers navigate day-to-day challenges and develop strategies to reduce the impact of ongoing stress on their physical and mental health.

As a practicing clinical psychologist, I often recommend *A Caregiver's Guide to Dementia* to those clients struggling with the practical and emotional aspects of having become a family caregiver. Many of them report that the opening chapter and the chapter vignettes helped them understand they are not alone. The worksheets and reflective writing prompts at the end of each chapter helped them organize their thoughts and observations, as well as evaluate their strategies to prevent or reduce difficulties.

I remember trying to introduce my own mother, who was incapable of living alone, to her new residential facility. It took many trips to the assisted living facility, when the two of us sat outside and looked at the beautiful lawn and flowers, before I could get her to venture inside. When we finally made the move, she was angry and tearful, and she screamed at me as I walked away.

It was such a joy and relief when one day, after one of our frequent outings, she looked at me, smiled, and said, "I'm tired. I'd like to go home now." She meant her new home.

In this second edition, the author provides updated information about ways to create a healthy diet that matches the ability of a loved one to make safe choices, feed herself, and eventually, when the ability to chew and swallow diminishes, make the transition to handfeeding.

We come to know the differences among treatment, palliative care, and hospice, as well as how each of these choices may impact your life and the family member in your care.

In *The Caregiver's Guide to Dementia*, you will find current information regarding eligibility and access to Medicare, Medicaid, and Veterans Administration benefits. The ability to navigate these complex resources saves time and reduces frustration and stress.

Because of our ongoing COVID-19 pandemic, infection control—at home and in care facilities—has become an especially important topic. The author, a former microbiologist, presents simple ways to reduce the transmission of infectious illness between you and your loved one, as well as to other family members and the public.

I, both as a clinician and caretaker, was often struck with the honesty of Shagam's own emotions and those of others in her vignettes, which include anger, irritation, hopelessness, and oftentimes humor and fun. Her workarounds were absolutely ingenious and certainly give the reader creative problem-solving ideas.

A Caregiver's Guide to Dementia, beautifully written, is a thoughtful and comprehensive book that can make a bumpy road easier to travel.

Mary Ann Conley, PhD

FOREWORD

The fact that you're reading this book is a sign that you're already in a better position than I was when my wife, Ginny, started showing signs of dementia. At the time, I was unaware of what lay ahead of us and how all-encompassing caring for a loved one living with dementia can be.

We were having marital problems, and I was on the verge of asking for a divorce. I did not realize the behaviors affecting our marriage were some of the first signs of her dementia.

For example, we visited an Indian restaurant that we had been to a few times before. I recognized the hostess and called her by name. My wife questioned how I knew her. Ginny then said she'd never been to this restaurant and I must have been with another woman!

During this time, we were seeing a family therapist to help sort out things in our marriage. This, as it turned out, was a fortuitous first step. The therapist suggested that something else was the root of our difficulties. Our next step was an appointment with our primary care physician. The eventual diagnosis of dementia led to a years-long journey for the both of us.

The road to a diagnosis can be frustrating and complicated. Caring for a loved one living with dementia can last for many years or decades.

While Ginny was getting worked up from a medical perspective, I thought about her future care needs. I contacted a respected and nearby home care agency to get a home care aide to help out for a couple of hours a week and when I was away on business trips. Over time, we found many wonderful home companions.

But as time moved on, Ginny's needs increased and bigger decisions had to be made. I consulted with an eldercare attorney to help plan for the time when Ginny needed more care than I could provide at home.

This experience, though it ended up being a good one, started out a bit shaky. One of the lawyers I met with admitted that he was still relatively new to eldercare law. I was cautious, and he was empathetic. And after interviewing several other eldercare attorneys, I felt I trusted him so I took the risk and hired him.

As Ginny's dementia progressed and her safety at home became worrisome, I made the difficult decision to move her to a dementia care community.

The community I found provided a high level of care. Today the industry buzzword is *person-centered*, a caregiving concept that focuses on the resident's individual's needs. Of course, respect and dignity are part of the equation.

The benefits were many. Ginny could continue to engage in her favorite activities as well as socialize with people other than myself and her home care aide. Most important, it seemed like a weight was lifted off *her* shoulders, and not just mine. She just brightened and became more animated.

Years later, her dementia progressed to the point when it became necessary to consider hospice. I felt totally unprepared for what hospice means and the kinds of places that *are* hospices. I discovered many care communities will not, or cannot, honor your loved one's end-of-life wishes.

So even though hospice has general guidelines about the person's end-of-life wishes, the care community often controls the process. Knowing this type of information ahead of time can be extremely helpful.

It took several moves before I found a hospice willing and able to honor the wishes Ginny had expressed many years before.

As it turned out, Ginny was best served at a free-standing residential hospice. This hospice both recognized and understood Ginny's needs. It was emotionally hard for both of us, but it was a beautiful, loving, and meaningful way for us to say our good-byes.

In the first edition, Janet Yagoda Shagam very successfully translates her personal experiences with her mother living with dementia into a meaningful and authoritative guide. The information she provided was spot on.

While she maintains the personal theme, the second edition of *A Caregiver's Guide to Dementia: An Unintended Journey* contains updated information regarding new ways to predict and test for Alzheimer's disease, recent changes that define eligibility for services like hospice, and the ins and outs of Medicare, Medicaid, Social Security, and Veteran benefits. Most important, she has included timely information about infection control in assisted living facilities, as well as predatory fraud, scams, and elder abuse.

The second chapter "Together" contains several fictionalized vignettes based on interviews with families who experienced, or are experiencing, their unintended journey.

You will meet a sandwich-generation daughter caught between meeting her mother's needs while, at the same time, juggling her job and three adolescent children. You also meet husbands, sons, sons-in-law, several marrieds, and a sister.

Perhaps you will find yourself nodding in agreement over familiar and shared experiences.

I was so impressed with the first edition of the book that I contacted Janet. Since then, we have enjoyed many fruitful discussions and have completed several successful projects.

This updated version will prepare readers to proactively navigate the many unknowns along the road ahead for family members and their loved ones living together with dementia.

Kevin Jameson
Founder, President, CEO, and Volunteer
Dementia Society of America

Kevin Jameson is founder of the Dementia Society of America, a nationwide, all-volunteer nonprofit dedicated to increasing dementia awareness and support services to family members.

INTRODUCTION

The purpose of this book, *A Caregiver's Guide to Dementia: An Unintended Journey*, is to help family caregivers—and others, too—navigate the challenges and personal growth experiences that dementia care can bring.

Many of you are the adult child of a widowed parent. Others of you step in to help parents age safely at home or to give a brother or sister the support they need. A few of you are one of those extraordinary friends or neighbors who really mean it when you say, "Tell me what you need," and "How can I help?"

You will notice that throughout the book I call my mother "Dorothy." Using her first name gives me the ability to write objectively and make *A Caregiver's Guide to Dementia* more than just my story. In that way, Dorothy is your mother, sister, aunt, husband, or any other person in your life who has dementia.

Without question, providing care for a person who has dementia is a life-altering experience. It's impossible to emerge at the other end without a profound respect for those things that make us human and, even more specifically, for those subtle characteristics that make us the person we are.

Well, it's time to get started. I hope what you read in the following chapters will make it easier for you to be the caregiver for the person with whom you share a lifetime of memories.

1

MY UNINTENDED JOURNEY

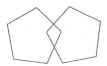

Woman, age seventy-two, pentagon.

This book is about my mother and our journey through dementia. It was a trip neither of us had planned on taking together.

Dorothy Yagoda was a furiously independent woman with an inordinately strong sense of privacy. Concern about how she might appear to others made it impossible for her to share intimacies with friends or to have frank conversations with her doctors and family. Everything was just fine until it wasn't. By that time, Dorothy could no longer make competent decisions or even comprehend that things were not okay.

It's hard to say when dementia became bigger than her quirky and difficult personality. Did the first sign occur when, in her mid-sixties, she was certain that family members were spreading lies? Was it ten years later when she informed me, that because of my presumed disloyalty, she would never speak to me again? Or was it a few years after that when she was unable to follow her doctor's written colonoscopy preparation directions? Maybe her inability to use the phone book was an early indication of cognitive decline.

Perhaps the first sign of dementia was her propensity to open cereal boxes from the bottom.

A few months after Dorothy's death, I asked the members of her neighborhood book club when they first saw changes. Looking back, they said, it must have been about twelve years earlier when she brought a reference book for them to consider for their next reading.

It is easy to explain the odd behaviors of people you see frequently without considering dementia. This is especially true when there are no big or sudden personality changes. The person is the same—only more so. You think, "This is just what happens when people get old."

Dementia slowly and silently crept into our family life. Without realizing it, we made accommodations to avoid confrontations and misunderstandings. We got into the habit of keeping conversations short and simple and never telling Dorothy about plans until the last moment. We expected to have to explain things to her over and over again. By the same token, we got used to hearing slightly muddled information from her over and over again.

Dorothy was very good at giving plausible reasons to explain strange situations. The print in the phone book was too small, we had forgotten what she had said, or she fell because a nameless woman pushed her off the stairs. Dorothy was an expert at inventing her own reality and shifting the responsibility for her misinterpretations to others.

Her fall, in combination with osteoporosis and compressed vertebrae, caused pain that intensified to the point where Dorothy could no longer walk. A three-week hospitalization to reduce back pain and inflammation and several more weeks in a rehabilitation facility did get her back on her feet; however, the time in unfamiliar surroundings made Dorothy increasingly confused, belligerent, and combative. An evaluation of her memory and ability to make decisions showed that she could no longer live in her home without assistance. Incontinence, a problem we had long suspected, was another difficulty she could no longer hide. The doctors suggested that we place her in a nursing home. One doctor told Dorothy she needed to use a walker. Her response: "I'd rather kill myself."

It didn't take long to see that a nursing home wasn't the right place for her. Based on discussions with other family members, and against the advice of a medical social worker, I agreed to take on the major responsibility of moving Dorothy back to her house and overseeing her care. It seemed like the right thing to do, and certainly it would be better for her and possibly easier for me.

Getting the house ready for her arrival was revealing. It was sad to find the soiled underwear she had hidden in the bathroom. It was frightening to discover a melted tea kettle and numerous blackened pots and pans concealed behind less damaged cookware. And it was unsettling to think about my future and my ability to keep up with work, my home, and the possibility of ever again having any free time.

I wrote this book as both a daughter who needs to tell her story and a medical writer who knows there is a story to tell. Of Dorothy's two children, I am the youngest. And as is often the case, the responsibility of caring for a family member who has dementia often falls on the shoulders of one person.

The reasons are many. Location—some family members live too far away to take on the responsibility of daily care. Others have their own problems that take precedence. And some don't know how to care.

I'm not sure when my role as a caregiver first started. By some criteria, it might have happened when the death of my father required that I take on responsibilities beyond my thirteen years. Maybe caregiving began in 1988 when my mother opted to move roughly a mile from my house rather than to the city where her other daughter lived. Maybe it began when a daily phone conversation was my solution to maintaining Dorothy's emotional stability. And without question, my life as a dementia caregiver began in summer 2007, when a nameless woman became Dorothy's scapegoat for anything that defied explanation.

My personal story is a real one. It's painful. It's exhausting. My story also describes a process rich in personal growth. And yes, if I knew then what I know now, I'd do it again; however, unlike my first experience, I would know how to handle many of the situations that make dementia challenging. I would also know to take better care of myself.

Dementia care is a hazardous occupation. In addition to learning how to safely transfer an uncooperative adult into and out of a bathtub, studies show that family caregivers are at increased risk for depression, anxiety, heart disease, and stroke. The same studies show that elderly dementia caregivers are more likely to die than people of the same age who aren't responsible for another's care.

As dementia progresses, it gets more and more difficult to see your family member and dementia as separate entities. Dementia robs people of their education, careers, and their personal history; however, as a matter of respect to the person you once knew, you do your best to remember them as people of accomplishment who at one time could smile, crack a joke, or maybe make a homemade pie.

Because I owe you more than just my story, you will read about the experiences of other family caregivers. Some of them, rather than taking care of a parent, are responsible for a grandparent, aunt, uncle, or perhaps a sibling, spouse, or partner.

You can take advantage of the research I accumulated in my role as a medical writer that I had neither the time nor the fortitude to do while being an active caregiver. You will learn to think ahead and make arrangements to become your parent's power of attorney (POA) or, if necessary, their guardian and conservator. You will also read about the advantages and disadvantages of hiring agency caregivers as well as learn how to find helpful community resources. Other topics, such as behavior management, food, clothing and bathing issues, medication, and the eventual need for palliative and hospice care, will also be presented in a sensitive and approachable manner.

At the other end, when death overtakes dementia's hold, you will read about a new journey—the transition from caregiver to mourner and estate manager. The end result is a book that I hope will give you the emotional support and the practical information you need to make healthful and meaningful decisions for yourself and the family member in your care. But before you get started, take a look at table 1.1—and then look at it again on those unbearably long and difficult days.

Table 1.1.   A Caregiver's Ten Commandments

I must be mindful of my physical and emotional health.
I may accept the assistance of others.
I deserve time for myself.
I give myself permission to delegate tasks.
I recognize it is not always possible to keep my promises.
I recognize it is sometimes necessary to bend the truth.
I am mindful that my feelings of anger, guilt, and depression are normal.
I give myself permission to seek counseling.
I take comfort in knowing I have done the best I can.
I know in my heart that "thank-you" is often spoken without words.

2

TOGETHER

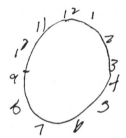

Man, age fifty-six, clock, 9:10 a.m.

Each year, more than sixteen million Americans provide more than 18.5 billion hours of unpaid care for family and friends with Alzheimer's disease and related dementias. Yes, this a very impressive number; however, this very big number doesn't describe the impact dementia and caregiving have on physical and emotional health, family dynamics, and the ability to juggle the responsibilities of family, home, and work. This very big number doesn't have much to do with you and your day.

Soon you will meet people, individuals, who will bravely tell you how dementia changed the way they live. Some stories are remarkably uplifting, and, sadly, some are just the opposite.

Their stories, although true in spirit, are fictionalized here to protect privacy. While each person has a unique story, you will discover that common themes run through their accounts. Perhaps you will even find yourself nodding in agreement over familiar and shared experiences.

DIANE: SOMETIMES THINGS COME IN PAIRS

I could tell by how my mother spoke on the phone that something wasn't right. My father—he didn't sound so good either; however, it was a phone call from one of their neighbors that made it clear that my husband John and I needed to fly to Connecticut.

It was kind of a shock. The house was messy with dirty clothes on the floor, an unmade bed, and a stinky bathroom. I cannot tell you how much that is unlike my neatnik mother.

My father, even though it was late afternoon, was still in his pajamas. In fact, it looked like he hadn't gotten dressed in several days. He smelled like he needed a shower. His feet were swollen.

John and I looked at each other, and without even saying a word, we knew some big decisions were just over the horizon.

During dinner, we discussed our options. Should we move my parents from their condominium into a local assisted living facility? Maybe having them live with us was a better solution. Eventually, we decided our best option was to move them into an assisted living facility near our home. It was obvious that having them nearby would make everything so much easier. That meant no more long-distance caregiving plus the ability to include them in family activities and celebrations.

It wasn't until my father fell that they were willing to move from the town they had lived for close to fifty years. I guess his fall got both of them scared.

It would take at least a week before their new apartment would be ready. John and I took them shopping so they could pick out dishware and other things to make their apartment feel like home.

Before the week was over, my father was hospitalized—congestive heart failure, they said. Meanwhile, my mother was totally freaking out. She couldn't understand why my father wasn't with her, and she had no idea where she was.

My father—he died in the hospital. Without my father to keep her grounded, my mother quickly worsened. We hoped having her live with us, rather than in the assisted living apartment, would slow her decline. Both of us had recently retired, and we believed taking on this responsibility was doable.

John and I learned to manage her scary hallucinations and the side effects of medications used to quiet them. We installed handrails in the bathroom. Eventually, incontinence became a twenty-four-hour-a-day challenge.

John and I agreed that it was inappropriate for him to help with my mother's personal care. Nevertheless, he was more than willing to do the grocery shopping and many of the chores associated with running our house.

Even though we made a great team, it didn't take long before the combination of exhaustion and the unrelenting stress made it all too easy to get angry with one another.

For everyone's well-being we knew it was time. My mother lived the remainder of her life in a memory care facility. It was a hard decision—but it was the right one.

STEVE: A GOOD MARRIAGE

Margaret—Maggie to me—and I have been married for fifty-four years. Between us we have four wonderful children and nine even more wonderful grandchildren. We share lots of love and respect for each other. By all counts we enjoy a good marriage.

Now Maggie, the person I love, is gone. I no longer see her million-dollar smile, hear her musical laugh, or feel her wonderfully warm hugs. Now she spends most of the day curled up on the couch, face to the wall, and under a favorite blanket.

Her caregivers are wonderful people, and with their help, I can survive the day—and the night, too.

It took this illness to realize how much I depended on Maggie. I now do the grocery shopping. I take care of the laundry and manage to cook simple meals. I hope she can taste love in my attempts to make split pea soup that is as good as hers.

It takes two people to get her in and out of the shower. Her caregiver and I do it together. It takes two people to help her dress. With the help of the caregiver, I have learned how to manage the buttons and hooks that are a part of women's clothing.

Maggie and I still share our bed. I am there to calm frightening dreams. We keep each other warm.

CAROL: MAKE IT RIGHT BEFORE IT IS WRONG

A good friend said, "Make it right before it is wrong." At the time, I didn't understand the wisdom in her statement. Alzheimer's disease was something new to me. My mother, yes, she was a little cranky and forgetful—but nothing terrible. I figured taking responsibility for her care was something I could manage.

My brother said to call whenever I needed an extra hand.

It didn't take long before "a little cranky and forgetful" became "full-time angry and dangerously forgetful." Still, I felt I could manage the situation.

I didn't notice when my watchfulness morphed into devoting the entire day to her care. Running errands with her became impossibly difficult. It was a major accomplishment to get her to doctor appointments without one of us having a major meltdown. Aside from bathroom accidents, her refusal to take a shower, falls, and hallucinations, her mood swings went from angry to inconsolable weeping in seconds. Soon, I was spending the night in her home.

I declined a promotion because it required frequent travel. I still feel bad about that. Aside from a big raise, I missed out on an exciting and interesting opportunity.

It's not that I'm complaining. My mother sacrificed a lot to make sure my brother and I got an education. She didn't have those same opportunities. I am happy to give her the help she needs. All I am saying is that I am exhausted—and I need some help, too.

And my brother—where did he go? He always said that he was too busy, couldn't drop what he was doing, or had long-standing vacation plans. Maybe what he really meant by his seemingly generous offer was I should let him know things had become difficult at Mom's house. Maybe the extra hand wasn't going to be his.

I guess you can tell I am angry. Seething might be a better way to describe how I feel. Even though it's been more than five years since *our* mother's death, I still carry the emotional burden of my brother's behavior.

"Make it right before it is wrong." Now I get it. In the very beginning, my brother and I owed each other a conversation. Maybe, if I had asked, he would have been willing to manage our mother's finances or be responsible for car maintenance. If he really couldn't help he should have said so.

MARC: CARING

I am just beginning to get my head around the fact that my mother has dementia. For so long, my dad and I thought she was having another bout of major depression. That's what her doctors told us. Then they said pseudo-dementia.

Her doctor really didn't explain what pseudo-dementia means. I had to look it up online. The best I can figure is pseudo-dementia seems like dementia, but it only happens to people who are in very deep depression. The doctor told us this was temporary. It sounded like treatment with the right drugs would make her better.

Another doctor told us that my mother, without question, has both—deep depression and Alzheimer's disease. He also said that depression is a risk factor for Alzheimer's disease—and it works the other way around, too.

Her doctor tried many medications, and all seemed to make her worse. Some medications made her totally crazy. Other medications left her confused or anxious, or they turned her into a zombie. When she talks, it's all mixed up. Sometimes she makes up words. It's hard to figure out what she needs or how she is feeling. I hope she can tell I am listening.

Once in a while a sparkle of my ol' mom peaks through the fog. Sometimes it's an "I love you" smile. One time she asked, clear as a bell, "What's for lunch?" That was totally unexpected—and kinda funny, too.

At first, my mother lived in an assisted living facility that looked more like an upscale hotel. As they say, looks can be deceiving. It wasn't a horrible place; it was just that my father and I felt she would do better at home. Our ability to have twenty-four-hour paid care made this possible.

I am self-employed, which gives me the flexibility to stop by for lunch or just to sit with her. While there, I attend to the details of running a house— you know, like paying bills and fixing stuff. My dad is still working. I hope he will retire soon. My wife, a lawyer, pitches in on the weekend. Our teenage daughter needs attention.

My mom is such a kind person. She was our rock. My mom was a medical social worker who made so many people become whole again. She had unfailing love for my father and, of course, her granddaughter and wonderful daughter-in-law.

My mother is suffering. Sometimes I wish I will wake up one morning to hear my father say his lovebird quietly died in her sleep. It's scary to have those thoughts and even scarier to say them out loud. Watching a life unwind can make you think and say things like that.

RUTH: MY FATHER AND HIS SON-IN-LAW

My first husband and my father never got along. I don't know why—they just didn't like each other.

The story completely changed when I married Chuck, a Vietnam-era fighter pilot. My father spent his college years protesting the war. Back in those days, Chuck and my father wouldn't have been friends. Now, they are best buddies. There is great love, respect, and camaraderie between the two. Hard to believe—but lovely to see.

A few years ago, it became obvious my father was becoming forgetful and easily confused. The doctor said, "Alzheimer's disease"; however, she felt that with minimal assistance Dad could continue living in his apartment. That was until he had a stroke.

The stroke made it hard for my dad to communicate, let alone get out of bed without assistance. No discussion needed—my father came to live with us.

Then incontinence became an issue. Incontinence is something I am sure is difficult for everyone, and especially for a father's daughter. I didn't have to ask. Chuck took care of that. I guess their years of love and respect made it possible.

PRICILLA: MY LOVE

Twenty years ago I met the love of my life. I don't know, maybe God brought the two of us to this small Colorado town. For the most part, Danielle and I kept to ourselves. The stares and comments made doing something as simple as going to the grocery store difficult.

I wish others could just see two people who love one another and not transgender freaks.

Then came two diagnoses. Danielle had stage 4 colorectal cancer. Another doctor told us I was beginning to show signs of dementia.

Maybe that's why I am always getting lost.

Those most awful moments made our love even stronger. Maybe the Good Lord was testing us.

Neither Danielle nor I have blood family. My parents, now deceased, booted me out years ago. With the exception of one brother, my siblings disappeared. I haven't seen my brother in more than twenty-five years, but on rare occasions he does call. My grandchildren have never met their grandfather, and I suspect my great-grandchildren don't know I exist.

It's a little different for Danielle. She and her wife never divorced. Danielle's children do remember their father and send birthday cards. Danielle, when necessary, could make herself appear like the person whose former life never felt like the right one.

Okay—too much about this stuff. You asked about how we, a transgender couple, managed in the world of straight-person medical care.

To make things easier for herself, Danielle morphed back to David, the person who appeared on her driver's license. Of course, she was still my Danielle, but to her oncologist and surgeon she was David. I guess they pretended not to see her other surgery. Maybe they thought Dave's strange-looking companion was the kindly neighbor lady who often forgot to bring Danielle (David to them) to her appointments. I have to say everyone was respectful.

Danielle died 372 days after her diagnosis.

My friend—my friend-family—helped me find this new apartment. It's funny. No more trips to the grocery store. Now, all I have to do is walk down the hall to get my dinner.

LINDA: BETWIXT AND BETWEEN

My mother was forty years old when I was born. My sister, thirteen years older than me, was a college freshman the same year I entered kindergarten. Sounds strange, but even though we had the same parents, the both of us were "only" children.

I wanted to be a young mother, and by the time I was thirty-five, I had three children. The eldest was in sixth grade, and my mother was a widow.

I don't know if it was my father's death or something else that made my mother seem so different. My kids no longer wanted to go to her house. They said Grandma smells bad. My eldest, now in high school, told me Grandma made some awful-tasting muffins—like she had mixed up the salt and sugar.

My mother calls me all day long. She needs help with this, she cannot find that, and someone stole her keys. I am pretty sure she has dementia.

I do the best I can to help her. But geez—I have a job, and on the weekends it's soccer, music lessons, and scouts. I am spread so thin I feel invisible.

I am the caregiver for my elderly mother and the mother of three teenaged children. I guess that makes me a member of the sandwich generation.

JUDY: WIFE AND CAREGIVER

Just three years ago, like two adventuresome kids, we took off for a world tour. No travel agent, no package deal—just Bill and me and two backpacks. The only hard part was finding a house sitter who wasn't allergic to cats.

We did it fifty years ago, so why not do it one more time?

Now, Bill is angry with me. He says there is nothing wrong even though his doctor says otherwise.

While Bill got dressed, Dr. Blake and I chatted in a private area near his examination room. Dr. Blake was confident Bill was close to mid-stage Alzheimer's disease. He suggested that Bill see a neurologist for more testing.

Of course, Bill refused. I told him to just go to this other doctor so he could prove me wrong. Nothing better than an "I told you so!"

Well, I guessed right: "I told you so" was his answer.

Since then, things have gotten worse. I try to keep Bill busy. He helps me make dinner and does attempt to clean up afterward. That's okay; however, I do wish he would put things away in a place where I can find them later. Sometimes it's so strange, it's funny.

He wanders around the house trying to fix things that aren't broken. Now, none of the door knobs work.

Bill does like to use the gym at the City Multigenerational Center. But, because of COVID-19, it's closed. We cannot go out for lunch nor do any of those other things to help break up the day. We are totally stuck in the house. I wish I could spend an hour reading a book.

I am so glad we took that crazy trip. Those memories are what keep me going.

CAROLYN: MISS GOLD DUST EYES

It's not fair to say my brother Everett was a womanizer. But there were lots of women in his life. Three marriages produced five daughters. In between the marriages, there were several partners. One of them I call Miss Gold Dust Eyes.

She was beautiful in a Barbie doll kind of way, and my brother loved showing her off. It was all very odd as my Everett was a flannel shirt guy who loved to build furniture.

Maybe Barbie would have been a better name, but it was money—not the flannel shirt guy—she wanted.

Miss Gold Dust Eyes showed up between wife number two and wife number three. She stayed with Everett long enough to get mixed up in his bank accounts. Sometimes she contributed to paying the utility bills. Then she took off with another man.

Wife number three and I got along well enough to call each other by name. Cindy was good to my brother. Most of all she was patient and able to manage his increasingly odd behavior.

Cindy called to tell me Everett saw big-eyed bunnies with blood dripping from their mouths. He was terrified they'd bite him while he was sleeping.

Cindy asked if I would help her make next-step decisions. A week-long visit lasted nearly two months.

The doctor felt that, because of the hallucinations, Everett probably had dementia with Lewy bodies. I'd never heard of that one before. His doctor wrote a prescription for Risperdal. He thought that might stop Everett from seeing things.

Then wife number two showed up. On her own, she decided Everett was taking too much Risperdal.

I already knew that Everett had named me as his durable and health care power of attorney (POA). What I didn't know was that he had also named his daughter from his first marriage. She and I made it work. And in the end, it was helpful to have my niece in charge after I returned home.

Everett died in 2012—five years after his diagnosis. Now, it's 2020. We are still trying to settle his estate. Miss Gold Dust Eyes claims she is Everett's common-law wife and therefore owns the house.

Thank God wife number one is the executrix of the estate.

LYNN: THE RIGHT WORDS

I just got off the phone. The lady up the street died. Weird, but I already knew that. I was thinking about her just a few days ago. I wondered if her family would call as it has been many years since we visited.

Receiving this kind of news always takes one back to another time and place.

I had a favorite dress—my hieroglyphics dress. The pattern was just like the ones that decorate the inside of a pharaoh's tomb. Back in those days, I dreamed of becoming an Egyptologist. I wore that dress until the waist moved several inches above mine. It was a nerdy dress by any measure, and the kids at school made sure I knew that.

Out of the blue, the lady up the street said she liked my dress. I don't know if she *really* liked my dress. But you know what? It doesn't matter.

Dementia robs people of their memories. But many of those memories are yours to keep.

3

WHAT'S GOING ON?

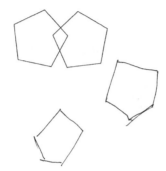

Woman, age seventy-eight, pentagon.

When I was a child, one of my favorite things was hearing Dorothy's stories about the old days. I learned that at one time all cars were black, chicken was very expensive, and only rich people had store-bought clothes.

Dorothy was born in 1911. She was seven years old when the flu of 1918 entered her home. My grandmother stayed up all night taking care of Dorothy, as well as her two sisters and four brothers. She checked their temperature, gave cool baths to reduce fever, and made a paste out of mustard and water to make it easier to breathe. Dorothy said her mother applied the mixture, called mustard plaster, on their chests. It was hot and, if left on too long, caused skin burns. Unlike many other families, everyone in Dorothy's household survived.

In 1918, doctors understood that an unidentified microbe was the cause of this frightening illness; however, when it came to behavioral illnesses, it would be many years before clinicians understood the physical connection between the brain and behavior. Clinicians, well up through the 1950s, thought many kinds of "insanity" were the person's fault and a sign of weakness.

Dementia was considered a behavioral condition that affected older people. Even with Alois Alzheimer's 1906 discovery of the brain changes that we now associate with Alzheimer's disease, many clinicians did not link one to the other.

As a young woman, Dorothy was a histopathologist at the New York Cancer Hospital. She could see the cellular changes that accompanied lung cancer. Even back then, there was the feeling that smoking caused lung cancer. Nevertheless, she, like many others, believed dementia was largely a behavioral malady. That my grandmother, Dorothy's mother-in-law, often wandered away from home was somehow related to her emigration from Eastern Europe. And many years later, when a good family friend could no longer live safely at home, Dorothy said it was because her recently widowed friend had been too dependent on her husband.

I don't believe Dorothy knew anyone who had what we call dementia. But she did know people who, through their own failings, could no longer take care of themselves.

Now medical imaging assessments, as well as laboratory studies, unquestionably link brain changes to illnesses such as schizophrenia and depression—and, yes, to the many kinds of dementia.

DEMENTIA IS A SYNDROME

A syndrome? Yes. Dementia is a syndrome because dementia is a collection of identifying signs and symptoms. The operative word is *collection*. For example, memory and word loss, as well as diminished ability to perform complex tasks, are symptoms all forms of dementia have in common.

If you have reason to read this book, you are probably already aware of the ten warning signs of dementia. These ten warning signs are the collection of the in-common symptoms. The ten warning signs do not identify a specific kind of dementia (see table 3.1).

Characteristic brain changes and reactions to certain medications can differentiate Alzheimer's disease from other kinds of dementia such dementia with Lewy bodies.

Other kinds of dementia include vascular dementia, frontotemporal dementia, and dementia with Lewy bodies. Many people, particularly those who are very old, have mixed dementia or dementia caused by more than one kind of brain disease. Because it often requires an autopsy to make a confirmed diagnosis, many health care providers simply say "senile dementia" to cover all possibilities.

WHY DOES IT MATTER?

Hearing that your family member has dementia is hard enough. But the other parts—it's progressive and incurable—can make you wonder why it is important to know dementia is an umbrella term for more than one disease. As it turns out, the different dementias do not take the same path as they progress from beginning to end. For example, delusions and hallucinations tend to occur in mid- to late-stage Alzheimer's disease but are an early symptom of dementia with Lewy bodies. It is also true that some medications that relieve Alzheimer's symptoms can worsen symptoms associated with other types of dementia; therefore, knowing about the different kinds of dementia can give a forewarning of expectations and needs, give your family member with dementia the opportunity to talk about their care and end-of-life wishes, and help them take advantage of the medications and clinical studies that may relieve symptoms and improve quality of life.

CLINICAL STUDIES

Clinical studies related to dementia include a wide range of subjects. As expected, investigations to assess the ability of medication to slow the progression of Alzheimer's disease or modify behavior are the majority.

Other studies include patients who also take medications for other conditions. In this case, these studies determine if the combination improves, worsens, or has no effect on the patient's health.

In addition to behavioral studies, researchers are interested in the effects of medication on brain function. These investigations usually require a long-term commitment and willingness to donate one's brain for inclusion into a research brain bank.

Before becoming a study subject, the individual must be competent and able to understand the requirements of the study. In addition, the research project itself undergoes a rigorous evaluation to ensure both its safety and merit. You can learn more about research safety on the Office for Human Research Protections website.

Quality of life is another area of active research. Here, the emphasis is on the effect of such things as art, music, or gardening programs on patient behavior. You might be interested to know that quality-of-life studies also include caregivers. These studies focus on ways to reduce stress and improve resiliency.

Not everyone may join a clinical trial. Many dementia studies require that the participant not have any other illnesses, such as diabetes or cancer.

Others may state age requirements or distance from the research site. Other factors include assurances that the participant can follow directions or that there is a family member or another person who can monitor the participant and take responsibility for transportation.

Doing an internet search using the keywords "clinical trial" and "dementia"—and perhaps the location and type of dementia—will link you to many studies. Your doctor and the Alzheimer's Association are other resources. In addition, you can inquire at local medical research facilities, such as those located in teaching hospitals.

MEMORY AND AGING

It can be difficult to separate the normal aging process from conditions where age, in combination with genetics, lifestyle, and environmental exposures, is a risk factor. Examples of truly age-related changes include thinning and graying hair, sagging skin, and alterations in vision, hearing, and taste. Other changes, such as incontinence and certain types of memory loss, are not a normal part of aging.

Memory is the ability to retrieve information from specific areas of the brain. Long-term memory is classified into two types: declarative and nondeclarative. Declarative memory, based on conscious recall, is the storage and retrieval of learned facts and associated memories. For example, we learned in school that Washington, DC, is the capital of the United States. And because of a childhood family vacation we also remember that Washington, DC, summers are hot and humid. The ability to remember facts and past experiences allows us to use "our mind's eye" and travel back and forth in time.

Nondeclarative, or implicit, memory is our collection of learned skills and procedures. Riding a bicycle, typing, and tying shoelaces are implicit memories because we can do these tasks without thinking about the process. The ability to retrieve and use our store of "built-in" skills allows us to live independently.

When disease processes affect our declarative and nondeclarative memory banks, we may forget our address or our birth date, and we may no longer remember how to drive to the store or prepare dinner. When we lose access to our collection of learned information and built-in skills and procedures, we require assistance to live safely at home.

Other terms used to describe memory include *working memory* and *remote memory*. Working memory is the ability to retain small bits of recently learned information, such as phone numbers, login codes, and street addresses. In contrast, remote memory is the ability to access events that occurred in the distant past, such as the Kent State riots.

The normal aging process may affect memory by changing the way the brain stores and retrieves information. While normal aging does not affect long-term memory, it may affect short-term memory by making it difficult to remember such things as the name of a new acquaintance. Occasional word-recall lapses are another symptom of normal aging (see worksheet 3.1).

Memory problems that aren't a normal part of aging include the following:

Experiencing frequent memory problems
Forgetting how to do things
Having difficulty learning new information or skills
Repeating questions and conversations
Having difficulty making decisions
Experiencing difficulty handling money
Losing track of daily events

MILD COGNITIVE IMPAIRMENT

The forgetfulness associated with normal aging includes minor lapses like misplacing a pair of reading glasses or forgetting a website login. Conversely, having continuous problems with remembering doctor appointments or regularly scheduled social events, or having significant word-finding difficulties may be more serious than the memory gaps associated with normal aging.

Mild cognitive impairment affects approximately one out of five people aged seventy or older. Studies show that mild cognitive impairment is a risk factor associated with Alzheimer's disease. Each year, approximately 10 to 15 percent of individuals who have mild cognitive impairment progress to Alzheimer's disease. But some people who have mild cognitive impairment remain stable, and a few may improve.

People who have mild cognitive impairment may seem quite normal and have adequate life skills. Sometimes a family member or coworker may notice memory difficulties. For those who have mild cognitive impairment, the outcome of tests used to evaluate their cognition may be slightly lower than for people of the same age and background.

Recognizing that mild cognitive impairment often transitions to early Alzheimer's disease makes differentiating this condition from normal aging especially important. In addition to giving patients the opportunity to participate in the clinical trials designed to determine if newly developed drugs or other treatments can delay or prevent dementia, early diagnosis also gives patients and their families the time to plan for future health care needs (see Helpful Resources).

ALZHEIMER'S DISEASE

Alzheimer's disease is the most common kind of dementia. Researchers estimate that as many as five million people living in the United States have this type of dementia. Although scientists have found various genetic and environmental factors that may increase the likelihood of having Alzheimer's disease, age is the most important risk factor.

In the United States, about 1 out of every 20 men and women between the ages of sixty-five and seventy-four have Alzheimer's disease. The frequency for this disease nearly doubles every five years beyond age sixty-five. Researchers believe that nearly half of all people older than eighty-five may be in various stages of the disease. According to the Centers for Disease Control and Prevention, Alzheimer's disease is the fifth most frequent cause of death for adults aged sixty-five years and older.

While it is hard to say what actually causes Alzheimer's disease, we do know the deposition and accumulation of fibrous proteins in the brain accompanies irreversible brain damage. These insoluble proteins form β–amyloid plaques that disrupt brain architecture, alter how brain cells use energy, and promote cell death. The result is a slow and progressive decline in memory, thinking, and reasoning skills. Eventually people lose the ability to swallow and breathe in a coordinated fashion. Pneumonia is often the cause of death when Alzheimer's patients inhale food into their lungs.

Alzheimer's disease comprises a spectrum rather than a defined set of characteristics. People who have Alzheimer's disease do not decline at the same rate and often may express a collection of behaviors associated with one or more different stages. Therefore, the amount and type of caregiving depends on many factors that include their safety and your ability to meet their needs or to find and pay for caregivers. Life expectancy after an Alzheimer's diagnosis can be anywhere from four to twenty years. Often people die from other causes, such as cancer, kidney failure, and cardiovascular disease.

At first, Alzheimer's disease signs and symptoms are subtle and hard to differentiate from normal aging; however, eventually, people become more debilitated and lose the ability to live without assistance.

Be sure to communicate your concerns and observations to other members of your family. Eventually, you may need their support when discussing

Table 3.1.   The Ten Warning Signs of Alzheimer's Disease

Signs	Examples
Memory loss that disrupts daily life	Forgetting important dates or events; asking for the same information many times; depending on others to do things once done without assistance
Difficulty in making plans and following directions	Having a hard time running errands or doing simple math, such as making change or following a recipe
Difficulty in completing familiar tasks	Forgetting how to knit or use woodworking tools
Confusion with time or place	Losing track of time, dates, seasons; being unable to drive to a familiar location
Trouble understanding visual images and spatial relationships	Experiencing difficulty in judging distance and interpreting facial expressions
New problems with finding words and conversation	Having trouble following a conversation; making inappropriate comments; repeating conversations; using made-up words to cover for lost words
Tendency to misplace things and the inability to use logic to find them	Putting things in odd places (e.g., leaving a pair of scissors in the refrigerator); being unable to retrace steps to find things like missing keys
Increased poor judgment	Giving charge card numbers to phone solicitors
Withdrawal from work or social activities	Losing interest in hobbies and social activities
Changes in mood or personality	Experiencing confusion, belligerence, and/or depression; exaggerating former personality traits

memory difficulties with your parent/other family member and their doctor (see table 3.1).

After reading table 3.1, you might think, "How are these behaviors different from what everyone does at one time or another?" The difference is the frequency and the ability to make self-corrections.

Everyone misplaces their car keys; however, unlike a person who has Alzheimer's disease, we know we did get home so the keys must be somewhere in the house. We may then recall rushing to answer the phone or leaving a heavy bundle on the washing machine. Retracing our steps, we find the car keys in our coat pocket, on a table, or in the laundry room. A person who has Alzheimer's disease cannot do this. Instead, they assume their keys were stolen or, when found, purposely hidden.

Dorothy had many of the Alzheimer's warning signs. She often called to tell me that numbers were missing from the phone book. Frequently, she gave my phone number, rather than hers, as a callback number. One incident that still stands out today involves Dorothy's difficulty in understanding her sense of place.

Walking together from the parking lot, she complained that I had parked too far away from the store. A few moments later, a tree blocked her vision, and she turned to me and said, "The store isn't here. Where are you taking me?" What is striking is that this event occurred many years before dementia was something we even thought about.

Health care providers often use staging to describe the progression and severity of diseases such as cancer, kidney failure, and dementia. Slow progression, rather than sudden change, is often the key to differentiating Alzheimer's behaviors from those associated with other kinds of dementia. The following staging criteria will help you understand your family member's condition and plan for future caregiving needs.

Mild or Early-Stage Alzheimer's Disease

In this first stage, people experience memory loss, have difficulty remembering newly learned information, and have trouble completing complex tasks like planning a family event. Personality changes such as uncharacteristic anger, increasing difficulty in finding the right words, getting lost, or misplacing items are other common signs. With help, your family member may still be capable of independent living.

Moderate or Mid-stage Alzheimer's Disease

During this phase, people may confuse family members with close friends, forget personal history details like where they went to school or where they were born, and need help with dressing and personal hygiene. Some people may become restless, suspicious of others, and confrontational. At this stage, your family member will need close supervision and assistance during the day and perhaps a caregiver during the night.

Severe or Late-Stage Alzheimer's Disease

During this last stage, people lose the ability to speak coherently and need help with eating, dressing, using the bathroom, and walking. Eventually, late-stage Alzheimer's patients lose the ability to swallow and control their bladder and bowels. During this final stage, the individual will need 24/7 care either at home or in a dementia care facility.

While staging Alzheimer's disease can help you make day-to-day decisions, it isn't a confirmed diagnosis. Today, a postmortem inspection of the brain, as well as using a microscope to see the presence of brain plaques, is still the only reliable way to make a confirmed Alzheimer's disease diagnosis.

Therefore, even when the behavioral clues add up to Alzheimer's disease, many doctors prefer to say "presumed Alzheimer's disease" (see Helpful Resources).

VASCULAR DEMENTIA

Vascular dementia, accounting for 12 to 20 percent of all dementias, is the second most common age-related dementia. Unlike the gradual progression of Alzheimer's disease, the onset of vascular dementia symptoms is often abrupt and often occurs when a heart attack or a stroke dramatically reduces blood flow to or through the brain.

Vascular dementia can also have a slow progression. This happens when the accumulative damage of transient ischemic attacks—often called TIAs—cause many small areas of brain damage and, eventually, noticeable symptoms. The descriptive name *multi-infarct dementia* is the term health care providers use to describe this kind of vascular dementia. Multi-infarct dementia is the most common type of vascular dementia.

Vascular dementia can produce a spectrum of physical, behavioral, and emotional changes (see table 3.2). Examples of physical symptoms include shuffling or walking with small rapid steps, weakness of an arm or leg, and incontinence. Behavioral symptoms range from slurred speech to difficulty navigating in familiar surroundings and following instructions.

Without question, the way Dorothy walked showed that vascular dementia was part of her picture. Her gait, similar to that of a toddler first learning to walk, was because of her insistence on wearing high-heeled shoes. She walked this way barefooted and on those rare instances when we convinced her to wear "those cute flats."

Table 3.2.   Some Signs and Symptoms Associated with Vascular Dementia

Mental and Emotional	Physical	Behavioral
Slowed thinking	Dizziness	Slurred speech
Forgetfulness	Leg or arm weakness	Difficulty finding the right word
Mood changes	Tremors	Difficulty navigating familiar places
Hallucinations and delusions	Walking using rapid, shuffling steps	Laughing or crying at inappropriate times
Confusion	Difficulty with balance	Difficulty following instructions
Loss of social skills	Loss of bladder or bowel control	Difficulty performing familiar tasks

As you can now appreciate, telling the difference between Alzheimer's disease and vascular dementia can be difficult. If the changes appear rapidly, vascular dementia, resulting from a stroke or heart attack, is the likely culprit. If the changes appear to have developed over time, Alzheimer's disease and vascular dementia multi-infarct dementia are possible causes. To make things even more complicated, many people have both Alzheimer's disease and vascular dementia (see Helpful Resources).

MIXED DEMENTIA

As the name implies, mixed dementia describes a condition in which characteristics of more than one type of dementia occur simultaneously. The combination of Alzheimer's disease and vascular dementia is the most common form of mixed dementia.

Alzheimer's disease, described by the deposition and accumulation of fibrous proteins, accompanies irreversible brain damage. Memory loss is one of the first symptoms of Alzheimer's disease.

Vascular dementia is most often caused by the cumulative effects of "warning" strokes (TIAs), as well as actual strokes that create areas of brain damage. Symptoms of vascular dementia depend on both the location and amount of brain damage.

The combination of dementia with Lewy bodies with Alzheimer's disease is another kind of mixed dementia. Characteristics of dementia with Lewy bodies include hallucinations and delusions, as well as alterations in sleep, heart rate, and digestion. It is possible for people to have a mixed dementia that includes all three—Alzheimer's disease, dementia with Lewy bodies, and vascular dementia.

Parkinson's disease is another neurological disorder that affects the brain. The classic symptoms that include tremors, slow movements, rigidity, and poor balance are the result of the brain making insufficient dopamine.

After ten to fifteen years, some people who have Parkinson's disease develop Parkinson's disease dementia. Some of the symptoms of Parkinson's dementia include confusion, moodiness, hallucinations, disorientation, and memory problems (see Helpful Resources).

FRONTOTEMPORAL DEMENTIA

In 1892, the German neurologist and psychiatrist Arnold Pick described a case involving an elderly patient with progressive loss of speech and dementia.

Later, when the patient died, the autopsy showed that certain parts of the brain had shriveled. Unlike the diffuse shrinkage associated with Alzheimer's disease, this type of dementia appeared to target the frontal and temporal lobes.

The two frontal lobes, one located on the front of each side of the brain, contain the structures that control our executive functions, including planning, organizing, and solving problems. The frontal lobes also control behavior, emotions, and personality.

The two temporal lobes, one located on each side of the brain just above the ear, give us the ability to perceive and recognize faces and objects and transfer short-term memories into our long-term memory banks. Table 3.3 contains information that links structural brain changes to easily observable behaviors.

It is not surprising to discover that people who have frontotemporal lobe dementia may no longer seem like the people we once knew. A parent who was once friendly, polite, and careful about their appearance may say and do socially unacceptable things like becoming sexually aggressive. Emotional blunting, or the inability to express verbal and nonverbal feelings, is another characteristic of this type of dementia.

Another clue that can indicate frontotemporal dementia is difficulty in using and understanding spoken and written language. Language difficulties include repeated mispronunciations, such as "sork" for "fork," and the inability to make appropriate associations between names and objects. If your family member has this particular kind of language difficulty, or aphasia, they may point to a sandwich and say they want a baseball. Frontotemporal lobe patients may use words and phrases like "this," "that," and "over there" in place of specific nouns and descriptions. People who have frontotemporal dementia are not aware of how they have changed.

Table 3.3.   Magnetic Resonance and Frontotemporal Lobe Dementia (FTD)

MR Finding	FTD Subgroup	Description
Bilateral frontal atrophy	Behavioral variant	Inappropriate behavior: disinhibition, neglect of personal hygiene, altered language function
Left hemisphere atrophy involving both the frontal and temporal lobes	Progressive nonfluent aphasia	Deterioration of language function, occasional increase in artistic and musical expression
Temporal lobe atrophy, sometimes bilaterally	Semantic dementia	Loss of word-meaning connections, word-finding difficulty, reduced fluency

Note: Adapted from Howard S. Kirshner and Jasvinder Chawla, "Frontotemporal Dementia and Frontotemporal Lobar Degeneration," *Emedicine*, updated June 18, 2018, accessed June 6, 2020, https://emedicine.medscape.com/article/1135164-print.

Scientists do not know the cause of frontotemporal lobe dementia; however, research demonstrates that genetics often plays a role in its development. Some studies show alterations in genes that code for specific brain proteins in nearly 45 percent of people who have family members with certain types of frontotemporal lobe dementia. These altered proteins form insoluble deposits in brain neurons and in some way either cause or are associated with frontotemporal lobe atrophy. But it is also important to remember that for more than 50 percent of patients with frontotemporal lobe dementia, genetics either does not play a role or is not yet an understood factor (see Helpful Resources).

DEMENTIA WITH LEWY BODIES

In 1912, Friedrich Heinrich Lewy, a neurologist and contemporary of Alois Alzheimer, described the disease that bears his name. Dementia with Lewy bodies, also called Lewy body dementia, is a spectrum disorder characterized by a precipitous decline in the patient's cognition and behavior. Hallucinations and delusions, as well as alterations in sleep, heart rate, and digestion, are other characteristics of dementia with Lewy bodies. Certain types of Lewy body dementia cause people to experience shaking, rigidity, and balance difficulties. The presence of Lewy bodies—abnormal brain deposits composed of several proteins—located throughout the brain is the postmortem diagnostic hallmark.

Unlike Alzheimer's disease, dementia with Lewy bodies does not have predicable stages. Early symptoms of the disease vary. Some people first experience cognitive and memory changes similar to those associated with early Alzheimer's disease. For other people, first symptoms may include shaking and a shuffling gait. Sometimes hallucinations are a first symptom. Therefore, a thorough medical exam plays an important role in ruling out other causes, such as Parkinson's disease, Alzheimer's disease, or the side effects of medications. Dementia with Lewy bodies is a rapidly progressing disease. Death usually occurs within five to seven years of diagnosis (see Helpful Resources).

TRAUMATIC BRAIN INJURY

Traumatic brain injury (TBI) may occur when external force, such as a fall or a blow to the head, causes extreme pain and is often accompanied by a short or a long period of unconsciousness.

The skull, plus a layer of cerebral spinal fluid, protects the "squishy" brain from relatively minor impacts like bumping the head against a kitchen cabinet;

however, strong impacts may jostle the brain and cause it to knock against the hard and inflexible skull. The resultant bruising and swelling is the difference between a painful bump and a traumatic brain injury.

Football players and boxers are at increased risk for dementia later in life, as are people who have experienced combat. The shock wave originating from a grenade blast can cause the brain to slam against the skull. Researchers believe this kind of brain injury may be one of the causes for post-traumatic stress disorder (PTSD) (see Helpful Resources).

PARKINSON'S DEMENTIA

Parkinson's disease causes tremors and loss of coordinated movements. Some kinds of Parkinson's disease make it difficult to start walking or cause the person to freeze in mid-step. Another symptom is loss of affect, or the loss of ability to show feelings through facial expressions like smiling, frowning, or grimacing.

Some people who have Parkinson's disease also experience Parkinson's dementia, or PD. Symptoms include depression, hallucinations, memory loss, and sleep disturbances (see Helpful Resources).

HORSE OR ZEBRA?

The expression, "When you hear hoof beats, don't look for zebras," is one that some medical professors use to tell students that it is more important to look for a frequently encountered rather than exotic cause for illness. Alzheimer's disease, vascular dementia, mixed dementia, dementia with Lewy bodies, frontotemporal lobe dementia, and Parkinson's disease dementia are "horses"; however, don't forget, "zebras" do exist!

Wernicke–Korsakoff Syndrome

Wernicke encephalopathy and Korsakoff syndrome are different brain disorders that usually occur together. Wernicke encephalopathy is the first step in the development of the combined syndrome. Vitamin B1 (thiamine) deficiency is the origin of both illnesses.

Confusion, poor muscle control, abnormal eye movements, and double vision are common symptoms of Wernicke encephalopathy. Intravenous vitamin B1 may reduce or reverse symptoms. Even with vitamin B1 treatment, Korsakoff psychosis often follows.

Permanent damage to the parts of the brain responsible for converting short-term memory into long-term memory is the cause of Korsakoff psychosis. Other symptoms include personality changes and difficulty in acquiring new information and learning new skills. People who have Korsakoff psychosis may find it difficult to concentrate, anticipate and plan ahead, make decisions, and solve problems.

A diagnosis of Wernicke–Korsakoff syndrome is the outcome when a detailed medical history, a thorough physical exam, and an assortment of laboratory tests and medical imaging studies fail to rule out other causes for the patient's signs and symptoms. Treatment usually consists of giving the patient oral or intravenous vitamin B1 to manage psychosis, as well as medications to treat the underlying cause for Wernicke–Korsakoff syndrome. Without treatment, Wernicke–Korsakoff syndrome worsens and can lead to death (see Helpful Resources).

Multiple Sclerosis Dementia

Multiple sclerosis (MS) is a progressive disease that affects the brain, spinal cord, and the optic nerves. Multiple sclerosis occurs when the immune system attacks the protective sheath that surrounds the nerve fibers, disrupting communication between the brain and the nervous system.

The first symptoms of MS often start between the ages of twenty and forty, and include fatigue, clumsiness, blurred or double vision, poor bladder and bowel control, pain, and depression. Researchers believe that approximately 50 percent of people who have MS experience some degree of memory loss.

Generally, the degree of memory loss is less severe than it is for other kinds of dementia, such as Alzheimer's disease. Rather than dementia, clinicians describe the memory loss associated with MS as "cognitive impairment" or "mild cognitive impairment." People who have MS usually have difficulty remembering information learned in the past and are less able to learn and work when distractions are present (see Helpful Resources).

AIDS Dementia Complex

Human immunodeficiency virus (HIV) is the infectious microbe that causes acquired immunodeficiency syndrome (AIDS). The virus is transmitted from person to person by exposure to HIV-contaminated blood and other body fluids.

Many of the signs and symptoms of early-stage AIDS—headache, sore throat, fever, swollen glands (lymph nodes), and achy muscles—seem more flu-like than serious. Nevertheless, as the disease progresses to late-stage AIDS, many people experience neurological symptoms, such as confusion, memory loss, and depression. Together, these AIDS-related neurological symptoms are called AIDS dementia complex or ADC. Fortunately, the introduction of highly active antiretroviral therapy (HAART) nearly twenty years ago has greatly reduced the incidence of ADC.

Behaviors that increase risk for HIV infection include sexual contact, multiple partners, and illicit drug abuse. When properly used, condoms (male and female) reduce risk for infection; however, condoms do not provide 100 percent protection.

As the name suggests, the virus attacks the immune system and makes people susceptible to other infectious diseases as well as an array of autoimmune diseases. HIV can increase risk for certain kinds of cancers.

Older people are less likely to receive a diagnosis of HIV when still in the early stages of the disease. You may be surprised to know that in 2013, people aged fifty and above accounted for 21 percent of HIV cases and more than 25 percent of AIDS diagnoses in the United States.

There are many reasons why older people do not receive a diagnosis earlier in the course of the disease. AIDS progresses more rapidly in older people than it does in people younger than fifty years of age. In addition, the symptoms of early-stage AIDS overlap with the symptoms of other, often less serious, illnesses older people experience. Stigma and the unwillingness on the part of patients *and* their doctors to discuss sexual activity also contribute to the failure to consider AIDS as a cause for the patient's symptoms. Taken together, late diagnosis with rapid progression both increases the likelihood of transmitting HIV to others and increases the risk for AIDS dementia complex. HIV does not discriminate. Anyone can get AIDS (see Helpful Resources).

Creutzfeldt–Jakob Disease Dementia

Creutzfeldt–Jakob disease (CJD) is a rare and rapidly progressing type of dementia. In 2017, the Centers for Disease Control and Prevention (CDC) received notification of a total of 511 cases. It is quite likely this is an underestimation as CJD is not on the list of CDC-reportable diseases.

Early symptoms, including failing memory, behavioral changes, lack of coordination, and hallucinations, at first mimic a more common type of dementia, such as Alzheimer's disease. Conversely, unlike other forms of dementia, CJD rapidly progresses to increased mental deterioration, blindness, and involuntary twitches and jerks, as well as the inability to make voluntary movements. Death usually occurs within a year of the onset of symptoms.

A proteinaceous infectious particle (a prion) appears to be the cause of CJD. Research shows the particular kind of prion proteins that cause CJD are ones that clump in and around brain nerve cells and thereby cause overwhelming brain damage.

Ruling out a treatable cause for the patient's symptoms, such as meningitis, is often the first step a physician takes when there is reason to suspect CJD or other causes for dementia. Standard diagnostic tests include a spinal tap to assess the presence or absence of substances linked to certain types of dementia. Patients may also undergo an assortment of brain imaging evaluations that can provide visual and functionality kinds of evidence. There is no treatment that can cure or slow the progression of CJD. The current treatment is to use medication to alleviate symptoms and to make the patient as comfortable as possible (see Helpful Resources).

Huntington's Disease Dementia

Huntington's disease (HD) is an inherited brain disorder that affects the part of the brain that controls thinking, emotion, and movement. Most people who have the disease begin to see symptoms between the ages of thirty and fifty.

Symptoms include poor memory, depression, and eventually the inability to perform fine motor skills, such as those needed to use buttons, zippers, and eating utensils. Other symptoms include involuntary twitches and jerks. People who have Huntington's disease eventually lose the ability to walk, talk, and swallow.

Dementia can occur at any stage of the disease. In addition to memory loss, symptoms include poor judgment and reduced problem-solving and abstract-thinking skills.

Physicians often prescribe a number of medications to help reduce the emotional, cognitive, and movement difficulties associated with HD. It is important to remember that. while there are medicines that help keep these clinical symptoms under control, there are no treatments that stop or reverse the course of the disease (see Helpful Resources).

IT'S CONFUSING FOR EVERYONE—CONFABULATIONS, DELUSIONS, AND HALLUCINATIONS

One of the first things we notice about people who have dementia is a marked change in their perception of the world around them. Some will say things and respond to events that are clearly untrue or unrealistic. Others will have an uncanny way of making truly strange things seem quite plausible.

For many family members, adjusting to changes in their loved one's thought processes and perceptions is one of the most difficult aspects of caring for someone who has dementia. Despite the challenges, it's important to remember that these tall tales and odd visions are part of their disease. Their brain is playing tricks on all of us.

Confabulation, when people fill in missing details with plausible information, is an interesting phenomenon. For people who have dementia as well as other mental illnesses that distort memory, the fill-ins are often fanciful and usually contain detailed embellishments.

I have to say that Dorothy was a grand confabulator. You have already heard about the nameless lady who pushed her off the stairs, and you may have wondered about Dorothy's persistence in telling others about her back surgery. Dorothy was also quite sure that her caregivers were entertaining men on her front lawn.

All these stories are based on a flash of truth, and all were Dorothy's way of explaining her situation to herself and others. The nameless lady did not push her off nonexistent stairs but was the person who found her semiconscious by the door. And yes, we did discuss back surgery, but all decided it was too risky for a person of her age to undergo the procedure.

During her years at home with caregivers, Dorothy often talked about her back surgery in the context of eventual recovery and freedom from household help. Telling her that she didn't have surgery always produced a moment of quiet and a strange expression. Pursuing the topic further with, "Can you see a surgical scar?" would cause her to say something like, "Isn't the weather wonderful?" or "Did you read the newspaper today?"

Looking back, telling Dorothy that a back surgery never happened was neither right nor kind. It would have been better if we had been the ones to make a redirecting comment about the weather.

Although seemingly similar, there are some fundamental differences between confabulation and delusions. While confabulation involves many fanciful and forever-changing details contained within a kernel of truth, delusions are vague and usually do not have a truthful element to them. Your family member may say people are out to hurt them, strangers are hiding things, or that someone is talking behind their back. Asking about the "who, what, or when" will not produce more specific information. Trying to convince them of their safety will often make them argumentative.

Confabulation and delusions are persistent phenomena. You might be under the impression that because of your superlative caregiving skills you single-handedly fixed the situation. You believe that because of what you said or did your family member now understands that she fell, and was not pushed, off of her neighbor's stairs; however, I can assure you that confabulation and delusions are just below the surface, and with the right trigger, they instantly reemerge.

Hallucinations involve sensory activity where there is no stimulus. Your family member may say that they see blood on the wall or the faces of long dead relatives. They may also report hearing voices or that bugs are crawling on their skin. Understandably, some hallucinations are terrifying. Other times your family member, perhaps recognizing the oddity of the situation, will not feel scared. The point is that hallucinations are sensory tricks. The individual sees, hears, or feels something without the stimulus of light, sound, or touch.

Confabulation, delusions, and hallucinations are all important clues that help clinicians diagnose and stage dementia. Nevertheless, for caregivers, learning how to respond to and report these behavioral manifestations of dementia can make the difference between a good day and a disaster. You will learn about ways to manage this aspect of dementia behavior in chapter 4.

FREQUENTLY ASKED QUESTIONS

1. Are the altered brain proteins and insoluble deposits associated with Alzheimer's disease and dementia with Lewy bodies the same or different?

Each disease is associated with distinctly different brain deposits. The brain pathology used to verify Alzheimer's disease is the presence of senile (neuritic) plaques composed of a tangle of dying nerve cells surrounding an amyloid protein core.

The structures associated with dementia with Lewy bodies contain alpha-synuclein. Lewy bodies are found throughout the outer layers of the brain (cerebral cortex) and deep within the midbrain and brainstem.

2. Why "associated with" rather than "caused by"? Don't these altered proteins and odd deposits cause dementia?

Before medical researchers can say with certainty that β-amyloid deposits cause Alzheimer's disease, they have to design and perform experiments that show that statement is true. At this time, finding β-amyloid deposits only confirms the patient has Alzheimer's disease. The production of β-amyloid plaques may only be a byproduct of the actual disease-causing events.

3. I live far away from my father, but I do make efforts to visit every two or three months. Lately, it seems as though he doesn't keep his house as clean as he once did. He seems isolated and doesn't make efforts to visit with friends. I often find rotted food in the refrigerator, and he smells like he doesn't change his clothes often enough. Are these signs of dementia?

Yes, these are signs of dementia; however, they are also signs of depression. Worksheet 3.1, provided at the end of this chapter, may help you evaluate his situation. And don't forget the importance of a thorough medical exam to help make a diagnosis and to provide the most appropriate treatment.

4. In the "Memory and Aging" section, you state that dementia patients "lose access to [the] collection of learned information and built-in skills and procedures." Does this mean that people who have dementia still have all that knowledge but are simply blocked from accessing it?

What an interesting question. Unfortunately, unlike amnesia, no one recovers from having Alzheimer's disease or other types of dementia. It's an untestable experiment, and considering dementia actually destroys the brain, it seems unlikely that information recovery is possible.

WORKSHEET 3.1:
Age-Related Changes

Everyone experiences age-related changes. Some changes, such as gray hair and occasional forgetfulness, are a normal part of aging. Frequent memory lapses, repeated conversations, and getting lost while traveling to familiar places are not normal age-related changes. The following tasks and questions will help you understand your family member's situation. Use your worksheet findings to organize your thoughts and, if need be, guide conversation with other family members and health care providers.

1. Make a list of four to six words that describes your family member's personality and behavior as you remember him or her five or more years ago.
2. Make a list of four to six words that describes you family member's personality and behavior as of one or two years ago.
3. Make a list of four to six words that describes your family member's personality and behavior today.
4. After reviewing your lists, write one sentence that summarizes the change in your family member's personality and behavior. For example: Over the past five years, my mother went from being a friendly and independent woman to one who is now forgetful and angry and does not bathe often.
5. Are there extenuating circumstances—such as debilitating or chronic illness, medication, a move to a new community, or the death of a spouse—that could be affecting your parent/family member's personality or behavior? If so, list those potentially influencing factors.
6. Describe the incident that made you feel that dementia may be something you now need to consider.

4

WHAT COULD THIS BE?

Diagnosing Dementia

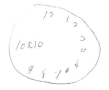

Dorothy, age ninety-six, clock, 9:50 a.m.

Dorothy's diagnosis came in bits and pieces. Or maybe it would be better to say my ability to connect dementia to the Dorothy in front of me was a gradual process.

Because of worsening confusion, her first evaluation occurred while convalescing in the rehabilitation hospital. The psychologist said, "Such a lively and remarkable lady."

I asked for a reevaluation. This time he said, "She is one of the most manipulative people I have ever encountered." And from him, I learned a new word—*confabulate*. Dorothy had false memories or perceptions about herself and her environment. To us confabulations seem like lies, but to a person who has dementia, confabulations are truths. Because a variety of brain disorders—dementia included—cause people to confabulate, a neuropsychologist was her next visitor.

She wondered why "that man" asked her to count backwards or make drawings. She said some of the things he wanted to do "were silly beyond words." She refused to answer some of his questions or do certain tasks. The words *senile dementia, confused, memory impaired,* and *unable to follow directions,* became an official part of her medical history. Dorothy's scores indicated that she was close to mid-stage dementia.

Okay, dementia. That makes sense. And of course, it didn't take a PhD neuropsychologist to tell me that she couldn't follow directions or remember what she had said just a few moments earlier. But seeing the word *dementia* on paper is different than a self-made diagnosis. It makes the potential for Alzheimer's disease jump out from the background. It makes you think about how much worse things might get. Seeing that word next to your loved one's name makes you wonder if dementia will be your fate as well.

A few months later, Dorothy began to experience hallucinations. An anxious morning pointing out blood spots on the walls and bugs crawling on the carpet provided an entryway to the University Hospital psychiatric clinic; however, getting her to agree to see a psychiatrist first involved a call to the police department and then a long, awkward wait until the Critical Intervention Team (CIT) arrived.

The appointment took longer than expected, but when Dorothy, wearing her best two-inch heels, finally shuffled out of the psychiatrist's office, she triumphantly announced, "I am fine. I answered all of his questions." The psychiatrist said otherwise—adding that the sedatives her doctor prescribed were not a likely cause of her hallucinations. It was reassuring to hear that he agreed with the medication Dorothy was already taking.

A few days after our experience in the psych unit, Dorothy's primary care doctor showed me the results of her clock-drawing test—an easy-to-administer evaluation that shows a patient's ability to anticipate and organize. The figure at the beginning of the chapter shows Dorothy's attempt at illustrating how ten minutes before ten might appear.

For some reason, that clock face was the concrete information I needed. Dementia wasn't just an interesting article about brain tangles and disintegrating cognition and behavior. I now understood that dementia controlled my mother, my family, and my day.

DIAGNOSING DEMENTIA—WHY IT'S IMPORTANT

Many wonder why it is important to diagnose dementia. After all, without a cure there is nothing you can do but watch and wait for the inevitable. The possibility the behavior changes you see may be caused by something other than dementia is probably the most important reason. What if your loved one's confusion was actually the result of having an ongoing bladder infection or perhaps a side effect from a medication used to treat another condition?

On the other hand, if testing does reveal dementia, then you and other family members can begin planning for next steps. If early-stage dementia is the diagnosis, then your family member may want to be included in these discussions. Your family member may still have realistic opinions to offer about driving, long-term care, and end-of-life wishes; however, don't be surprised if anger, rather than a willingness to engage in a discussion, is their response.

In the long run, knowing your family member's feelings about these important issues early on will make things easier for you when they adamantly state that they are just fine and that all of you are totally wrong.

You might find it interesting to know it is often a close family member who reports changes in behavior to the doctor. And yes it is true; your loved one's doctor may not notice these changes without your help. Remember, even if your parent or spouse is a long-time patient, their doctor does not see the "day-to-day" person in the examination room.

People who have dementia can be amazingly good at hiding their difficulties. If the doctor does not ask the kinds of questions that can reveal an inconsistent or unrealistic story, your family member may present herself as a charming, although somewhat eccentric, oldster. The "yes" responses to questions like "Can you prepare your own meals?" or "Do you pay your own bills?" do not tell the doctor that dinner is tea and crackers and that important mail is often lost and forgotten.

The reasons for this are many. Patients are often unwilling or unable to self-report memory-related changes. Some physicians are either unfamiliar with the physical symptoms or behavioral signs of dementia, or they feel that, without effective treatments, a diagnosis is a waste of time.

Sometimes, rather than a family member or clinician, your loved one's dental hygienist, hairdresser, or barber are the first to notice the first inklings of dementia. Unlike a doctor's appointment, these interactions are informal, chatty, and nonthreatening.

The dental hygienist may note such things as repeated conversation, odd responses to simple questions, and memory lapses in the patient's record. Should you ask, the hairdresser or barber may have some insightful things to say.

MEMORY LOSS DOESN'T ALWAYS MEAN DEMENTIA

With memory loss and dementia frequently in the news, it's no wonder people assume forgetfulness always foretells a diagnosis of an Alzheimer's-like disease. Nevertheless, before jumping to that conclusion, it is important that your family member receives a complete medical evaluation that includes a detailed medical history, physical exam, and an assortment of urine and blood tests to rule out other causes for their behavioral changes. The doctor may also request medical imaging procedures, such as an MR (magnetic resonance) evaluation, to see if structural changes in the brain are the source of symptoms.

ASSESSING COGNITIVE FUNCTION

It is important to assess your loved one's cognitive and daily living skills when the results of a thorough medical exam do not reveal other reasons for memory loss and behavioral changes. The purpose of evaluating cognition and daily living skills is to link brain function to the kind of assistance the person in your care may need. Sometimes these appraisals can reveal behaviors associated with specific types of dementia.

The Mini Mental Status Exam

The Mini Mental Status Exam (MMSE), often called the "mini mental," and the clock-drawing test are two assessments of cognitive function. Your family member's primary doctor may administer these tests as a part of a medical exam or make a referral for your family member to see another health care specialist, such as a neuropsychologist.

The mini mental evaluates orientation, recall, and various attention, calculation, and language skills. The examiner asks a standard set of questions that include such things as "What is today's date?" and "Can you tell me the name of this hospital/clinic?" In addition to answering questions, your family member will be asked to perform simple tasks, such as repeating a sequence of words, counting and spelling backwards, writing a sentence, and copying a drawing. Although interpretations of the patient's overall score out of a possible 30 points can vary, many clinicians use the following assessment breakpoints:

24 to 30: essentially normal
20 to 23: possible early-stage Alzheimer's disease
10 to 19: mid-stage Alzheimer's disease
0 to 9: late-stage Alzheimer's disease

The mini mental is an easy test to administer; however, the test does rely on the patient's ability to read, write, and make verbal responses. People who do not read well, who are visually or hearing impaired, or who have other communication difficulties may perform poorly on the exam without the accompanying declines in cognition. Refusal to participate is another issue. Some people, in attempting to hide their deficits, may refuse to participate or only respond to questions they feel they can answer correctly.

When communication and cooperation problems are not factors, the mini mental reliably differentiates between people who have cognitive impairment from those who are cognitively intact. Repeating the mini mental test as a part of follow-up visits helps the clinician make well-founded decisions about such things as the patient's ability to drive a car or their need for assistance at home.

The Clock-Drawing Test

The clock-drawing test is another screening tool used to assess people for Alzheimer's disease and other types of dementia. The ability to draw a clock face that shows a specific time, such as ten minutes past eleven, tests for a spectrum of cognitive, motor, executive, and perceptual function skills. Common errors found with patients who have Alzheimer's disease include counterclockwise numbering, missing numbers, repeated numbers, odd spatial arrangements of clock-face features, and the absence of clock hands. Dorothy's clock drawing, located at the beginning of the chapter, illustrates many of these features.

Although drawing a clock face may seem deceptively simple, it is a remarkably powerful tool. Clocks are nearly universal, and drawing a clock face avoids many language and cultural barriers. And unlike the Mini Mental Status Exam, patients find the test less threatening and are therefore more willing to participate.

Researchers from the Royal Victoria Infirmary and the Newcastle University Medical School found good correlation between mini mental and clock-drawing test scores. These same researchers suggest that, because dementia is both a universal and an underdiagnosed syndrome, the clock-drawing test could become an important addition to the annual physical exam.

The Blessed–Roth Dementia Scale

Unlike the Mini Mental Status Exam and the clock-drawing test, the Blessed–Roth Dementia Scale relies on daily living skills as the basis for evaluation. In this case, a family member or caregiver rates the patient's ability to perform household tasks, handle money, and recall recent events. The Blessed–Roth Dementia Scale also ranks the patient's ability to eat and dress without assistance and evaluates bladder and bowel continence. This evaluation helps determine the level of care your family member may need at home or at a care facility (see worksheet 4.1).

Remember, the Blessed–Roth evaluation tool reveals the skills that your family member *can* perform as much as it shows areas where they may need assistance.

Susceptibility to Scams

Research studies show the inability to pay bills and make change, as well as susceptibility to fraud and scams, may be an early indicator of cognitive impairment. Many family caregivers, recalling a stack of unopened envelopes and odd credit card payments, may say, "Of course, now it's perfectly obvious."

It was Dorothy's incredibly heavy purse that was one of the many "of course" clues. Yes, women do carry a surprising amount of stuff in their purse, but not several pounds of nickels and dimes. My only explanation was Dorothy, unable to count change, paid with dollar bills and dumped the change into her handbag.

Susceptibility to scams is another heads-up clue. In a six-year study, the Rush Memory and Aging Project showed that people who lost the ability to identify scams and fraudulent behavior were more likely to develop Alzheimer's disease than people able to spot deception.

DAILY LIVING SKILLS AND HOME SAFETY

The Blessed–Roth evaluation helps align daily living skills with home safety and the type and amount of assistance needed. To improve home safety, consider installing automatic shutoff timers on appliances like the toaster oven. Replace the overhead microwave oven with a countertop model. Install a smoke detector and a carbon monoxide alarm. Remove tripping hazards and improve household lighting. Adjust the thermostat on the hot water heater to a lower temperature. Mount handrails in the bathroom. Install safety locks on the cabinets that contain toxic cleaning supplies. Remove door locks to prevent entrapment in the bedroom or bathroom.

Another approach to creating a dementia-safe home is installing assistive technologies that help disabled people live as independently as possible. Smartphone apps, as well as televideo and other kinds of monitoring systems, can let you know if your loved one is as active as expected or has left a certain area, or if an appliance remains on. Other smartphone apps can remind your family member to take medication, give verbal instructions on how to use an appliance, find misplaced items, and help keep track of day and time.

Your internet browser and the keywords "home safety," "assessment," and "dementia" will bring up many excellent online resources. Another option is to arrange an inspection by an eldercare home safety consultant. The consultant can suggest where to buy safety equipment and, if need be, people to install such things as handrails. Use the phrase "eldercare home safety consultant" to find online home safety services. Be sure to include the location where the person in your care lives.

MEDICAL IMAGING: LOOKING INSIDE THE BRAIN

The doctor may refer your family member to a medical imaging facility to have either a CT (computed axial tomography) scan or an MR (magnetic resonance) scan. The doctor may also request a more specialized procedure, such as a PET (positron emission tomography) scan. The PET scan can reveal the presence or absence of normal brain activity. Conversely, CT and MR procedures are the ones your family member will most likely receive.

The CT and MR procedures involve taking many pictures from the surface of the body. The end result is a sequential series of images or image "slices" showing the area of interest from various different angles and depths. Sophisticated computer software combines the stack of slices into a 3-D representation of the internal structures contained within the brain or other parts of the body.

What Is a CT Scan?

A CT scan, also called a CAT scan, uses X-ray energy to visualize internal anatomical structures. Conversely, unlike the familiar box-shaped X-ray machine, the CT machine is shaped like a large doughnut, and the patient lies on a platform that slowly moves through the doughnut hole. A motor turns the doughnut ring so that the X-ray emitting part of the machine revolves around the patient. Each revolution of the machine scans and records an image representing a narrow horizontal slice of the body. Usually, only a specific area of the body, such as the head or the torso, undergoes a CT scan.

The radiologist may look at a series of image slices, or use computer software to reconstruct the individual slices into a 3-D picture. A CT scan can show evidence of brain atrophy, strokes, and TIAs (transient ischemic attacks).

In addition, a CT scan can identify changes to the blood vessels that affect blood circulation, as well as the accumulation of cerebral spinal fluid and blood that can increase pressure within the brain. Although the symptoms mimic those associated with dementia, surgery to reduce intracranial pressure may restore memory loss and reverse confusion and personality changes.

What Is an MR Scan?

Unlike a CT scan that uses X-ray energy, an MR (magnetic resonance) scan uses an extremely strong magnet and radio waves to create detailed images of the soft (nonbony) organs. For some people, the exam can be a difficult experience.

First of all, the presence of metal on or in the body can cause imaging problems, and it can be dangerous. A radiologic technologist will ask your family member to remove all jewelry, pierce hardware, and any clothing that has metal parts, such as zippers or buttons. The radiologic technologist will also want to know if your family member works with metals or has wounds caused by shrapnel. People who were once machinists or dentists, or who have old shrapnel injuries, may have small bits of metal in their eyes or in other parts of the body. Entering a strong magnetic field may cause these bits of metal to move and cause damage. The magnetic field can damage credit cards and digital cameras, so do not bring those items into the examination area.

The technologist will ask if your loved one has any "indwelling hardware," such as a heart pacemaker, bone pins, aneurysm clips, skull plates, dental implants, or joint replacements. Having certain kinds of metal implants may still make it possible to undergo an MR study.

Your loved one should have received an ID card from their health care provider that lists information about their surgically placed hardware. If you cannot find the ID card, your loved one's surgeon or the hospital may have the information you need.

The design of the MR machine adds other elements of discomfort and difficulty to the procedure. The patient, positioned on a moveable table, enters the scanner bore—a tunnel roughly twenty-four to twenty-eight inches in diameter and nearly six feet in length. Some short bore machines can scan the brain with just the upper part of the body in the bore; however, confinement in a small dark space causes many people to feel claustrophobic.

Noise is another difficulty. In the course of creating the strong magnetic field, the machine makes tremendously loud and rapid hammer-like noises. Patients receive earphones so they can listen to soothing and distracting music. The earphones and a microphone facilitate communication with the radiologic technologist operating the machine.

The MR scan may show a spectrum of potentially treatable conditions, such as brain tumors, accumulated spinal fluid, and head injury damage. An MR study can sometimes show the brain changes associated with certain types of dementia.

Vascular dementia and frontotemporal lobe dementia are two types of dementia where a scan can help confirm a diagnosis. In the case of vascular dementia, the damage of many small strokes leaves a path of easily observable white spots or hyperintensities. An MR scan may help correlate the behavioral changes associated with frontotemporal lobe dementia to smaller than normal frontal and temporal lobes.

Unfortunately, MR scans do not reveal the tangles and plaques associated with Alzheimer's disease. There is some data that indicate a smaller than usual hippocampus—the region of the brain that converts short-term memory into long-term memory—may be a structural clue associated with early-stage Alzheimer's disease. An MR study may show the gross structural changes associated with late-stage Alzheimer's disease.

CONTRAST MEDIA

Contrast media are substances used to make selected anatomical features appear either dark or light as compared to the surrounding tissue. In other words, contrast media improve contrast and the ability to see details. For brain imaging procedures, the patient receives the contrast media through an injection into a vein.

CT and MR scans use similar contrast agents. Typically, they contain gadolinium, a naturally occurring element, and iodine. Contrast media make it easier to see blood vessels and the damage to the blood-brain barrier that strokes and head injuries may cause.

Some people are at risk for contrast media side effects. The radiologic technologist needs to know if your loved one has kidney or heart disease, epilepsy, a shell fish allergy, or asthma. Having any of these conditions may increase the likelihood of having a reaction to gadolinium, iodine, or both substances. Side effects can range from nausea, dizziness, and rashes to low blood pressure, irregular heartbeat, and seizures.

It is important to discuss the various risk factors during your loved one's medical exam. That way the doctor can choose the medical imaging procedure least likely to cause problems.

A FEW WORDS FROM THE MEDICAL IMAGING FACILITY

Radiologic technologists are professionals who have the education and training to work in a medical imaging facility. In addition to scanning patients, the radiologic technologist is also responsible for preparing patients for the procedure, positioning for optimal views, and performing other tasks to ensure the radiologist receives a high-quality image to evaluate.

According to a 2019 U.S. Census study, more than 23 percent of the population is aged sixty-five years or older. For radiologic technologists, this statistic means that many of the patients they see each day are older people who may have an assortment of age-related problems, for example, hearing and vision loss, arthritis, and balance difficulties. These age-related changes can make managing and positioning patients who also have dementia a considerable challenge. Having dementia impairs the ability to understand and remember complex instructions. Patients who have dementia often are fearful, apprehensive, and may need more assistance than other older patients.

"Please," says one University of New Mexico Health Science Center radiologic technologist, "do not drop your mother off at the front door and leave!" As surprising as this may seem, this happens frequently.

Radiologic technologists find that patients who are accompanied by a family member or another caregiver are less fearful and more cooperative. Having you or the caregiver available to help with examination gowns, to ask or answer questions, to translate instructions, and to take your loved one to and from the bathroom can make the difference between a successful medical imaging procedure and an all-round disaster. And when the exam is over, helping them dress and then accompanying them to the discharge area will give the radiologic technologist the time they need to prepare for the next patient.

GENETICS AND DEMENTIA

Early-onset Alzheimer's disease that affects people as young as thirty years of age has different genetic risk factors. Changes to genes located on chromosomes 14 and 21 affect the majority of people who have the early-onset version. In either case, this information makes it possible to test people who may be at greater risk for developing Alzheimer's disease.

For the most part, the altered genes do such things as change how the body processes cholesterol and other blood lipids. It's not surprising to find that high cholesterol is another risk factor associated with Alzheimer's disease.

Having an inherited risk factor does not mean that you will get Alzheimer's disease. It's a subtle distinction, but people who have an altered gene have inherited only the increased risk and not the disease itself. On the bright side, knowing that you have an inherited risk factor gives you the opportunity to do those things known to reduce Alzheimer's disease risk—maintain a healthy weight, refrain from smoking, exercise, eat a heart-healthy diet, and engage in socially and intellectually satisfying activities.

Testing for the presence of genes associated with increased risk for dementia is available. Nevertheless, making the decision to undergo testing is often difficult. It is important to consider how you and other family members might feel if you should receive positive results for an inherited dementia risk factor. Will knowing make you feel anxious, relieved, or empowered? Will other family members also want testing? How might this information affect family planning for you or your children? Will having a positive test for dementia risk factors influence your career plans?

Anyone would find these and many other questions difficult to answer. Often, people find talking with a genetic counselor can make the decision to test—or not—easier. The genetic counselor, by explaining the technical and emotional issues associated with genetic testing, can help you make a personally comfortable decision. Afterward, the genetic counselor can explain the test results to you and suggest any further steps you may want to take.

You can find genetic counselors at most medical centers and university hospitals. Your loved one's doctor may know of local options, or you can check with the local Alzheimer's Association office. The National Association of Genetic Counselors and the American Board of Genetic Counselors are additional options.

JUST OVER THE HORIZON: A NEW WAY TO DIAGNOSE DEMENTIA

A group of simple blood tests hold promise in someday helping clinicians screen patients for Alzheimer's disease in the examination office. Researchers working in the United States and elsewhere are in the process of developing blood tests that can predict the onset of Alzheimer's disease and other dementias years before the patient experiences symptoms. These same blood tests may also identify people who show signs of mild cognitive impairment or are in the early stages of the disease; the tests also may predict those likely to suffer a rapid decline in cognition and other skills. A group of National Institute on Aging scientists is in the process of readying a blood test that can predict the onset of disease ten years or more before Alzheimer's disease symptoms occur.

You may wonder why it's important to predict Alzheimer's disease as much as ten years before people will experience symptoms. A decade seems like a very long time to carry the burden of such significant worry.

Research studies indicate that predictive information may make it possible to prevent or, at least slow, the brain damage dementia causes. In many ways, a blood test to monitor Alzheimer's risk is similar to monitoring cholesterol blood levels that predict increased risk for heart disease and stroke.

The long-term goal is to package easy-to-use tests that patients can undergo in their health care provider's office. The hope is to have these tools available within the next five years.

In addition, an Alzheimer's blood test can help identify people eligible to participate in various kinds of Alzheimer's research studies. An internet search using the keywords "clinical trials," "Alzheimer's," and "dementia" will bring up a treasure trove of useful information.

FREQUENTLY ASKED QUESTIONS

1. What is a screening test, and what is its purpose?

Screening tests are simple procedures that do not require the expertise of a laboratory technologist. Usually performed in the doctor's office, screens are an effective way to identify patients who need more time-consuming and expensive tests. An example of a commonly used screening test is the urine dipstick test. Relying on color matching, this assessment tool can indicate if the patient has higher than normal amounts of substances in their urine associated with such conditions as diabetes or kidney failure. It would be a waste of time and money to send every patient to the laboratory just to identify the relatively few people who might have diabetes or some other disease reflected in the chemical composition of their urine.

2. What do you mean by "risk factors," and what does risk have to do with dementia?

Risk factors, such as high blood pressure, heart disease, and family genetics, don't cause dementia but make it more likely that dementia will become a part of a person's medical history. It takes careful medical research to identify statistically validated risk factors. For example, you may have read that cooking food in aluminum pots or using baking powder or anti-perspirants that contain aluminum may increase risk for dementia. Although this risk factor gets a lot of press, research has yet to confirm a link between aluminum exposure and dementia.

3. My father's doctor wants him to have an MR scan. My father wonders why and says he won't go. What can I say or do so I don't create more problems?

One way to approach this difficult situation is to ask the doctor if having an MR scan is likely to change your father's treatment plan. If not, and if the doctor feels the procedure is an option, then you might consider forgoing the scan; however, if your parent's doctor says an MR exam is crucial to your father's treatment, then do what it takes to minimize your parent's anxiety. One way is to simply limit discussion about his upcoming MR evaluation or suggest going out for lunch afterward. You might also mention that the test doesn't hurt and that Medicare will pay for it. Often, pain and cost are the reasons why people try to avoid medical imaging procedures. Be sure to discuss your father's concerns with his doctor. He or she may have other suggestions, such as medication, to reduce your parent's anxiety.

4. What is the difference between "treating" and "curing" a disease?

It's a subtle difference, made more difficult by people often misusing the words *treat* and *cure*. When doctors treat a disease, they prescribe medicine, perform surgery, or recommend physical therapy to manage symptoms. The term *cure* means to restore a patient to their original health. Doctors prescribe antibiotics to cure infectious diseases like strep throat and pneumonia.

5. What is a genetic counselor, and how can I find one where I live?

Genetic counselors are medical professionals who have a graduate-level degree in genetic counseling. As part of their degree requirements, they take classes in genetics, psychology, ethics, and counseling. They also intern in an approved medical genetics center. After graduation, they must pass a national board exam.

Genetic counselors help people understand their risk for inherited diseases, such as early-onset dementia, and explain the range of possible options; therefore, rather than telling families what to do, counselors help families make decisions that are compatible with their personal beliefs.

WORKSHEET 4.1:
The Blessed–Roth Assessment

The Blessed–Roth Assessment does not diagnose dementia but will help you to evaluate the type and level of assistance the person in your care may need. Consider repeating the Blessed–Roth Assessment every four to six months.

Changes in Performance of Everyday Activities (yes/no)
Is able to do household tasks _____

Is able to count money or make change _____

Is able to remember a list of items (e.g., grocery store needs) _____

Is able to navigate around home or other familiar buildings _____

Is able to navigate on familiar streets _____

Is able to interpret surroundings (i.e., can recognize if at home or in a hospital) _____

Is able to recall recent events (e.g., outings and visitors) _____

Tends to dwell in the past _____

Changes in Habits (yes/no)
Eats neatly and uses proper utensils _____

Is messy and tends to use a spoon only _____

Eats hand-held foods (e.g., crackers) _____

Requires feeding _____

Dressing (yes/no)
Dresses without help _____

Needs limited help with buttons, bra, stockings _____

Dresses in the wrong sequence, forgets items _____

Is unable to dress _____

Bladder and Bowel Control (yes/no)
No accidents _____

Occasionally wets bed or self _____

Frequently wets bed or self _____

Has neither bladder nor bowel control _____

WORKSHEET 4.2:
Assessing Help Needs

Use this worksheet to summarize the kinds of help your family member needs to live in their own home, your home, or in some type of assisted living facility. Consider repeating this assessment every four to six months.

1. After reviewing your responses to worksheet 4.1, list the daily life skills your family member *can* accomplish:

   a. competently or reliably
   b. with some help
   c. on their own

2. Review your lists and consider your family member's needs in the context of safe, independent living, what you can realistically provide in your home, or what is available in an assisted living facility.

5

FAMILY DYNAMICS

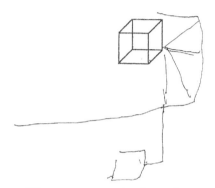

Woman, age seventy-nine, cube.

Many years ago, Dorothy said I was her favorite child. I am quite certain my sibling instinctually knew this without Dorothy saying so. I am also quite certain this situation made it difficult for my sibling to participate in our mother's care.

As I have said before, I had been Dorothy's caregiver for much longer than the period defined by her dementia diagnosis; however, the day her doctor informed me that Dorothy was no longer capable of independent living made it all official. It took me a while to understand the larger significance of his clinical findings.

An internet article published by the Area Agency on Aging (AAA), responsible for Pasco and Pinellas Counties, Florida, helped me understand that becoming a caregiver is a process that happens in stages. The AAA article describes stage 1 as the time when you recognize the impact of caregiving on your life and learn how to be a caregiver. Stage 2 is the period when you accept help from family and friends. The AAA article describes stage 3 as a phase of "heavy care" and a time to protect your own health. Stage 4, the final stage, is the phase when you resolve relationships, make end-of-life decisions, and make plans for when you are no longer a caregiver.

What the Pasco-Pinellas County AAA report states is both true and useful; however, I remember the first stage as one filled with horror and turmoil. It sounds silly now, but I felt that Dorothy had lied to me again. She wasn't as healthy as she claimed; she didn't have the insurance she promised; and because she didn't sign a health power of attorney (POA), her "easy-care" assurances weren't true either.

Horror and turmoil gradually evolved into the belief that I can do this, I am the right person for the job, and—gosh-darn-it—I am going to be a great caregiver. I didn't exactly feel euphoria, but I certainly had a feeling of heightened purpose and resolve.

Sadly, although quite realistically, stage 2 was short-lived. In truth, I hated this caregiving business. I was a lousy caregiver. In stage 3, I had what can be best described as feelings of abandonment and betrayal. There weren't enough hours in the day. I wasn't getting the support I needed. Dorothy's behavior, an exaggeration of her usual self, was wearing me down. And when would this end? Aside from having dementia, she was a healthy ninety-eight-year-old woman. Stage 3 was unbearably long.

Stage 4 was the one when the knot in my stomach quieted and I could take an occasional deep and cleansing breath. I found great caregivers. Medication was making Dorothy's behavior manageable, and the caregivers and I had figured out ways to make things run as smoothly as possible.

Much too soon, a change in Dorothy's health heralded the arrival of stage 5. The difficult decisions associated with end-of-life care and the logistics of moving Dorothy from her home to a dementia care facility was another period marked by self-doubt and stress. I felt I was a failure. The knot in my stomach returned, and feelings of abandonment crept back into the picture. I ruminated about Dorothy's explicit and unrealistic end-of-life instructions. I worried that moving her to a dementia care facility would prove I wasn't a trustworthy daughter. And again—when would this end?

Stage 6, marked by the few days before and after her death, was a peaceful stage. I prepared myself for Dorothy's death, as well as the practicalities associated with her funeral and my transition from power of attorney to representative of the estate. During those twilight days, I felt I could at last express a calming gentleness. It was especially wonderful to be present for her last coherent words—utterances that helped make up for those long and terrible years. I am grateful for stage 6.

The publication of the first edition of this book caught me at an odd place. Feelings of anger and stress remained. An incoming phone call still made me jump.

Now, many years later I remember Dorothy before dementia defined our life together. I now feel comfortable that we all did the best we could under the circumstances.

A POINT OF VIEW

This chapter on the interrelationships between and among individual family members is in contrast from the largely objective information found in the other sections of this book. Rather than offering ways to solve problems, this chapter poses questions for you and your other family members to consider and perhaps discuss.

Point of view is an interesting part of the family dynamics puzzle. Where do you feel you belong in this complex drama? Are you the team player, the family leader, the one who makes things easy for themselves, or the one who gets stuck doing everything? While you may feel that you understand the role you play, your family may have a different impression of you. Sometimes, by taking another person's perspective into consideration you can discover ways to alleviate conflict.

It seems that much of what health care professionals lump under family dynamics boils down to point of view. Of course, there are exceptions. Anyone can see that the son who embezzles money from his mother is a thief and the daughter who hurts her father is abusive.

The intent of this chapter is to get you and other family members thinking about better ways to work together.

WHERE FAMILY DISHARMONY BEGINS

Disharmony—when family members cannot agree on a fair and equitable division of caregiving duties—is a situation that can tear families apart. Often, family members don't notice the problem until pent-up anger makes it impossible to feel comfortable with one another. Unresolved childhood animosities resurface and color conversation. "You were Mom's favorite," is a common one. Then, there is the sibling who can list every good deed he or she performed over the past fifty years and now states, "It's your turn."

Occasionally, it is differences in age between oldest and youngest children that make fairly shared caregiving difficult. The oldest sibling may be retired but has health problems that make it difficult to be the primary caregiver. The younger siblings may still be working and have adolescent children living at home.

In some cases, the difference in age between the oldest and youngest is so great that they don't really know one another. If you never shared a bathroom or house chores with your sibling, learning how to share dementia care responsibilities is a very steep learning curve.

Where your brothers and sisters live is another consideration. It is difficult to share responsibilities when one sibling lives nearby and the others live far away; however, it is easy to find examples where it is the distant sibling who makes the long drive to visit and to oversee her mother's care.

One person I spoke to lost several years of weekends and wore out three cars when her brother, who lived less than five miles away from their mother, chose to ignore the situation—or so she said. Perhaps, in reality, she was a stoic personality who made it difficult for her brother to do his share. As they say, you cannot have it both ways.

Sometimes, the loss of parental influence is the force that makes sibling cooperation and collaboration impossible. Many parents, using not-so-subtle hints, unwittingly referee behavior long after their adult sons and daughters have left home. When dementia prevents a mother from orchestrating behavior, the daughter may no longer phone her brother, the son does his best to avoid his sister's bossy and overbearing ways, and the siblings settle into a meant-to-be relationship. At another extreme, some parents make the favorite child all too obvious, or rather than respecting their children's individual strengths, they focus on weaknesses.

THE DILEMMA OF THE POWER OF ATTORNEY AND PRIMARY CAREGIVER

Your parent has chosen one of their children to be their power of attorney (POA), as the person responsible for making decisions when they cannot. In chapter 7, you will learn about the power of attorney and other legal designations.

Often, the POA is the oldest one or the son or daughter who lives closest to their parent. Other times, the parent chooses the child they trust or feel especially close to.

The lawyer will want to list one other person on the POA. This other individual can take over POA duties should your parent revoke the POA or if the first-named person declines or is temporarily unavailable. Often the alternate is another adult child. But it could also be a son- or daughter-in-law or a nonfamily member, such as a lawyer, accountant, or even a close friend.

Speaking to my lawyer about writing my own durable power of attorney papers gave me a better understanding of the intent of this important set of documents. Because all my children are in the early stages of careers, homes, and families, I felt it was unfair to impose POA responsibilities on just one of them. And, as I explained to the lawyer, I wanted to take advantage of the individual strengths each could bring to my care. "No," she said. "Someone has to be in charge." So indeed, the role of POA is similar to that of a project manager.

Unfortunately, siblings may assume that the POA has agreed to do everything. They may also believe that living at a distance makes it impossible to provide help.

If you are the one who provides the majority of your parent's care, make sure your brothers and sisters know there are things they can do. In other words, don't wait for them to contact you. All that does is increase your anger as you count the days of silence.

And if you are the other sibling, there are things you can do to make things easier for your brother or sister. Your sibling needs to know that you appreciate his or her efforts. Call, text, or e-mail on a regular basis. In addition to asking about your mom or dad, also ask how your brother or sister is doing. Be prepared to hear and then respond with honest answers.

Your sibling may tell you she is exhausted and feels sad and abandoned. Or she may say that she feels overwhelmed, frustrated, and depressed. Don't take these responses as personal criticism. But do offer an empathetic ear and suggest things you can do to lighten the load.

For example, you could order clothes for your parent online or from a catalog store, pay bills, help manage your parent's finances, or take the car in for an oil change. Make efforts to visit your parent, and at the same time, give your sibling a few hours or days of respite. Saying "thank-you" and "I appreciate what you are doing for all of us" can do a lot to prevent hard feelings.

If you are your parent's primary caregiver, be prepared to accept that your siblings may be neither willing nor able to give you the help you need. It's a hard place to be, but sometimes it does happen. Although you make efforts to think of reasons why your sisters and brothers cannot be more helpful, your mind wanders to feelings of desertion. It's easy to take their lack of support as a personal affront; however, it's healthier to think of your siblings as people who, for one reason or another, cannot do any better. Yes, accepting that reality is another one of those things that is easier said than done.

TAKING A CLOSER LOOK AT OURSELVES

We all have words and phrases we use to guide our actions, temper our thoughts, or calm our frustrations. Before becoming Dorothy's caregiver, my mantras were "I can fix anything," "I make things happen," and "I can always do more."

Without realizing it, I had set myself up for failure. Dementia doesn't abide by any of these self-made rules. Dementia isn't a fixable disease. Dementia behaviors rule the day. Dementia care is more than a full-time job.

And to make matters even worse, my long history of approaching other challenges in this very same way made some people believe I am truly capable of doing anything and everything. Fortunately, I had friends and immediate family who knew better. It just took me a while to understand their wisdom and to appreciate their concern for me. Without question, dementia care is both a humbling and an enriching experience.

Taking a few moments to objectively evaluate the day's events can alleviate stress and reveal the behaviors that lead to family discord. Reflective writing is a self-assessment tool that many people use (see worksheet 5.1). As an added benefit, reflective writing allows you to have a grand monologue without wearing out your friends and family. Be sure to review your writings from time to time. Doing so will help you see past mistakes, appreciate progress, or give important insight about best next steps. Use worksheet 5.2 to get started in your reflective writing venture.

WORDS TO GUIDE ACTIONS

"Make it right before it is wrong." What a wonderful expression! Rich with so many positive overtones, it gives a moment's pause and helps us consider the influence of our own actions on others. "Make it right before it is wrong" gives us the courage to ask the right questions, to clarify ambiguity, and to make difficult decisions.

Rather than bringing Dorothy home from the rehabilitation hospital, I had arranged for her to go into a nursing home facility that also included assisted and independent living apartments. I needed more time to get her house ready. I also hoped she would like living there and would get well enough to transition into the assisted living wing.

But just the opposite happened. She refused to eat and became even more confused. In other words, Dorothy was failing. I knew I had to give her the gift of living in her own home for as long as possible.

My sibling and I discussed the situation. Location made it obvious that I would be our mother's primary caregiver. My sibling offered to "do what I can to help."

Had I known to "make it right before it is wrong," I would have asked, "And what will you do to help?" The response, whatever it might have been, would have told me what to expect. Some years later, I realized that my sibling had other struggles, and "do what I can to help" was a realistic and honest response.

DON'T MAKE ASSUMPTIONS

As you see, "don't make assumptions" is the flip side of "make it right before it is wrong." In the above example, I assumed that the other person understood the difficulties of being a caregiver; however, in many situations this is not the case. Differences in personality, perceptions, and circumstances mean that you cannot assume another person has the ability to step into your shoes.

Taking the situation beyond first assumptions helps make the situation understandable and easier to accept. It also makes taking next steps, such as hiring caregivers, an obvious priority. And don't forget to take into consideration the things you might have done or said that may make it difficult for your brother or sister to feel they can offer help.

THANK-YOU

Wishing for help is one kind of problem. The other kind of problem is the family member who offers unwanted help. Often this person is full of suggestions and may cause considerable confusion when they do things without your knowledge.

Sometimes, the primary caregiver assumes this person's actions are a form of personal criticism. But before making that assumption, take a moment to consider what the too-helpful person has to say. Maybe they are right. After all, it is easy to make mistakes when you are overworked and exhausted. Maybe with discussion, the two of you will come up with an even better solution. It is important to listen closely, evaluate carefully, and respond thoughtfully.

Of course, the opposite may also be true. What your family member says may be truly off the wall. They live two thousand miles away, haven't visited, and don't have a clue about dementia or what it takes to be a caregiver.

In either case, you can stop both the too-helpful and the clueless family members in their tracks simply by saying, "Thank-you, I will consider your suggestion." It's hard to believe, but those simple words almost always work!

SOME CHALLENGING FAMILY SITUATIONS

No matter how well you and your family get along, adding dementia care to the mix can reveal new behaviors or magnify ones that had been previously easy to ignore. Additional challenges, such as in-law relationships, the difficulties of divorce and the creation of blended families, the complications significant others bring to the mix, and the know-it-all sibling, are examples of situations that test our ability to stop, think, and respond calmly.

The scenarios below are fictionalized versions of real events. Their purpose is to help you apply what you read earlier about "make it right before it is wrong," "make no assumptions," and saying "thank-you" to the kinds of situations that can easily move attention away from your parent's care. Use worksheets 5.1 and 5.2 to help develop strategies likely to reduce the influence of these commonly encountered stumbling blocks.

SONS- AND DAUGHTERS-IN-LAW

Often a marriage begins with kind words to welcome the new son or daughter into the family. Then, with time, the in-law relationships develop. Perhaps we feel as close, or even closer, to the in-law parents as we do our own. And maybe we enjoy spending time with our brothers- and sisters-in law—or not.

With a little luck, we have had a thirty- or forty-year history with our in-law family before dementia enters the picture. The impact of the disease on the entire family can be more widespread than you might think.

A husband who was once helpful around the house may now spend all of his free time with his father. The normally even-tempered wife is now constantly heard arguing with her brothers about their mother's care. A daughter-in-law has to step in when her mother-in-law's children cannot or will not provide care. A son-in-law becomes the family arbitrator when his wife stops talking to her sister. And sometimes, the daughter-in-law who thought she was a member of the family discovers that she is an outsider.

BLENDED FAMILIES

According to a U.S. Census Bureau researcher, roughly 50 percent of all marriages in the United States eventually end in divorce. Of these failed marriages, nearly 45 percent involve couples who have children. Many people do remarry and, as a consequence, create a blended family where one or both spouses have children by a previous marriage. Sometimes, in addition to having "his and her" children, "our" children are part of the mix. The U.S. Census Bureau estimates that 65 percent of all people living in the United States are a stepparent, stepchild, stepsibling, or a stepgrandparent.

Complex issues arise when blended families face a chronic illness like dementia. The cost of care may be more than what the disabled spouse can afford. Many states, and the Veterans Administration (VA), do not consider prenuptial agreements when families investigate eligibility for Medicaid and various VA assistance programs. As a consequence, the healthy spouse may be responsible for all of the medical expenses. Sometimes people who haven't sheltered their assets discover that divorce is the only way they can protect their life savings.

Another challenge for blended families is naming the most appropriate person to make decisions for the ill parent or stepparent. Children from the first marriages create a blended family when their biological mother and father remarry. The adult children may still harbor anger and resentment over the divorce or may feel closer to one family over another, or there may be a long history of discord. It is also possible the biological adult children may already be coping with the challenges of chronic illness in their other blended family.

One might think that an "our child" might be the best choice to be the POA. Or maybe the best choice for POA is the sibling who is a natural diplomat and peacekeeper. More than likely, the best way to prevent family discord is for your parent to name another relative, a family friend, or her lawyer as her POA.

WHEN MOM OR DAD HAS A SIGNIFICANT OTHER

It can be a big surprise when, shortly after your mother's death, your father introduces his girlfriend to the family. "Gosh, that was quick," you silently think. But to your father, you say polite things and go through the formality of getting to know your father's new friend.

Sometimes you discover an interesting and charming person. Other times, the new friend is demanding and does not give you the time your family needs together. Even when the situation is less than wonderful, you make efforts to believe that your father's girlfriend is good for him—he isn't lonely, and after all those years of caring for your mother, he can now enjoy himself.

When a chronic or debilitating illness enters the picture, the relationship between your father's significant other and the family may change. Some companions, out of love, friendship, and loyalty, do everything they can to help the adult children care for their father. Others are quick to say they already have taken care of one sick and dying husband and disappear. But, sometimes the girlfriend interferes, demands attention, and does purposefully annoying things.

OH NO, NOT AGAIN!

Like clockwork, the phone rings. No need to guess who it is. Blah, blah, blah, blah. I don't want to hear about hospice care again. I don't care that my sister is a nurse. She keeps on yakking about dignity, but as far as I am concerned, hospice is just another way to say, "Pull the plug." What I really want her to do is to stop talking and leave me alone.

Having very different views about end-of-life care and treatment is a frequent cause of sibling arguments. These fights, often originating from deep-set personal views, are hard to resolve once changes in your parent's health bring these difficult decisions to the forefront.

Particularly if your parent has not discussed their end-of-life wishes, it is especially important to talk with your siblings long before the need arises. Doing so makes you realistic rather than making you morbid or overly focused on death. It may also be possible that your brother or sister is not ready to accept that their mother or father will die soon.

AFTERWARD

It's hard to imagine, but someday all of this will be over and your parent's care will no longer be the focal point of your day; however, this time of relative quiet is also the time when you, your family, and your siblings need to get reacquainted.

Sadly, the years of dementia care can damage family relationships. A Caring.com survey showed that 80 percent of respondents said their caregiving responsibilities put a strain on their relationship or marriage. And of those respondents, nearly all said that caregiving made them feel as though they were drifting apart from their spouse or partner; however, even those who reported stress also said the experience made their relationship stronger. For couples, there is something powerful and bonding in having weathered difficult times together.

Repairing sibling associations can be more complicated. Childhood histories color adult relationships. Another factor is adult siblings usually don't live together. And at the end of the day, siblings return their attention to their own families. Basically, when it comes to maintaining contact with one another, adult siblings have less at stake than husbands and wives or partners do.

Some siblings report that the caregiving experience was so embittering they no longer speak to one another. Other siblings say they are polite to one another but do not go out of their way to see each other outside of the usual family gatherings.

If you find yourself in either of these situations, taking a break from each other might be a good idea. Give yourself time to decompress and let memories of any good moments replace the unpleasant memories. Before taking a break, it might also be a good idea to tell your sibling of your plan so they don't think you are ignoring them. Both of you need time to recover and to evolve from bitterness to acceptance.

It's also important that your parent's grandchildren are not made to feel stuck in the middle. Your children and your sibling's children need to remain friends. And remember, someday your children may become your caregiver. Give them a positive model to follow.

FREQUENTLY ASKED QUESTIONS

1. I am my mother's POA and primary caregiver. It seems that every time I travel for work my sister suddenly decides to take a vacation. Although my mother does have a paid caregiver, I would feel better if a family member were available to help with any emergencies. What should I do?

Rather than wait for the expected, ask your sister if she, too, has travel plans when you tell her about yours. Be sure to tell her how much you appreciate her willingness to be the contact person in your absence; however, it is always a good idea to plan for surprises. It's a good idea to make sure the caregiver knows how to reach you or another family member.

2. My siblings and I don't communicate. I try, but it always ends badly. What should I do?

Judging by the second part of your question, it sounds like you and your siblings do speak to one another but have different ways of communicating. Take a few minutes to think objectively about your different communication styles. Doing so may help you figure out some better ways of talking to them.

It may also be helpful to consider how you discuss difficult or complex topics with workplace colleagues. As you would at work, define a meeting time and place and inform your siblings of the topics you wish to discuss. Tell them you are looking forward to their input. Timing is another important factor. People are more likely to become upset when they are tired or feel you are barging in. Meeting in a public location—a coffee shop or a restaurant, for example—rather than at home is another way to improve everyone's manners.

3. It seems like we argue about money more than we talk about our mother's care. My older brother, our mother's POA, feels we should spend whatever is necessary to keep her as healthy and happy as possible; however, my younger brother tells us that we are doing nothing more than throwing our inheritance into a deep hole. As the middle child, I don't want to take sides. I just want the arguing to stop.

Having money available for your mother's care is a good problem; however, as you are well aware, people have strong feelings about the most appropriate ways to provide care for a person who has an untreatable and progressive disease. Hopefully, respect and dignity are always part of the equation.

Some adult children feel comfortable with using the money their parents earned and saved to pay for dementia care services. These adult children remember it is the responsibility of the POA to act on their parent's behalf.

It is also important, however, to spend money wisely so funds last as long as possible. And yes, it is true that the money not spent on dementia care may someday become your inheritance.

Feelings that come with managing your parent's money are complex and often conflicted by a lifetime of emotional baggage. It might be useful to have an impartial person, such as an estate lawyer, psychologist, or a social worker, help you and your brothers understand your respective points of view. Having a professional available to guide discussion will help the three of you develop a mutually agreed upon dementia care philosophy.

4. You mention that when you were trying to decide who you wanted to be your POA, your lawyer said that "someone had to be in charge." Is that for legal reasons?

Though not a legal requirement, having "someone in charge" helps your family keep their focus on your parent's care. Even with differences of opinion, things will run more smoothly if one of you is your parent's care manager; however, you should list one or two other people who can take over when needed.

5. My fifteen-year-old daughter needs a summer job. I was thinking of paying her to help me with my mother's care. Is this a good idea?

I am glad you asked. One needs to be careful about giving the grandchildren more caregiving responsibility than is appropriate for their age. Several medical social workers told me about cases where much younger children, sometimes as young as eight or nine years old, were responsible for their grandparent's care while their own parents were at work or, for other reasons, not at home. The list of reasons why this is wrong is a long one—but abusive and unsafe care are two that quickly come to mind.

That being said, having young children participate in activities with their grandparent who has dementia is enriching for both the child and grandparent; however, it is imperative that a responsible adult is present to supervise. A young child should never be left alone with a grandparent who has dementia.

Some young adolescents can assume some types of caregiving responsibilities. Perhaps taking their grandparent for a walk would be appropriate as long as they have a cell phone to call you or another adult. It might be nice for all concerned if your daughter is able and willing to be your helper for a few hours per day. Puzzles, craft projects, gardening, reading aloud, and time to laugh and talk together are all activities both she and her grandmother might enjoy; however, your nearby presence is important for everyone's safety. Your daughter could also help by running errands, buying groceries, doing household chores, or by cooking simple meals. Your daughter should not be responsible for doing such things as giving your mother medication or helping her bathe or use the toilet.

It's also important that your daughter have time to spend with her family and friends. So, to answer your question, paying your teenaged daughter can be a good idea as long as she isn't working for more than a few hours per day, the tasks are age appropriate, and an adult is available to supervise. Oh—and you need to make sure your daughter feels comfortable taking the job. If she isn't, do not force the issue.

6. I am my mother's primary caregiver. My mother lives in my home along with my three children. My children are struggling to adjust to the person their grandmother has become. It is especially difficult for my youngest child, who is often on the receiving end of my mother's anger and frustration. What can I do?

You have hit upon an important and often forgotten topic—dementia and the grandchildren. It's important that your child understands that what has happened to his grandmother isn't his fault and that a disease controls, but does not excuse, her behavior.

Dementia behavior is something we all find difficult. It's especially hard to make an appropriately controlled response when a parent or grandparent, even when they are ill, becomes angry and says or does hurtful things.

As a family, it might be helpful to discuss what to do when your mother becomes angry. Another strategy is to help your child recognize behaviors that come before an outburst. That way your child can walk away or call to get help, and you can address your mother's distress before it develops further.

Since it appears that your mother targets your youngest child, it's important that he is not left alone with her without a plan of "self-protection." Most likely this would involve a nearby adult interceding in his behalf.

Many grandchildren do enjoy reading, playing games, or doing craft projects with a grandparent who has dementia. In the long run, the time your child spends with his grandmother will enrich his life; however, your child must feel comfortable in knowing that you or another adult is nearby should he need assistance or protection.

If the situation does not improve, a few meetings with a psychologist, counselor, or medical social worker can give your family and the targeted child the tools to develop better ways of coping with your mother's behavior.

7. My sisters and I are our mother's caregivers. We share most of the work but have difficulty discussing who pays for what. We also realize that eventually we will need to hire caregivers or place her in a dementia care facility. Our mother doesn't have much in the way of savings, and her only income is a monthly Social Security check. That means my sisters and I make financial contributions to her care. One of us has college-aged children, and another has a big mortgage payment. Of the three of us, I am the most financially comfortable; however, I am also doing most of the day-to-day work. What can we do so money doesn't become a sore point between us?

This might be a good time for the three of you to make a small investment in your relationship. Scheduling a meeting with a financial advisor, an elder law attorney, or a geriatric consultant will help you sort out an equitable way of dividing the financial responsibilities associated with your mother's care. The Alzheimer's Association is another resource you can use.

These professionals can help you find other sources of income for your mother. For example, if your mother owns a home, a reversible mortgage may provide the money she needs. Renting her home may make placement in a dementia care facility possible. It's also possible to convert life insurance policies into long-term care insurance.

WORKSHEET 5.1:
Self-Assessment

Learning to recognize family challenges before they become an overwhelming problem can help prevent family disharmony from escalating to anger. Make a list of the family challenges that cause you and your siblings to feel angry or frustrated with one another. For each one, describe things you can do to improve sibling communication and cooperation.

_____

_____

_____

_____

_____

_____

_____

_____

_____

WORKSHEET 5.2:
Reflective Writing

Reflective writing is similar to keeping a diary; however, rather than writing by long-hand in a small book with an easily opened lock, create a folder to save your word-processed daily musings. Like diary writing, it is important to relax and write whatever comes to mind. Don't worry about editing. The important thing is to periodically review what you have written. Reading earlier entries can reveal many surprises, for example, the progress you have made, areas that still need improvement, and clues to improving relationships.

6

MANAGING BEHAVIOR

Theirs, Yours, and That of Others

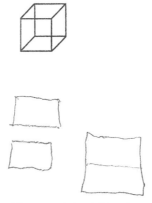

Man, age sixty-eight, cube.

Understandably, Dorothy did not like the rehabilitation hospital. She did not like those people who asked her strange questions. She found physical and occupational therapy exhausting and confusing. The food was terrible. One day she told me, in a matter-of-fact way, that a nurse had given her insulin by mistake. Then, Dorothy said, the nurse gave her a piece of chocolate to cover up the error.

Of course, I looked further into her accusation. What if Dorothy was correct? As it turned out, Dorothy had overheard a conversation about her roommate's condition. Difficult-to-control diabetes necessitated that the woman receive a late-night insulin injection.

Dorothy had a long history of saying odd things like this: a bit of truth reshaped into something plausible but not truly reasonable. Many years ago, I had learned the necessity of looking further into whatever Dorothy might say. I also learned that a nonspecific response, such as "I spoke with the head nurse who assured me she would look into the situation," was the best approach.

Difficult behavior was making it hard for Dorothy to improve her daily living skills. The physical therapist said Dorothy refused to use her walker. The occupational therapist said Dorothy did not pay attention and wasn't learning the skills she needed to dress herself.

The psychologist suggested giving her a low dose of an antianxiety medication. While at first Ativan® (lorazepam) made her a little drowsy, it did reduce Dorothy's anxiety, and within a week, she was able to go home.

Unfortunately, the calming effects of Ativan® lasted only for six weeks. Gradually, the agitation returned. She did not like having strangers in her home, and more specifically, she did not like "those ladies." Dorothy was quite certain that back surgery—which she truly believed was the reason for her hospitalization—had worked. Obviously, she no longer needed any help.

Her primary care doctor suggested that we replace Ativan® with Seroquel® (quetiapine), an antipsychotic often used to treat schizophrenia and bipolar disorders. Now, this is where my background as a medical writer got me into trouble. It didn't take long for me to discover that using Seroquel® to manage dementia behaviors is a controversial topic. Among other things, taking this medication would put Dorothy at a higher risk for a heart attack, stroke, and sudden death. I wondered if medicating her was ethical and maybe more for my convenience than for her benefit.

Her home caregivers were threatening to quit if I didn't do something. After many e-mail conversations with Dorothy's very patient doctor, I decided Seroquel® was worth a try. And what a difference it made! It gave her moments where she could enjoy listening to music or go to the store with a caregiver. And the caregivers said they would stay.

HOME AGAIN

After spending nearly two months in various hospitals and a few weeks' stay in a continuum of care memory unit, Dorothy returned home. She was, of course, very happy, and for a few days, she cooperated with me and her caregiver. Sadly, it didn't take long before her good mood gave way to the frustrations imposed by her new lifestyle. Nearly every day Dorothy told the caregiver not to come back tomorrow. She was also very angry with me and was certain that I had ganged up against her.

WHO IS THIS PERSON?

Some people find their family member almost seems like a stranger—perhaps morphing from a kind and helpful person to a combative and vulgar one.

Other times, dementia seems to magnify personality traits. When this happens, people often say, "It's my father, only 'more so.'" It's not so bad if a formerly cheerful and upbeat person becomes an exaggeration of their former self. But it can be a considerable trial if a difficult loved one becomes "more so."

Why dementia causes personality change is a complex question. The disease alters and destroys brain structures. As a result, the brain loses the ability to accurately process and relay information. Memory loss is a symptom associated with all types of dementia. Other brain changes release the censorship mechanisms that control anger and prevent people from being impolite or doing socially inappropriate things.

I worry about my children if dementia should become my fate or, perhaps more accurately stated, if my dementia becomes their fate. In preparation, I have already apologized for any difficulties I may cause. They also know I expect them to do what is manageable under their circumstances and to share the responsibility of my care. One friend told me that my consideration shows that if dementia should overtake my life, I won't be one of the difficult ones. I hope she is right.

WHO IS IN CHARGE?

Dorothy wasn't the kind of person who could listen to, much less consider, the advice of others. Now with dementia in the mix, talking to her about long-term care was impossible. In response to my obvious frustration, one of the rehabilitation hospital doctors asked if I would do everything a three-year-old child demanded; however, the doctor's rhetorical question did not take Dorothy's real age into consideration. Her demands to manage her own finances and drive do not compare with a toddler demanding another cookie. The doctor's response shows he did not understand the difficulties family caregivers face.

Managing behavior is the crux of dementia care. The truth of this statement is supported by an Alzheimer's Association survey that shows caregivers are more interested in medications that improve behavior and daily living skills than they are in medications used to improve cognition. Many of the people I interviewed say the drugs that improved cognition can make dementia care more difficult when their family member cannot understand why they must live in your home or with caregivers.

Basically, nearly everything you do in your caregiver role—from the legal hurdles to providing a safe home for your loved one—all boils down to your loved one's behavior and how they respond to you and their new situation.

The behaviors associated with early stage dementia are sometimes the most difficult. Your loved one is fighting the imposed changes the diagnosis has brought to their life. Your loved one does not want your help, cannot understand why you insist on paying the bills, and certainly doesn't want to move. And you, the family caregiver, do not have the experience to both calm your loved one and cope with the disquiet this new relationship brings into your life.

Sometimes the normal pressures and tensions that have now fallen on your shoulders can lead to behaviors that you may regret. Out of frustration, you anger easily. And much to your dismay, you begin to feel like a raging adolescent. Your loved one doesn't listen and manipulates what you say to serve their purposes. Nothing makes sense, nothing works, and more than anything you want your old life back.

Dementia behaviors may also include some weird and scary things. More specifically, your loved one may experience hallucinations and delusions. How you respond to these new and unexpected behaviors has the potential to turn uncomfortable moments into situations that may necessitate assistance from your local police department or a trip to the emergency room.

BUGS ON THE WALL AND
PICNICS ON THE FRONT LAWN

In chapter 3, you read that confabulations, hallucinations, and delusions often go hand in hand with dementia. Academically, and even philosophically, all are interesting phenomena. What happens that causes the brain to create fanciful stories, believe others are doing or saying hurtful things, or see things that are not there?

For caregivers, it is not enough to know that these aberrations are just the brain playing tricks on all of us. Caregivers need practical information. They need to know how to respond so the person in their care does not become even more fearful and agitated. Caregivers need strategies to avoid arguments and never-ending conversation about things that do not exist—or at least do not exist in our world.

Recognizing that bugs on the wall are real to your family member is an important first step. Something has happened that allows the brain to create and respond to false stimuli. Think how you might feel if your spouse insists you caused the car accident and not the person who ran the red light. You would be angry, confused, and quite sure your husband was mistaken. This is exactly how a person who has dementia feels when we try to make their reality match ours.

Fanciful stories were part of Dorothy's history long before dementia entered her medical chart. At first, I believed everything she said. Then, with time and experience, I developed the habit of checking with the people who might know something different. After all, most of her stories did have a seed of truth to them. What if Dorothy's sister was in fact spreading tall tales? And certainly, I would have been remiss if I did not look further into the insulin episode at the rehabilitation hospital.

Later, when dementia was unquestionably part of our day, I had to be extra careful about separating fact from fiction. What if Dorothy's caregiver had indeed abandoned her at the senior center? Or was Dorothy's inability to distinguish between five minutes and two hours the actual root of the problem?

Inquiring into these matters had to be done with utmost care. It was imperative that I speak with her caregivers with respect for their professionalism; however, as you will read shortly, elder abuse is a common problem. I needed to keep that possibility in mind, too.

I learned the hard way that people who have dementia cannot follow or accept rational explanations. Dorothy no longer had the capacity to listen, reason, adapt, or understand. If anything, reasoning made a trying situation worse. I found that joining her in this different world worked best.

In response to Dorothy mentioning her caregiver frequently had picnics on the front lawn with strange men, it was better that I say, "Gosh, that is terrible; I'll look into it," rather than, "Don't be silly." My vague, yet affirmative reply told her that I was listening, respecting her concern, and responding in an appropriate manner. I found that making an effort to speak in an affectionate and reassuring tone made everyone, including me, remain calm.

More often than not, I would again hear about the picnic and strange men a few minutes later. Sometimes the only way to stop Dorothy's "broken record" was to distract her with a comment about the weather or the possibility of an afternoon snack. Health care professionals call this tactic "distraction and redirection."

There are situations when it is important to report behaviors like hallucinations and delusions to your loved one's doctor. Having new, increased, or more fearful sensory events might be a drug side effect. This is especially true if your loved one now takes new medication or a different dose of an established one. A simple adjustment in timing or dose may be all it takes to relieve your loved one— and you—of these troubling symptoms.

Reporting hallucinations and delusions also may help your loved one's doctor distinguish Alzheimer's disease from frontotemporal lobe dementia. As stated in chapter 3, hallucinations tend to occur in mid- to late-stage Alzheimer's disease and very early in the course of frontotemporal lobe dementia.

Hallucinations are often frightening. Seeing bugs crawling on the walls or odd-looking people dancing in front of your face would terrify most people.

It's also true that hallucinations can be comforting. Your loved one may tell you about a pleasant visit with a long-dead relative. There is no need to say that the sister who stopped by for a most enjoyable chat is dead. Instead, just affirm that it must have been very nice to see your sister after all these years.

Again, when hallucinations become a problem, consider how you might respond if someone told you that the bugs you see really aren't there. I can tell you what Dorothy did—she went into survival mode and somehow managed to call an exterminator. Even though Dorothy had not used the phone for nearly two years, the caregiver said she was unstoppable.

To make matters worse, the extermination company was very willing to sell an expensive year-long contract to someone who was obviously incompetent. It took many phone calls and a letter to corporate headquarters to undo what had happened during those frenzied moments.

To prevent a difficult situation from escalating into survival mode behavior, you might say something like, "I cannot see what you see, but I am sure it is very scary." You might remind your loved one that you are there and that you will make sure they are safe. Sometimes a hug or a gentle touch will have a calming effect.

If that tactic doesn't work, you can consider pretending to call the exterminator to rid the house of bugs or the police to make those strange people go home. Other times, when hallucinations cause overwhelming fear, the only thing you can do is take your loved one to the emergency room.

A VERY DEEP SLEEP

Many people have mentioned the difficulty their family member has in separating from their dreams upon waking. Occasionally, Dorothy's caregivers would report similar observations in their daily notes. If the dream involved an argument or some other difficulty, the anger associated with that dream would continue many hours afterward. It was especially difficult if the dream was about something terrible that I or one of her other caregivers did. It's much easier to apologize than to explain the terrible thing never happened—it was just a dream. If the dream was a scary one, then similar to calming a hallucination, a soothing voice, an assurance of safety, and a comforting hug or touch is often helpful.

WHEN THE SUN GOES DOWN

Agitation, confusion, anxiety, disorientation, and depression are symptoms frequently associated with having Alzheimer's disease, as well as other kinds of dementia; however, for some people who have dementia these symptoms worsen late in the afternoon or perhaps somewhat later after the sun sets. Sundowner's syndrome is the name used to describe this cyclic behavioral pattern.

The extreme agitation and confusion associated with sundowning can make it especially difficult to manage your loved one—particularly since you or other the caregivers may be tired and short tempered by the end of the day.

Medical researchers don't know what causes sundowner's syndrome. Some clinicians feel these behavioral changes reflect a late afternoon dip in the patient's ability to communicate, an increase in confusion, or perhaps a strong response to frightening shadows. Others believe hormonal or other physiologic changes that disturb the normal sleep cycle are what cause sundowning behaviors.

Demonstrating that sundowner's syndrome comes from the brain may eventually help clinicians develop new and better ways to manage the behavior. Meanwhile, in the absence of drug therapies that specifically target sundowning, clinicians and caregivers rely on medications that treat agitation and other difficult behaviors. Be sure to inform your family member's doctor if sundowning becomes a regular occurrence. The doctor can prescribe medications to reduce symptoms (see table 6.1).

Sometimes doctors prescribe sleeping pills, such as Ambien® (zolpidem), Lunesta® (eszopiclone), and Sonata® (zaleplon), to make sure your loved one falls and stays asleep. The National Institute on Aging warns that people who have Alzheimer's disease should not use sleeping pills on a regular basis as taking them may increase risk of falls (see table 6.2).

WANDERING OR ELOPEMENT

It seems we regularly hear news alerts about an elderly family member who wandered away from their home or care facility and is now lost. Some people seem compelled to escape while others get lost and just keep on going. If not located within twenty-four hours, up to half of these people are found

Table 6.1.   Strategies That May Ease Sundowning Symptoms

Identify and remove possible triggers, for example, shadows and low lighting.
Limit caffeine and sugar to early parts of the day.
Plan activities to increase exposure to sunshine.
Place nightlights throughout the house.
Serve dinner early.
Serve the largest meal at noon.
Maintain a structured routine throughout the day.
Encourage an afternoon nap.

Table 6.2. Medications Used to Modify Dementia Behaviors

Medication Brand Name (Generic Name)	Things to Know
Ativan® (Lorazepam)	Helps people relax and reduces agitation Can make people drowsy, confused, and prone to falling
Celexa® (Citalopram)	Reduces depression and anxiety May take four to six weeks to work Sometimes used to help people sleep
Depakote® (Sodium valproate)	Used to treat severe aggression and to reduce depression and anxiety
Klonopin® (Clonazepam)	Helps people relax and reduces agitation Can make people drowsy, confused, and prone to falling
Remeron® (Mirtazapine)	Reduces depression and anxiety May take four to six weeks to work Sometimes used to help people sleep
Tegretol® (Carbamazepine)	Used to treat severe aggression and to reduce depression and anxiety
Trileptal® (Oxcarbazepine)	Used to treat severe aggression and to reduce depression and anxiety
Zoloft® (Sertraline)	Reduces depression and anxiety May take four to six weeks to work Sometimes used to help people sleep

Note: Adapted from National Institute on Aging, "Caring for a Person with Alzheimer's Disease: Your Easy-to-Use Guide," accessed March 17, 2021, https://order.nia.nih.gov/publication/caring-for-a-person-with-alzheimers-disease-your-easy-to-use-guide?_gl=1*ay8x90*_ga*MTI1NDc1ODU4NS4xNjA3NDYxNTkw*_ga_TK3CE80DBZ*MTYxNjUyNjExMy4xMi4xLjE2MTY1MjYzNDEuNjA.

seriously hurt or dead. According to the Alzheimer's Association, about 60 percent of people who have dementia wander.

People who have dementia often say they are on their way to the grocery store, the bus stop, or to see a friend. Therefore, many dementia care professionals prefer the word *elopement*, rather than *wandering* to indicate a purposeful, rather than random, behavior.

It's hard to determine why people who have dementia elope. It may be a way to express or cope with anxiety or anger. It may be an attempt to find a familiar place, do a familiar activity like going to work, or escape from things wrongly interpreted as dangerous or scary.

Perhaps, like sundowner's syndrome, researchers will discover that brain chemistry changes are what make some people compelled, as we might say, to get out of the house.

Many dementia care facilities accommodate elopement by incorporating a circular path in their floor plan. The patient can walk, perhaps socialize with other residents, and eventually return to their starting point. Meandering garden paths are another feature you might see in some dementia care facilities.

But what can you do at home to prevent elopement? One simple tactic is to encourage physical activity to curb restlessness. Taking a walk together, perhaps with a purposeful destination, will be a refreshing break for both of you. If your family member or spouse tends to leave at the same time each day, a planned physical activity, such as a simple craft or baking project, gardening, setting the table, or folding laundry, might quiet the urge.

Another suggestion is to provide a safe place for your family member to walk. In the house, remove rugs, extension cords, and other tripping hazards. For nighttime walkers, install night-lights and place gates at stairwells to prevent falls. A gated yard that contains various interesting stopping points may give your loved one the ability to safely leave the house on their own time. Exposure to sunshine, an added benefit, may lessen sundowner's symptoms later in the day.

SAFE TRAVELS

Even with your best efforts, it may be impossible to prevent your family member from walking away from home. Therefore, it is important to build safeguards into their home environment. First of all, many people who have dementia use their car as a means of escape. If taking the keys away is impractical or impossible, disconnect the battery cables or sell the car.

Other safeguards include placing a pressure-sensitive mat by your loved one's bed. A light or a buzzer will inform you when they get out of bed and leave their room. Installing childproof doorknob covers on the doors and touch pad combination locks can prevent your loved one from leaving the house without your knowledge. Some people go as far as to camouflage or hide doors with wallpaper or curtains.

Finding a lost loved one is not the same as looking for a lost hiker. Unlike the hiker, people who have dementia often don't know they are lost. They don't call for help or respond to searchers. Once found, people who have dementia may not know their name, phone number, or address.

Enrolling your loved one in the Alzheimer's Association's safe-return program can be a literal lifesaver. The program supplies your loved one with an identification bracelet, and you receive access to twenty-four-hour support.

"Comfort Zone," an Alzheimer's Association GPS tracking system, is another way to locate people who have dementia.

The Dementia Society of America offers the Operation KeepSafe ID kit. The kit includes several kinds of physical identification, as well as an online profile to help first responders, and other people, locate your loved one.

The Silver Alert, a public notification program, is another resource you can use. Silver Alerts use television, radio, and the internet to broadcast missing person information. Notification banners posted on overhead LED street signs that warn drivers about weather conditions and road accidents can help locate people who may be wandering along highways and other major roads. More than forty states and several cities have Silver Alert or similar programs that target missing adults who have dementia or other cognitive disabilities (see Helpful Resources).

Inform your neighbors and nearby businesses about your family member who has dementia. Keep a daily record of the clothes your loved one is wearing so you can give an accurate description to your neighbors, the police, or to your local radio or TV station. These simple tactics may make the difference between a safe return and a tragedy.

But the bottom line is to alert your neighbors, local authorities, and any safe-return programs as soon as you realize that your loved one is missing. A search should begin immediately. The Alzheimer's Association suggests looking within a five-mile radius of where your loved one was last observed.

IT'S EMBARRASSING FOR EVERYONE

For many family caregivers, dealing with toileting accidents is one of the hardest aspects of dementia care. It's embarrassing. It's smelly, and it signifies a complete reversal of the relationship you once shared with your loved one.

Gender differences, such as an adult son being the primary caregiver for his mother, can make toileting issues particularly difficult. Under these circumstances, it might be best to have a female family member, or a female paid caregiver, responsible for your mother's toileting needs.

Keep in mind that your loved one did not soil themselves on purpose. They cannot prevent and may even be unaware of their mishap. Punishment for a toileting accident is never appropriate, and kindness and tact are of the utmost importance. Rather than saying "It looks like you wet your pants again," you might say, "Let me help you change your clothes, it looks like you spilled something on yourself or sat in something." For many families, the arrival of incontinence means the difference between home care and moving their loved one either to an assisted living or a dementia care facility.

Sometimes Dorothy just couldn't make it to the bathroom in time. Other times, being upset seemed to make it harder for her to control her bladder. There were occasions when she was unaware of her toileting accidents; however, it didn't take long for us to discover that certain foods always caused Dorothy to have accidents. Chocolate, graham crackers, and vegetables like spinach always led to problems.

We also learned that despite her modesty, we had to take charge of the cleanup to prevent the mess from spreading further. Even though Dorothy didn't say much, I know she was terribly embarrassed. Afterward, she just wanted to be by herself.

With the onslaught of obvious dementia, Dorothy truly believed each bathroom accident was an isolated event that would never happen again. Because she couldn't remember any previous accidents, she refused to wear absorbency products. To keep her as dry and clean as possible we frequently reminded her to go to the bathroom—"just in case."

We washed her clothes and sheets in Odo-ban® plus regular washing machine detergent. Lysol spray helped remove odors from chairs and her plastic mattress cover. Using these products sometimes replaced one odor with another that was a little sickeningly sweet.

Dorothy didn't like to see us clean *her* house. To keep her in as good a mood as possible, we scheduled laundry and housecleaning around naps, the evening news, or after she had gone to bed for the night.

WHY DOES INCONTINENCE HAPPEN?

The effects of dementia, as well as many other conditions, can make it difficult for your loved one to control their bladder and bowel. Because many causes of incontinence are treatable, it is important to discuss this aspect of your loved one's health with their doctor. Some causes of these are bladder infections and the side effects from medications used to treat anxiety. Other causes include an enlarged prostate gland (men), pelvic floor dysfunction (women), and the urgency both men and women may experience.

Many bladder control treatments require the ability to follow directions or cooperate with postoperative rehabilitation efforts; therefore, having dementia may make treatment difficult or inappropriate for some patients. For these people, absorbency products may be the best option.

A Wake Forest University School of Medicine study showed that nursing home patients receiving medications to both modify dementia symptoms and improve continence lost the ability to perform basic daily living skills 50 percent faster than those receiving dementia medications alone. The authors conclude that simultaneous treatment for dementia and urgency reduced the effectiveness of both medications; therefore, it is important that family caregivers first consider nondrug treatment strategies.

Absorbency Products

Absorbency products include pads, panty liners, disposable briefs, and reusable incontinence products. While it might be tempting, and certainly less embarrassing, to buy mini-pads and sanitary napkins, these products do not keep urine away from skin. Using them without frequent changes may cause painful skin irritation, open sores, and infections. Disposable absorbency products absorb and retain urine, as well as minimize odor. In addition to items made for men and women, absorbency products also factor in such things as "high- and low-flow" situations, body weight, activity level and ambulation, and possible travel needs.

You can buy absorbency products at just about any store that carries health care goods. You can also buy absorbency products online. Using the keyword phrases "incontinence products," "urinary incontinence products," "absorbency products," and "adult disposable underwear" is an efficient and discreet way to make these purchases. Some online stores offer trial packages that include a variety of styles.

Controlling Odor

Making sure that your loved one has enough to drink each day can reduce body odor problems. Concentrated urine has a stronger and, therefore, a more noticeable salty odor than urine that contains enough water. Drinking sufficient water can also help lower the risk for bladder infections. Eating certain foods, such as asparagus, Brussels sprouts, and onions, can contribute to making odoriferous urine.

Skin Care

Avoid scrubbing and using harsh soaps to prevent making tender areas rough, sore, and prone to infection. A pH-balanced, no-rinse, fragrance-free, alcohol-free, and residue-free incontinence skin cleanser can help prevent this painful outcome. You can find out more about incontinence skin cleansers from your local pharmacist, hospital supply salesperson, or the internet. The phrase "incontinence skin cleansers" is a good way to begin your internet research.

While it's important to keep the urogenital area clean and dry, it's also important to do so in a way that maintains your loved one's dignity. As much as possible, maintain eye contact as you clean and never make comments about bad smells or use words related to babies or diapers. Even if your loved one may not understand what you are saying, distractive chat about baseball, the antics of the family cat, or spring flowers can make the situation easier for both of you. Always speak in a soothing and reassuring tone.

OTHER HELPFUL HINTS THAT MAKE TOILETING EASIER

One of the best things you can do to help your loved one manage their toileting is to stay calm. Rushing and creating a sense of panic will make having a bladder or bowel accident even more likely. There are many other things you can do to help your loved one maintain effective toileting behaviors for as long as possible.

Avoid clothing with buttons, belts, or other complicated closures. Keep the bathroom door open and always available for your loved one's use. You and the other caregivers should use a less accessible bathroom. Use night-lights to identify the path to the bathroom to make it easier for your loved one to find the bathroom throughout the day.

As mentioned earlier, it may be tempting to restrict liquids; however, it is important that your family member gets enough to drink. Dehydration can cause constipation, dizziness, and confusion. If bedwetting is a problem, you can consider restricting liquids four to five hours before bedtime—especially coffee, tea, and some carbonated drinks. Caffeinated beverages are diuretics and cause people to produce more urine. Taking your loved one to the toilet after meals or when they have that certain look on their face can help reduce the frequency of bowel accidents. Use waterproof pads to protect the sheets and the mattress.

Diet is another factor. Whole wheat and beans, and other high-fiber foods, are often a problem for people who have bowel incontinence. People who have dementia may not be able to distinguish the "pass gas" feeling from the "need to go to the bathroom" feeling; however, to prevent constipation, it's important keep some fiber in the diet. Discovering the amount of high-fiber food—and spicy foods, too—your family member can tolerate can reduce the number of toileting accidents. Adding yogurt to their diet may also be helpful.

BATHING

You might feel relieved to know that dementia and an aversion to bathing is a topic worthy of research studies and PhD dissertations. Researchers, usually nurses seeking an advanced degree in gerontology or eldercare studies, feel the reasons for this behavioral trait are related to fear of falling, the inability to recognize the person they see in the mirror, or an inborn sense of modesty.

Knowing that refusal to bathe is a typical dementia-related behavior doesn't make telling your loved one they need to take a bath any easier. The invasion of their privacy makes us feel uncomfortable. It also alerts us to the significant involvement we have in our loved one's daily care.

Asking Dorothy to take a bath was a little like playing cat and mouse. The direct approach usually resulted in something like, "I took a bath yesterday," or "I don't need one." The caregivers and I thought marking the days on the calendar that Dorothy did bathe might make her more receptive to our suggestions; however, the record keeping only provided documentation that she sometimes went as long as three weeks without anything more than a quick sponge bath.

The strategy that sometimes worked was preparing the bathroom, turning on the shower, and simply stating, "Your shower is ready, and it's time to get washed."

I have since learned that doing certain things, such as providing soothing music and removing the mirror, may make bath time less of a battle. I noticed that many dementia care facilities have replaced the bathroom mirror with a mural or another type of wall art and that baths are regularly scheduled events. Apparently, the "professionals" manage to convey a sense of authority that family and home caregivers cannot achieve.

In any case, it is important to make bathing as safe as possible. A shower chair and a hand-held shower head may prevent falls and injuries. You can buy a shower chair at a hospital supply store or at some of the larger drug store chains. A plastic lawn chair is a good alternative for stall showers. You can buy a hand-held shower conversion kit at most large hardware or home supply stores. Converting a regular shower head to a hand-held or a "telephone" shower head is not difficult. But even if you are handy with tools, call a handyman. You already have enough to do.

IT'S HARD TO IMAGINE

Daughters and sons, even when dementia is not in the picture, have a difficult time accepting their parent or other loved one as a sexual being and that dementia can impact sexual feelings and behaviors. The effects are unpredictable and depend on the parts of the brain altered by disease as well as by the medications used to manage dementia.

Some people who have dementia have little or no interest in sex. At the other extreme, some may experience a heightened interest in sex or may even become uncharacteristically sexually aggressive.

As you have read earlier, dementia can affect the ability to censor or inhibit socially unsuitable behaviors. Some people who have dementia cannot understand that it is impolite to touch or expose their private areas in public or make unwanted or inappropriate sexual advances; therefore, it is important to consider other reasons for their behavior.

Inappropriate sexual advances may occur if your loved one mistakenly identifies another person as their husband, wife, or partner. On the other hand, touching or undressing may simply mean your loved one wants to use the toilet or that their clothing is uncomfortable.

As difficult as this may seem, it is important to approach these situations without making your loved one feel fearful or embarrassed. If you are caring for a widowed family member or one whose partner is either infirm or living elsewhere, exercise, a craft project, a board game, or other distractions can ease the situation.

Be sure to talk to your loved one's doctor if you feel threatened by overt sexual behaviors. Medications are available that can stop sexually aggressive behavior and thereby protect you and others from this uncomfortable situation.

BEHAVIORAL MANAGEMENT STRATEGIES

In the best of worlds, managing the difficult behaviors without resorting to medication is a lofty goal. Managing behavior without medication takes time, patience, and ingenuity. Health care providers and the people you meet in support groups can offer suggestions. They can tell you the tricks that work for them; however, what works for the person in their care may not be as effective for you. Sometimes medication is truly the best solution.

Probably one of the most important ways to manage behavior is to avoid arguments. There is no need to set the record straight. It doesn't matter if your loved one fervently believes it's 1956. Arguments make everyone angry and make a stressful situation even more so. Dementia is a time to "go with the flow."

Body language is another important behavioral management strategy. Just as with anyone else, approaching a person with a happy face, a comforting hug, and a kind voice always works better than a frown and a harsh tone. Using body language to manage your loved one's behavior is a simple way to reduce anxiety and aggressive behavior, and it can reduce your own stress as well. After all, a smile makes everyone feel good.

Therapeutic deception, or what many laypersons call "creative lying," is a tactic that takes advantage of how well you understand your loved one's world. As you will read in chapter 8, I discovered it was better to tell Dorothy her new blouse was a gift from her granddaughter than to give her another reason to be angry with her overbearing daughter.

Distraction and redirection are other ways to soothe and diffuse difficult behavior. Often you can head off arguments by changing the subject or suggesting a favorite activity.

Sometimes difficult behavior reflects boredom, getting too much or not enough sleep, or the inability to use words to express the need to use the toilet or other physical discomforts. With time, you will learn how to translate your loved one's behavior into workable solutions. It's important that you discuss the pros and cons of medication with their doctor when behavioral solutions do not work.

WHAT ABOUT MEDICATION?

It's impossible to talk about dementia without also mentioning the medications. To prevent this important topic from becoming a visual and mental stumbling block, I will briefly discuss the difference between registered and generic medications.

The pharmaceutical company that developed the medication owns the registered name. *Brand name* is another, more familiar, term for registered name. The symbol ® differentiates the brand name from the generic product.

When the drug patent expires, usually after twenty years, other pharmaceutical companies can make and sell the medication under the generic name. As you probably know, generic medications are usually less expensive than their brand name counterpart.

To help you feel more comfortable with this two-tiered naming system, with the first mention, you will see the brand name first. The generic name will follow in parentheses; for example, Aricept® (donepezil) is a medication frequently used to reduce memory loss. Aricept® is the brand name, and donepezil is the generic name for the same medication. After the first mention of the drug, I will simply say, "Aricept® is a medication frequently used to manage early- to late-stage Alzheimer's disease."

MEDICATIONS USED TO MANAGE BEHAVIOR

The decision to begin using medication to modify dementia behaviors can be surprisingly difficult. You might hear some people describe the drugs to reduce behavioral challenges as a "chemical straight jacket." It sounds terrible, and immediately you envision a room filled with zombie-like elders. Hearing that phrase makes you feel certain that you would never use medication to control your loved one's behavior. Somehow, you believe you can do better than that (see table 6.1).

Eventually, it becomes obvious that your loved one is suffering. While your family member may not be in physical pain, they may be confused, fearful, angry, depressed, and belligerent. Your loved one may become so disturbed that it affects their safety and perhaps yours as well. Depression, another common symptom associated with dementia, also deserves medical attention.

Today, we are fortunate to have medications that relieve the suffering mental anguish causes. Medication extends the length of time your loved one can live at home and improves quality of life for everyone.

Dorothy took pride in the fact she, unlike other people, did not need many medications. It wasn't surprising that she questioned her doctor every time he wrote a prescription.

I knew we were headed for trouble when he said, "These pills will help you sleep better." Dorothy's doctor didn't know that Dorothy believed she did sleep well and didn't need what she believed was a sleeping pill. To head off a disastrous afternoon, I quickly interjected and said, "This medication will keep you strong." "That's right," said her doctor. "It will keep you strong." Health professionals call this behavior management tactic "therapeutic deception."

Just for the record, the pill was neither a sleeping pill nor was it one that would make Dorothy stronger. The prescription was for Seroquel®, the little orange pill used to reduce problems with agitation and hallucinations.

Encouraging Dorothy to take her medication was an ongoing challenge. If I or one of the caregivers didn't sit with her, we would later find her pills on the floor, in a pocket, or hidden under her breakfast or dinner plate. If she refused to take all or some of her pills, we'd say, "How about taking just the orange one today? It will make you strong." Other times, because of her poor short-term memory, we'd wait twenty minutes, give her a tasty snack, and try again.

ALZHEIMER'S DISEASE AND MEMORY-EXTENDING MEDICATIONS

You may have heard about drugs that improve memory and slow the progression of early-stage Alzheimer's disease to more advanced stages (see table 6.3). These medications take advantage of what researchers know about communication between nerve cells. Drugs like Razadyne® (galantamine), Exelon® (rivastigmine), and Aricept® (donepezil) help maintain brain cell communication.

Sadly, for Alzheimer's patients, the effect is often short lived. Clinical researchers use such factors as improvement in cognition, memory, self-sufficiency, and behavior to measure the effect of memory-preserving medications.

Table 6.3.   Medications Used to Slow the Rate of Memory Loss

Medication Brand Name (Generic Name)	Things to Know
Aricept® (Donepezil)	Delays or slows memory loss Used for early- to late-stage Alzheimer's disease Loses its effect throughout time Does not prevent or cure Alzheimer's disease
Exelon® (Rivastigmine)	Delays or slows memory loss Used for early- and mid-stage Alzheimer's disease Loses its effect throughout time Available as pills and skin patch Does not prevent or cure Alzheimer's disease
Namenda® (Memantine)	Delays or slows loss of memory and some daily living skills Used from early- to late-stage Alzheimer's disease Loses its effect throughout time Sometimes given along with other medications included in this table Does not prevent or cure Alzheimer's disease
Razadyne® (Galantamine)	Delays or slows memory loss Used for early- and mid-stage Alzheimer's disease Loses its effect throughout time Available as pills and skin patch Does not prevent or cure Alzheimer's disease

Note: Adapted from National Institute on Aging, "Caring for a Person with Alzheimer's Disease: Your Easy-to-Use Guide," accessed March 17, 2021, https://order.nia.nih.gov/publication/caring-for-a-person-with-alzheimers-disease-your-easy-to-use-guide?_gl=1*ay8x90*_ga*MTI1NDc1ODU4NS4xNjA3NDYxNTkw*_ga_TK3CE80DBZ*MTYxNjUyNjExMy4xMi4xLjE2MTY1MjYzNDEuNjA.

The long-term measure of drug effectiveness is the length of time it takes for the patient to transition from home care or assisted living to the memory care wing of the building. Side effects may include nausea, vomiting, diarrhea, dizziness, drowsiness, and shakiness (tremor). Many of these effects last up to one to three weeks and then lessen.

Namenda® (memantine) is another type of memory-preserving medication. Unlike the previously mentioned medications, Namenda® somehow slows the rate of brain cell death. Namenda® taken during mid- to late-stage Alzheimer's disease can preserve your loved one's daily life skills, such as dressing and toileting, for a few months longer than otherwise expected.

While the benefits may seem trivial, the medication does extend your loved one's quality of life and thereby makes your life a little easier, too. Side effects are rare but do include confusion, dizziness, drowsiness, headache, insomnia, agitation, and hallucinations. Be sure to refer to table 6.3 to see a summary of the medications used to slow memory loss.

INTEGRATIVE AND COMPLEMENTARY MEDICINE

Complementary medicine refers to health care practices that traditionally have not played a role in what clinicians and others call "conventional" medicine. Examples of integrative medicine are meditation, acupuncture, and massage, as well as the inclusion of herbs and dietary supplements. With evidence of safety, many physicians will now incorporate these therapies into their practice.

With regard to dementia, research shows the inclusion of creative and social activities as well as Tai Chi and exercise into the patient's care plan can improve behavior and overall quality of life. In many cases, these integrative practices can reduce the amount of medication the patient takes each day.

The clinical research data to support the use of herbals and supplements to manage or, in some cases, claim to cure dementia, however, is largely based on testimonials. Unlike prescription drugs, U.S. Food and Drug Administration (FDA) regulations do not require that supplements (such as omega-3 fatty acids) and herbals or "medicinal foods" (such as ginkgo biloba) undergo rigorous scientific research to determine safety and efficacy. The FDA regulates dietary supplements under a different set of regulations than those covering "conventional" foods and drug products.

Although some of the supplements and herbals may eventually become valid treatments, there are concerns about their use in place of, or in addition to, physician-prescribed medications. Some of these include unknown effectiveness and safety, lack of content standards, and dangerous interactions with other medications. It's important you inform your loved one's physician of any supplements, herbals, or over-the-counter medications they take. Many physicians, as long as these substances do not cause harm, will accept their use.

MEDICATIONS USED TO QUIET DIFFICULT BEHAVIORS

It's easy to think of psychoactive medications in terms of our benefit. Without question, our loved one's anger, combativeness, and hallucinations make for a long and stressful day. Eventually, these behaviors impact our physical and emotional health.

Even family caregivers who, in their professional life, are psychologists, psychiatrists, and social workers have a difficult time when dementia enters their personal space.

One must also to take into consideration how psychoactive medication can improve your loved one's mood and behavior as well as reduce the fear hallucinations cause. When used judiciously, psychoactive medications reduce suffering.

Of all the medications Dorothy took, the little orange pill was the most important one. What Seroquel® (quetiapine) did for her—what Seroquel® did for us—was take the edge off of what was becoming unmanageable anxiety and belligerence. As for hallucinations, it's hard to tell, but maybe hallucinations would have been more of a problem if Seroquel® wasn't a part of Dorothy's daily medication.

Many of the medications used to manage the behaviors associated with dementia are more typically used to treat other conditions, such as depression and schizophrenia. Off-label drug use indicates that the FDA approved these medications as safe to treat other conditions or groups of people who do not have dementia; therefore, one must take into consideration the overall risks and benefits of using off-label treatments. It is also important to take into account the risks of *not* giving medication.

One wonders if dementia patients who do not receive medication to quiet their anxiety, belligerence, and hallucinations are also at increased risk for strokes and heart attacks. One might also think that difficult-to-manage dementia behaviors could place patients at an increased risk for abuse.

Many studies and government organizations recommend using off-label medications to treat dementia-related behavioral problems only when behavioral strategies have failed.

As you read at the beginning of the chapter, giving Dorothy Seroquel® to modify her behavior was not an easy decision. The literature shows that giving elderly people who have dementia medications like Seroquel® may cause their death as a result of heart failure or stroke. The increase in risk for what researchers call premature death is small—but it does happen. Before giving your loved one a drug normally used to treat schizophrenia or bipolar disorder, it is important to discuss the benefits of this kind of treatment with their doctor.

Dorothy was nearly ninety-six years of age when her fall caused the cascade of events that eventually led to a diagnosis of senile dementia. At that age, what does premature death really mean? Most people don't live that long. Congestive heart failure was another diagnosis that was already a part of her medical chart. Would this situation make taking Seroquel® even more risky?

It's impossible to know if Seroquel® shortened Dorothy's life; however, Seroquel® did extend her ability to live comfortably and safely at home for four more years.

SOME IMPORTANT THINGS TO REMEMBER

There are medications that people who have dementia should take with caution or not at all. In addition to the off-label use of medications normally used to treat various mental illnesses, one should take a cautious approach to using antianxiety medications like Ativan® and antipsychotics like Risperdal®.

It's important that elderly people, especially those who have dementia, avoid anticholinergic medications, a class of medications that inhibit communication of nerve cell information to and from the brain. Research shows anticholinergic medications, such as Benadryl® (diphenhydramine), can worsen cognition and confusion. Atrovent® (ipratropium), used to manage asthma and bronchitis, is another example of a medication that people who have Alzheimer's disease should avoid. And just as a reminder, sleeping pills, drugs that induce sleep and keep people asleep for many hours, are another class of medication where a cautious approach is best (see table 6.4).

It's also important not to make any changes in your family member's medication without first discussing it with their doctor. Changes in dosage, particularly a sudden withdrawal, may cause seizures or significant mental and behavioral problems.

Table 6.4.   Medications to Use with Caution

Medication Brand Name (Generic Name)	Things to Know
Ambien® (Zolpidem)	Used to help people fall and stay asleep
	People with Alzheimer's disease should not use this medication on a regular basis
Lunesta® (Eszopiclone)	Used to help people get to sleep and stay asleep
	People with Alzheimer's disease should not use this medication on a regular basis
Sonata® (Zaleplon)	Used to help people get to sleep and stay asleep
	People with Alzheimer's disease should not use this medication on a regular basis
Ativan® (Lorazepam)	Makes people more relaxed, calms agitation
	Can cause drowsiness, confusion, and falls
Klonopin® (Clonazepam)	Makes people more relaxed, calms agitation
	Can cause drowsiness, confusion, and falls
Risperdal® (Risperidone)	Reduces aggression, paranoia, hallucinations, and agitation
Seroquel® (Quetiapine)	Reduces aggression, paranoia, hallucinations, and agitation
Zyprexa® (Olanzapine)	Reduces aggression, paranoia, hallucinations, and agitation

Note: Adapted from National Institute on Aging, "Caring for a Person with Alzheimer's Disease: Your Easy-to-Use Guide," accessed March 17, 2021, https://order.nia.nih.gov/publication/caring-for-a-person-with-alzheimers-disease-your-easy-to-use-guide?_gl=1*ay8x90*_ga*MTI1NDc1ODU4N4xN jA3NDYxNTkw*_ga_TK3CE80DBZ*MTYxNjUyNjExMy4xMi4xLjE2MTY1MjYzNDEuNjA.

MAYBE YOU COULD USE A LITTLE SOMETHING, TOO

I have to admit that there were occasions when I thought taking one of Dorothy's little orange pills might improve my day. For me, it was more of a humorous thought than something I would do; however, if you feel the need for "a little something," don't hesitate to discuss that option with your doctor.

Because of ongoing stress and social isolation, as well as the inability to attend to personal needs, many clinicians understand the family caregiver is a "sidecar" patient. Peter Vitaliano, a geriatric psychiatrist at the University of Washington, has published more than thirty articles that reveal the many ways caregiving impacts health and longevity. Many of his findings demonstrate that elevated stress hormone blood levels contribute increased risk for high blood pressure, diabetes, and a compromised immune system less able to provide protection from infectious diseases and cancer. Dr. Vitaliano likens caregiver syndrome to post-traumatic stress disorder (PTSD).

Knowing about the risks is important. But more important, knowing how to protect your health reduces the chances of having a serious illness while still responsible for your loved one's care. Good health also allows you to enjoy your free time with family and friends; therefore, you owe yourself an annual physical exam; breast, prostate, and bone density screens; and appointments with specialists, such as the eye doctor.

Many family caregivers find support groups and counseling help reduce stress, resolve pent-up feelings of anger and resentment, and lessen feelings of social isolation. You can find information about the support groups in your community by contacting your local Alzheimer's Association office and various city, county, and state services, such as the Agency on Aging and the Department of Public Health. The calendar section of your local newspaper may publish support group meetings, and many dementia care facilities and nursing homes encourage the public to take advantage of the support group services they provide for their clients.

The internet is another way to find and make community connections. Use keywords that include the name of your town, county, and state followed by "dementia, Alzheimer's, support groups" will provide an extensive list of local groups and services.

Support groups, best led by a person who has the training to manage group discussions, will introduce you to other people who face the same difficulties. Not only will you discover that nearly everyone in the group feels overworked and frustrated, but you will also find that your support group is a rich treasure trove of practical tips that only a person who is a dementia caregiver could possibly know. And that includes you—something you do to manage your family member's care and behavior may help make another person's day a little better.

Counseling is another way to help ease the emotional difficulties that become entwined in the family caregiver's daily life. Emotional difficulties are part of being human. We all feel angry or sad, or we have difficulty understanding the situations that befall us at one time or another.

The emotional difficulties associated with being a loved one's caregiver are extreme, unrelenting, and out of the ordinary. Making the effort to get a healthier perspective on your situation and learning ways to manage difficult situations is time well spent. It is costly, but most insurance policies do cover all or some of the expense. For those of you who are at least sixty-five years of age, Medicare is another option.

Look for a mental health professional who has knowledge about geriatric conditions and the impact they have on the whole family. Some counselors will state their areas of expertise on a website or on their business card.

These health care professionals have ways of directing conversation to help you become more insightful about your situation; for example, rather than hoarding pent-up anger about a relative who does not provide the help they should, you learn to improve the situation or perhaps develop a different kind of relationship with the difficult family member. After all, even if warranted, being furious with your brother, sister, or some other close relative isn't going to solve anything. You can put that "anger energy" to better use.

And face it—bending the ear of a professional can save your personal relationships. Your friends and family may be kind and supportive, but they don't really want to hear about your bad day every time they speak to you. Not only will the daily dementia report wear them out, it is better for you if time spent with family and friends is time away from dementia.

CAREGIVER SYNDROME: GIVING A NAME TO HOW YOU FEEL

Stress is just part of the picture. More than likely, you also feel exhausted, anxious, depressed, sad, or angry. And sometimes you are hostile toward people who wonder what they did to deserve your wrath; however, caregiving syndrome does more than affect your behavior.

For many reasons, it is important that family caregivers get relief from the overwhelming stress that comes from years of doing more than your abilities, circumstances, and resources would normally withstand.

IF I HEAR THIS ONCE MORE!

Think about the kinds of caregiving situations that put you on edge. Is it the constant repeating of the same stories, same questions, and same demands? Or maybe it's those mean or "button-pushing" things your family member says that create instant anger. Sometimes, in retrospect, you realize a little planning may have helped avoid behavioral difficulties. Self-assessment, education, and planning ahead are all ways to prevent potential flash points from escalating into unfortunate situations (see worksheets 6.1–6.3).

Keeping in mind that many people who have dementia cannot censor their thoughts may make certain verbal behaviors easier to accept and perhaps even modify. Unlike other people who can keep off-color or impolite thoughts to themselves, everything and anything seems to tumble out of your loved one's mouth. At home, it is best to ignore the personal jabs your loved one might make about your appearance. Even when they say they hate you for taking over their life, try to remember it is the dementia, not your loved one, who is saying those words. In public, you hope others will see and understand that you are a loving adult child and not, as Dorothy often told strangers, her jailor.

The National Institute on Aging suggests printing a business-sized card with something like: "My mother has Alzheimer's disease. She may say or do things that are unexpected. Thank-you for understanding."

Many family caregivers find they need help with learning how to prevent pent-up feelings from eventually erupting as anger. If you feel this is your situation, consider talking to a psychologist, a medical social worker, or support group peers.

It is worthwhile to first consider some old-fashioned remedies. Counting to ten is a tried and true way to separate the emotion from the instant response. Simply walking away is another way to diffuse the feeling. Dorothy's caregivers said a quick trip to the garage helped them cool off.

In time, you will learn to anticipate the kinds of situations that tend to make you feel a little nuts. For me, taking Dorothy to the doctor was one of those situations. While she refused our help at the check-in counter, she was also unable to understand the intake questions, fill out the forms, or find her insurance and Medicare cards. Meanwhile, the people in line, as well as the front desk personnel, were showing their impatience, and I, trying to control how I really felt inside, made efforts to appear as the ever-patient daughter.

Calling the doctor's office before our arrival gave us the ability to take care of the paperwork over the phone. It also helped that the caregivers discovered that arranging Dorothy's wallet the evening before going on any planned doctor appointments made things considerably easier for everyone. Making sure her medical cards were visible and within easy reach gave Dorothy a moment of independence and reduced the tension of taking her to the doctor.

ELDER ABUSE

Several times in this chapter I have used a phrase "the normal pressures and tensions that fall on the shoulders of family caregivers." Gleaned from an interview with Dr. Jordan I. Kosberg, a retired social gerontologist, this phrase is a polite way to say that the pressures and tensions associated with dementia caregiving can cause each of us to become momentarily or even habitually abusive to the person in our care.

According to Dr. Kosberg, elder abuse within the privacy of a family setting can result in a "conspiracy of silence" that makes mistreatment difficult to identify and prevent. Family or paid caregivers are not likely to admit to such behavior. The dependent family member may deny abuse or lack the competency or ability to report it.

Kosberg states that elder abuse is one of the most invisible problems in society (see table 6.5). As part of his research, Kosberg has identified the characteristics of high-risk caregiving situations and caregivers. Many of these risk factors come from situations when families designate the least capable person as their loved one's caregiver. Family members often view this person as "needing something to do" and overlook medical or emotional problems, alcohol or drug dependencies, or situations of economic hardship.

Other high-risk caregiver characteristics include a stoic attitude that prevents the caregiver from asking for or accepting help, having received childhood abuse from the person now in their care, or, because of inexperience, having unrealistic expectations. Disharmony among family members with respect to shared responsibilities is another important factor that can lead to abusive situations.

Kosberg has developed a caregiver assessment worksheet to help identify high-risk caregiving situations. His worksheet takes into consideration such things as the older person's personality, caregiver and family characteristics, and similar views regarding the relationship between the loved one and their family caregiver. With his permission, I have adapted his "High-Risk Placement" worksheet to one you can use either for self-reflection or to open meaningful dialogue between family members (see worksheets 6.3 and 6.4).

Table 6.5.   What Is Elder Abuse?

Physical mistreatment (e.g., hitting, burning, or using restraints)
Verbal, emotional, or psychological abuse—teasing and insulting
Misuse of property or finances
Withholding food, water, and other daily living needs
Forced social isolation
Using fear and intimidation to control behavior
Enabling dangerous situations

One of the most important things you can do if you suspect abuse, neglect, or exploitation, is to call the Adult Protective Services hotline and Eldercare Services.

If possible, document the abuse, neglect, or exploitation. Documentation should include such things as photographs showing injuries or poor physical condition; written reports made by other caregivers, friends, or relatives; and bills showing inappropriate use of credit cards. In many states, Adult Protective Services must investigate reports of elder abuse, neglect, or exploitation within thirty-six hours of having received a report.

FINANCIAL ABUSE

Many of us have seen or read news reports about a well-known person exploited by an associate or a family member. Stan Lee, the ninety-five-year-old creator of Spider-Man and Hulk, was entangled in a legal battle against an associate and memorabilia collector attempting to control Lee's fortune. Buzz Aldrin, the second man to walk on the moon, claimed his youngest children were trying to gain control of his estate by alleging he has dementia.

A National Center on Elder Abuse (NCEA) report states that that financial abuse is becoming more of a problem as our population becomes increasingly more elderly. The report also states that financial abuse is an underreported and hidden crime. According to NCEA estimates, 90 percent of perpetrators are family members or other people close to the elderly person. Some of these are caretakers, neighbors, and friends. It's shocking, but there are lawyers, accountants, and court-appointed guardian services guilty of financial abuse.

According to a 2015 *Consumer Reports* publication, the cost of financial elder abuse ranges from $3 billion to $36 billion per year. There are many reasons for this huge discrepancy. Some of these include underreporting, how financial abuse is defined, and the assessment methodology. By any measure, the cost of financial elder abuse is a big number.

There are many ways to protect your loved one from financial abuse. Perhaps the most important is to plan ahead and encourage your loved one to designate their power of attorney (POA) while they are competent to do so. You will learn about POAs and related information in chapter 7.

Staying connected to your loved one through regular phone calls, visits, or e-mails will give you an ear for when things don't sound right. Along with that comes developing a relationship with your loved one's caregiver or the assisted living facility staff. Knowing that you are in the picture will reduce the likelihood of financial exploitation.

One of the best resources is "The Complete Guide to Elder Financial Abuse." Compiled by Medicare Advantage, the guide contains everything you need to know about financial abuse and ways to protect your family member from predation. Perhaps the most important sections are "Resources for Assistance" and a state-by-state compilation of relevant government and social service contact information.

FREQUENTLY ASKED QUESTIONS

1. What should I do if my mother refuses to go to the emergency room or see her doctor?
    This is a difficult question to answer. But you need to take into consideration your mother's competency. Can she make realistic decisions about her health and care needs? You also need to take into consideration your role and responsibilities as her medical power of attorney or possibly her guardian. If you decide taking her to the emergency room or doctor is indeed in her best interests, you can simply say, "Let's get dressed; we need to go out."
    Once, I did acquiesce to Dorothy's refusal to go to the doctor. It was time for her annual eye checkup, and she did not want to go. She had cataract surgery some years before, and it seemed that she could still see well enough. In addition, Dorothy believed wearing glasses made her look old. Taking her to the eye doctor would have been confusing to her and a waste of the doctor's time, and it would have created difficult-to-manage behaviors for everyone; however, the choice was not hers when she needed a blood transfusion to combat severe anemia.

2. What should I bring to the emergency room or to a doctor who has not seen my father before?
    First of all, prepare a grab-and-take travel bag. The bag should contain an assortment of snacks, magazines, and other items to occupy your parent while waiting. And should incontinence be a difficulty, include a change of clothing and undergarments, as well as absorbency products, bathroom wipes, and a spare plastic bag to store soiled clothes.
    Also bring an updated list of *all* medications he takes, a brief summary of his medical history, and the names and contacts for his primary care doctor. Try to make a list of any worrisome signs and symptoms, and prepare a couple of questions to ask the doctor. If possible have a friend, family member, or paid caregiver to accompany you. This makes drop-off and parking issues much easier and affords you the ability to have a few private moments with the doctor.

3. In the chapter you mention that when a parent claims they spent a nice afternoon with an old friend it is better to just tell them you hope they spent a nice afternoon together. What if my mother asks about her deceased husband?
    A friend, in a situation similar to what you describe, made the mistake of telling her mother that her husband of sixty years died several weeks earlier.

Her mother, responding as though it happened yesterday, wept and was angry that no one had bothered to tell her. My friend said it would have been better to say he was out of town visiting with his brother.

4. My father, who has dementia, is living in my home because my mother is no longer able to manage his care; however, when she visits, my father says he wants to sleep with her. How do I handle this, and what should I do?

First of all, talk to your mother. She may feel that it is not right to have sex with someone who is not competent or may seem like a stranger to her. If this is the case, suggest nonsexual contact, such as a massage, hugging, or dancing, so your father can feel her closeness. If your mother truly is interested in intimacy—give your parents the time and privacy they need. On the other hand, your father just might want to have company in bed—he just wants to sleep with her.

5. What can I do to make going to a restaurant or a store less stressful for everyone?

One of the first things is to limit excursions to your loved one's best time of the day. Because Dorothy was at her best mid-morning, we made efforts to schedule doctor appointments and trips to the store or library between 10 a.m. and noon. That way she could eat breakfast and get dressed without feeling rushed. Afterward, if she was still in a good mood, we could take her to a restaurant for coffee or lunch.

Another helpful tactic is to call ahead and explain your situation to the office, store, or restaurant manager. That way they can tell you the best time to avoid crowds, alert their staff to your special needs, or reserve a table for you in a quiet area.

6. My mother takes Aricept® and Namenda® to help improve her memory. While these drugs do seem to help her, they also make caring for her more difficult because she cannot understand why she has to stay at our house. We have noticed that our family life is much calmer on those days when she forgets to take her medicine. What should we do?

Many people find themselves in this uncomfortable predicament when memory medication makes their parent behave more like an early-stage Alzheimer's patient. You want to give your parent the best care—but without the increased behavioral difficulties that may accompany treatment. The best solution is to speak with your parent's doctor about the possibility of either discontinuing her memory medications or giving her additional medication to lessen her anger, anxiety, and belligerence.

7. I registered my father in the Alzheimer's Association safe-return program; however, he refuses to wear the bracelet. What can I do?

There are several things you can do. First of all, there is no rule stating that he must wear the bracelet on his wrist. While it's easier for others to see, you could pin the ID tag to his clothing or convert it to a necklace he can wear under his shirt; however, do notify the Alzheimer's Association of this change in the location of your father's identification information.

WORKSHEET 6.1:
Anger and Frustration

Learning to recognize your flash points is a good way to prevent the normal pressures and tensions of dementia care from escalating to anger. Make a list of the dementia-related behavioral challenges that cause you to feel angry or frustrated. For each one, describe the situation that often provokes the difficult behavior and then list or describe things you can do to defuse the behavior and modify your response to it.

WORKSHEET 6.2:
Reflective Writing

Looking back, were you able to apply your thoughts from worksheet 6.1 to a recent event? Did it work? If so, discuss how or why it was helpful. If not, consider what you might do to make it less likely that you will feel angry or frustrated.

WORKSHEET 6.3:
Honesty Part 1

Use this worksheet to initiate honest and sensitive conversation among family members. Consider having a disinterested third party, such as a counselor or a medical social worker, moderate discussion. Another alternative is to assign one family member the role of discussion moderator. The bottom line is that blaming, faulting, and arguing is not helpful.

If you do not have other willing relatives, use this worksheet to reflect upon your own ability to manage your loved one's care with or without the help of friends, neighbors, or paid caregivers.

Remember, no one fits the description of the perfect caregiver. We all have a history. It is also true that the family member in our care may also have a history that is difficult to overcome. Hopefully, by becoming aware of the risk factors, we can make efforts to modify our behavior and provide safe, loving, and humane care. It may also be true that, for any number of reasons, moving your family member into an assisted living or a dementia care facility is truly the best option.

Is your family member
- female?
- of advanced age?
- dependent?
- a problem drinker?
- difficult to get along with?
- a person who doesn't talk about feelings or wishes?
- known for favoring one family member over others?
- known to have been abused or abusive?
- stoic or someone who does not respond to joy, grief, or pain?
- isolated, with little need for friends or companionship?
- suffering physical impairments, such as poor vision or difficulty walking?
- irritating and tends to make others angry?

Any of the above traits puts your loved one at risk for abuse; however, understanding that your loved one has a difficult personality can give you the insight to modify your own behavior or to find paid caregivers best able to work under these conditions.

Does the caregiver under consideration (either a family member or a paid caregiver)
- have a drinking problem?
- abuse medication or illegal drugs?

(continued)

WORKSHEET 6.3:
Continued

- have dementia or is otherwise confused?
- have mental or emotional illness?
- have a physical illness?
- have caregiving experience?
- have problems managing their own finances?
- depend on others for money?
- have a history of childhood abuse?
- often suffer from stress?
- have few interests or friends?
- tend to blame others?
- tend to be an unsympathetic person?
- lack understanding?
- have unrealistic expectations of the caregiver's role?
- tend to be very critical?
- have a short temper?

Use the above questions and criteria to determine those among you who can best take on the day-to-day responsibilities. Other family members may be better suited to take on the responsibility of managing your loved one's finances, keeping track of paperwork, or being a willing source of short-term respite.

Does your family
- have a well-established support system?
- feel reluctant about taking on caregiving responsibilities?
- live in a crowded home?
- have outside interests and social activities?
- have marital conflict?
- have economic pressures?
- basically get along well with each other?
- prefer to place the family member into an assisted living or dementia care facility?
- understand dementia care and shared responsibilities?

These questions can help you and your family determine if your combined social, emotional, and practical resources are sufficient to withstand the likelihood of having to cooperate and collaborate for what could be several years.

WORKSHEET 6.4:
Honesty Part 2

1. If able, how might the person in your care describe the relationship they once had with you?
2. If able, how might the person in your care describe the relationship they now have with you?
3. How would you describe the relationship you once had with your family member?
4. How would you describe your current relationship with them?
5. Where does your family member want to live?
6. What are your preferences?
7. What kind of living situation would your family member consider ideal?
8. What is your perception of ideal placement?

These questions can serve as your reality check. Are you and your family member on the same page when it comes to perceptions about relationships, living conditions, and implied or assumed promises? These questions may reveal logical answers to hard questions.

7

ONE DAY AT A TIME

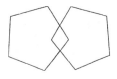

Man, age eighty-five, pentagon.

In my role as the family caregiver, I often felt there was too much to do and not enough time. The everyday tasks—groceries, bills, taxes, yardwork, doctor appointments, house repairs, and the paperwork involved in hiring and paying caregivers added up to another full-time job. In addition, there were frequent surprises that interrupted the flow of my normal work day. Some of those surprises included calming Dorothy's bad moods, dealing with hallucinations and delusions, and, on occasion, taking Dorothy to the emergency room. About a year into taking on the responsibility of Dorothy's care, I had, without realizing it, retired from my professional life.

For many family caregivers, the realities of dementia care mean opting to take a leave of absence from work, working part-time, or perhaps leaving the paid workforce entirely. The economic ramifications of becoming the family caregiver are immense. Not only are there added costs, such as paying for some or all of your family member's expenses, but the reduction in your income may eventually resurface as lower Social Security and retirement benefits.

Dementia care may also involve important long-term and end-of-life decisions. The likelihood of having to place Dorothy into a dementia care facility and the certainty of needing a burial plot and funeral service began to occupy my thoughts to the extent they dominated dinnertime conversation with my husband. Without question, I needed to do whatever it took to free up time and brain space.

My husband and I began to explore local dementia care facilities. Looking at these specialized care services and the people living there helped us understand that Dorothy, although difficult to manage, was not ready to leave her home. These field trips also opened the door to constructive conversation. We both agreed that the right time to move Dorothy to a facility would be when she no longer knew where she was living, had been discharged from a hospitalization, or had become so frail that the caregivers and I could no longer safely care for her.

We thought we were quite thoughtful and perhaps innovative in defining these boundaries; however, after talking with many other family caregivers, I now know all of us developed the same or similar criteria.

Eventually, I found a dementia care facility that seemed right for her. Defining that aspect of Dorothy's care meant there was one less thing to occupy my thoughts. When the time came, I wouldn't have to respond in panic mode.

Funeral and burial issues remained. For Dorothy, although she never spoke about her end-of-life wishes, I'd like to believe she trusted me to make the right decisions. I also knew my feelings about life, death, and whatever happens next were fundamentally different from hers.

Perhaps she would have preferred a burial alongside her husband in a cemetery nearly two thousand miles away from where we and the rest of her family lived. A distant burial and funeral seemed neither realistic nor cost effective. In the end, I purchased a plot and prepaid for a funeral that family and friends could easily attend. It just seemed like the right thing to do.

Defining those two benchmarks was such a relief. I had a plan to follow and could use the energy spent worrying about the nebulous future in other and more positive ways—and that made getting through each day so much easier.

WHAT'S DIFFERENT?

There is nothing new about family members helping loved ones as they age and eventually succumb to illness. This time-honored practice both mirrors our cultural and religious traditions and reflects our innate love and respect for our immediate and extended family. Nonetheless, the creeping impacts of societal change make it difficult for families to help one another as they once did.

Many of us leave our hometown to where our work and interests take us. Postponed childbearing makes it likely that some will have children at home at the same time when older loved ones need help. And unlike earlier generations, today nearly the majority of women work outside the home. The effect of needing two incomes adds another layer of difficulty when our loved ones require assistance.

We aren't the only ones who decide to live elsewhere. After living as long as fifty years in the home they bought as young marrieds, our loved ones may opt to relocate to a warmer climate or to a more affordable community. Sometimes our loved ones decide to move closer to another family member.

In either case—a move to a warmer climate or closer to family—having to learn about the community resources that support safe and independent living is something we usually put off until chronic medical problems occur. And when dementia enters the picture, the family is confronted with having to quickly learn how to navigate through the medical, legal, and emotional aspects of becoming their loved one's caregiver.

Advancements in medicine and public health affect longevity and how we age. Vaccinations, antibiotics, clean water, and workplace safety make it less likely that an infectious disease or an accident will claim our life. In 1900, when the average lifespan was forty-seven years of age, pneumonia was the most common cause of death. Today, we can expect to enjoy an average lifespan of seventy-five years. Cancer, diabetes, heart disease, and chronic illnesses have replaced infectious diseases as the top killers. Longer lifespan and lingering illness make it more likely that dementia will be part of the picture.

How long someone will live after receiving a diagnosis of Alzheimer's disease or another form of dementia is a difficult question to answer. Many studies compare age, gender, and level of disability caused by other conditions and diseases as a way to answer this question. Taking all of those factors into consideration, research shows that, on average, people who have Alzheimer's disease live between four to eight years after their diagnosis.

WHO ARE THE FAMILY CAREGIVERS?

The "typical" U.S. caregiver is a forty-six-year-old woman who works outside the home and spends more than twenty hours per week providing unpaid care to her mother. Therefore, in addition to the emotional issues associated with providing long-term care, the typical caregiver has significant work and family obligations. In all fairness, it is important to recognize the efforts of immediate and extended family as well as friends who assume significant caregiving responsibilities.

According to the most recent Alzheimer's disease factsheet, sixteen million family members and friends provide 18.6 billion hours of unpaid care to people who have dementia—an economic value of $244 billion. These staggering statistics illustrate the enormity of the challenge that promises to become even more so.

Looking back, it amazes me that people who have dementia, a life-threatening disease, receive so much of their care from well-meaning relatives and friends who, more than likely, do not have any health care training. One would think that, like childbirth classes, there would be more classes to teach family caregivers the skills they need to provide or oversee appropriate and safe home care for their parent or other loved one.

LEGAL CONSIDERATIONS

This may seem like an odd jump—going from the profile of the family caregiver to the legal aspects of dementia care—but in truth, it is difficult to get the help you need without papers that prove you have the legal right to intrude into your loved one's affairs. There are several approaches to getting the legal authority to manage your family member's medical and financial affairs—power of attorney (POA), guardianship, and conservatorship.

Although your family member's doctor appreciates speaking with you, they can neither respond to nor discuss your concerns without having a health POA document on file. This document assures the doctor that you, and possibly other designated individuals, have the authorization to receive confidential information and to make medical decisions on your loved one's behalf.

In addition, the general POA gives you—or perhaps another family member, an accountant, or a lawyer—permission to make financial decisions on behalf of your loved one. Without this document, you cannot sign checks, deposit or withdraw money from your family member's bank accounts, or use their credit card to pay their bills.

I was frequently in situations where having POA documentation allowed me to exchange information with the businesses and services Dorothy once used. To make these dealings as efficient as possible, I scanned her durable POA papers and saved them as separate PDF files. That way, I always had easy access to them. Depending on the situation, I either printed a copy to mail in a stamped envelope, or, if the recipient would accept an electronic version, I simply e-mailed the PDF. To save time when the recipient required a hard copy, I asked to e-mail the document with the promise of a hard copy to follow. Often the recipient was understanding and agreed to my request.

STEPS TO POWER OF ATTORNEY

The power of attorney is a legal document that states that your loved one voluntarily gives you the right to act on their behalf. Since only competent individuals can grant power of attorney to another person, it is important to discuss these issues well before the need arises. People who have early-stage dementia often do have the capacity to make decisions and therefore can sign power of attorney papers.

As with many legal procedures, the details vary from state to state; however, in the most general sense, becoming your loved one's POA involves a lawyer, witnesses, and a notary. The lawyer will ask your loved one a series of questions to determine their needs. Usually, obtaining a durable general power of attorney and a durable health power of attorney are sufficient. You are not present during these proceedings.

You may wonder about the word *durable*. Meaning "long-lasting" or "enduring," a durable POA is one that remains in effect even if your family member becomes incapacitated and can no longer grant the authorization described in the power of attorney document. Your POA role terminates when your family member dies.

Your family member can opt to designate more than one person to be their POA. This provides protection should travel, illness, or other situations interfere with your ability to fulfill your responsibilities. It is even possible for your family member to designate a partner or a nonfamily member like an accountant or a close neighbor. Having other people listed on the POA is especially helpful in situations where, for example, you and your parent live far away from one another.

It's important to know that your family member can rescind their power of attorney. Should this happen, their competency becomes the overriding factor, and you may need to consider becoming their guardian and conservator—a topic that follows shortly.

Each power of attorney document requires several signatures. The specific signatures depend on the state where your family member lives. Often, the only required signatories are your family member, one or more witnesses, and a notary. Yes, it does seem strange that you do not sign your family member's POA. In fact, your family member does not even have to ask if you are willing to take on this responsibility.

An advance directive, also called a living will, is another important document. Often included in the durable health POA, the advance directive is where your family member informs you of their end-of-life wishes in the event they become mentally or physically incapacitated. Here, they can state the conditions where they may or may not want tube feeding, cardiopulmonary resuscitation

(CPR), or other artificial life-sustaining measures. Your family member can appoint you, or another person, to make these end-of-life decisions. Resuscitation instructions—in the event of a heart attack, stroke, pneumonia, or another life-threatening condition—are another aspect of the advance directive. A DNR is the abbreviation many people use in the place of stating "do not resuscitate."

An advance directive does more than relieve you from having to make an emotionally difficult decision. Often, doctors, hospitals, and long-term care facilities will not treat or admit patients who do not have an advance directive on file. Liability is one reason; the other is to avoid conflict when family members do not agree on whether to prolong life with artificial life-sustaining measures.

Many people believe the person your family member designates as the power of attorney does all the work. Although in reality, this is what often happens, it is better to consider the POA role as one similar to a manager. Still keeping in mind the requirement to make decisions in your family member's best interests, it is permissible to delegate tasks to other people. Be sure to remind your siblings and other family members of this fact before you become frustrated and angry.

COMPETENCY

Competency is one of those hard to define concepts. Most people understand that competency has something to do with the ability to understand information and perform tasks to an acceptable level. In the work world we use the word *competencies* to describe the measurable behaviors, knowledge, skills, and abilities that make employees successful.

But what about competency as it applies to people who have dementia? It's probably easier to identify people who are clearly incompetent than it is to recognize those who have good-enough daily living and decision-making skills. To make matters even more difficult, people who have dementia are often very good at finding ways to hide their deficiencies.

Clinicians sometimes use the results of the mini mental status exam and the clock-drawing test (described in chapter 3) to support their opinion. But clinicians also know that environment, in this case a hospital or a medical office, can influence behavior and make it harder for patients to count backwards, remember three words, or draw a recognizable clock face.

In a presentation to the American College of Forensic Psychiatry, forensic psychiatrist Dr. Carla Rodgers urged colleagues to use their senses—sight, smell, touch, and hearing—when they evaluate patients for competency. She says that observing lack of eye contact, decayed teeth, low body weight, and the odors associated with poor hygiene are all indicators of questionable competency. Listening for appropriate vocabulary, ability to answer questions, or ability to speak without repetition is another way to assess competency; however, Rodgers does remind her colleagues to differentiate incompetence from treatable problems, such as depression, a bladder infection, and the confusion that some medications may cause. Other ways to assess competency include evaluating the patient's ability to understand their current condition, make reasonable decisions, follow directions, and perform certain tasks.

Competency takes into consideration the specific skills or tasks the patient needs to perform. If writing a will is the issue at hand, can the patient recognize and name their heirs and describe the nature and extent of their estate? Nonetheless, if the patient's ability to make sound self-care decisions is in question, does the patient realize they have a medical problem, know who is providing care, or understand the risks and benefits of receiving or forgoing treatment? The patient's ability to do such things as follow directions, remember to take medications, and prepare well-balanced meals can indicate the ability to live at home without assistance.

As you can see, something like competency is harder to unequivocally diagnose than something like a broken leg; therefore, to protect the patient from unscrupulous relatives and to assure a sound medical judgment, the patient must receive independent competency evaluations from two or more physicians.

WHAT TO DO!

Dorothy assigned me as her durable general power of attorney six years before dementia became obvious. She was proud of having made this decision and often told me that having this document would make it easier for me should she be in a car accident or have to undergo surgery. She was certain that she would need my help only on a temporary basis. Dorothy was unable to imagine a situation when she would be conscious yet incapable of taking care of her own affairs.

Her stay in the rehabilitation hospital revealed a missing piece in what she thought was a well-thought-out plan. Dorothy did not have a health power of attorney. Because she often told me that acquiring a medical alert system could wait until she needed it, I suspect Dorothy refused her lawyer's suggestion to prepare a durable health POA.

As you already know, a neuropsychologist had previously made a diagnosis of senile dementia. Her mini mental status exam score was low enough that no one questioned her need for home assistance. The rehabilitation hospital doctor assigned to her case told me that, because of her incompetence, she could not sign a durable health POA. He said my only alternative was to start guardianship and conservatorship proceedings.

An eldercare lawyer confirmed his statement, and I started the process of becoming Dorothy's guardian and conservator. I soon discovered that, unlike getting a POA, the guardian and conservatorship procedure was both lengthy and expensive. To make matters even worse, doing so involved a court hearing that included Dorothy and her court-appointed lawyer.

Even though her inability to make well-founded decisions and live safely on her own was obvious, I couldn't imagine taking my mother to court. Things were bad enough without this other point of contention adding to the mix. And what if on the morning of our court hearing she was back to her former difficult self? Today, I realize that is a totally laughable idea, but at the time, the prospect was too scary for words. I told the lawyer to stop the proceeding. She told me I was making a big mistake.

Maybe—but to me the emotional relief was worth every possible consequence. Besides, I had figured out a way to get around this awful situation. I found and spoke to the lawyer who had prepared her durable general power of attorney papers six years earlier.

The lawyer said he was willing to talk to her. He understood my situation and told me as long as she didn't claim that she was Napoleon, he would consider her competent enough to sign a durable health power of attorney document.

Before her appointment, Dorothy and I talked about the importance of signing a health power of attorney. She thought doing so was silly and unnecessary, but in the end, she agreed to meet with the lawyer. He must have said the right things to her, and she must have avoided claiming any Napoleonic tendencies. I now had a paper stating I was her designated durable health power of attorney.

At first, I thought the lawyer's Napoleon line was his way of using humor to indicate his willingness to help me out of a tough situation; however, I now have a better understanding of competency as a subjective quality based largely on observation and gut feeling. The lawyer had his way of determining competence, and he felt that Dorothy had a good-enough grip on reality to understand what she was signing.

Her advance directives opened another worry box. Dorothy had checked off the option stating: "I want my life to be prolonged as long as possible within the limits of generally accepted health care standards." While the second part of the sentence gave me and her doctor the room to make a humane decision, the first half of the sentence implied resuscitation. That issue became central to discussions with her home caregivers on how to handle emergencies and, some years later, with her nurses in the dementia care facility.

GUARDIANSHIP AND CONSERVATORSHIP

It took me a while to understand the similarities and differences between a guardianship and a conservatorship. Both a guardianship and a conservatorship involve making a court-appointed person, usually an adult child, responsible for their parent's care. Guardians see to it that the person in their care is safe and has food, clothing, and shelter. In contrast, conservators are responsible for paying bills and managing and protecting property and financial assets. Often the guardian is also the conservator.

You may wonder why it is necessary to take what might seem like a drastic step. What are the circumstances that may force you into taking your family member, usually a parent or a sibling, to court?

A common reason is the lack of competence and no previously signed power of attorney documents. Or maybe your family member rescinds their power of attorney because they believe you are stealing money or are planning on selling their home. When any of these things happen, you can choose to let your parent or sibling continue their struggle to live independently, or you can take them to court so they can receive the help they need. Both choices are difficult ones, but without the backup of a POA, you need to choose one or the other option.

The guardian and conservatorship process is a lengthy one. Usually the steps begin with a lawyer consultation. Based on the outcome of the meeting, your lawyer will file a petition with the court to designate an "ad litem" attorney, an attorney specifically appointed to represent your family member's interests. A different person, often a lawyer or a social worker, investigates the circumstances and files a report with the court.

Eventually you testify as to why you believe your loved one needs a guardian and a conservator. You also describe how you plan to manage their care and finances. Your family member and their lawyer are also present. Testimony to support or refute claims may come from your loved one's doctor, other family members, neighbors, and friends. Sometimes other family members intervene if they feel your efforts are unwarranted or perhaps motivated by greed. Family disharmony can draw out the processes and add significantly to the cost.

If the court finds your parent or other family member is incapacitated to the extent they can no longer take care of themselves or manage their finances, the court will issue Letters of Guardianship and Conservatorship and then delegate those responsibilities to you; however, the court remains in a position of oversight and requires that you submit detailed reports.

The specific responsibilities associated with becoming a guardian and conservator varies from state to state. Generally, the guardian is responsible for making decisions regarding living arrangements, as well as daily and medical care. Oversight and management is an integral part of the guardian's responsibilities.

As a conservator, you are responsible for managing your family member's property, savings, and investments. This can include the buying and selling of stock as well as selling the house and car. In some states, you must get permission from the court before you can buy or sell high-value items. Bills and taxes are another responsibility. In addition, you must keep your family member's estate separate from your personal property and financial holdings.

As you can see, the path to guardianship and conservatorship is lengthy, complex, expensive, and, from many perspectives, emotionally exhausting. The best way to avoid a conservatorship is to have POA documents in place before need arises.

I CAN'T DO EVERYTHING!

Remember you are the POA! And it's perfectly acceptable for a POA to delegate tasks to willing and trustworthy family members.

Working with relatives does have its own challenges and pitfalls—especially when money is involved. When taking that into consideration, it might be well worth the expense to hire an accountant who knows how to manage the finances and paperwork associated with a spectrum of home care scenarios. In addition to reducing your stress, you are less likely to receive letters from your state Taxation and Revenue Office.

It didn't take long for me to realize that keeping track of Dorothy's finances was more than I could or wanted to do. As it turned out, Dorothy had an accountant who prepared and filed her state and federal taxes. It made sense to work with the person who already understood her finances.

Our first meeting was a little painful. The accountant told me that for the last three or four years Dorothy could neither remember the location of his office nor follow his directions to get there. Sometimes, he or one of his colleagues waited for her on the street corner and walked alongside her car as she turned the corner and drove into the parking lot. Once we finished talking about Dorothy and dementia, he told me what he could do to help.

HELPFUL HINTS TO GET THROUGH THE DAY

There's grocery shopping, laundry, doctor appointments, and phone calls to Medicare. Your loved one may be living quietly with dementia, but you are more than busy keeping track of what seems like a million details. Managing your loved one's daily life has become an overwhelming task.

The following organizational tricks can make the day-to-day aspects of dementia care considerably easier: 1) create lists of regularly scheduled household chores; 2) prepare a one- or two-page directory of important names, phone numbers, and e-mail addresses, as well as the identification numbers that link your parent to such things as their medical benefits; 3) write a grocery and household supply check-off page you can use at home or through any number of internet delivery services; and 4) create a simple communications center.

Taking the time to do these relatively simple things will both streamline your caregiving efforts and make it easier for the other caregivers to work effectively and efficiently (see worksheets 7.1 and 7.2).

The communications center mentioned earlier doesn't have to be anything more than an agreed-upon place where the people involved in your loved one's care can read or leave messages for you or the other caregivers. A large calendar to keep track of appointments, a pad of paper, and a pencil are usually sufficient.

But you must protect your family member's personal information. "Need to know" is an important concept. Only those people listed on your family member's POA should have access to Social Security, Medicare, banking, and credit card numbers.

COMMUNICATING WITH CAREGIVERS

Effective and efficient communication with Dorothy's caregivers was something I learned the hard way. As you read earlier, I hired Dorothy's first independent caregiver from an agency. At first, it seemed the caregiver was a good mixture of kindness and no-nonsense; however, I soon discovered she was really an odd mixture of oversensitive and crazy-clean. She took many of Dorothy's insults as personal affronts, and she was easily embarrassed by

Dorothy's behavior in public places. I slowly became aware of these problems through the evening phone calls we made to each other to discuss the day's events. Those conversations made it clear Dorothy would be much happier with a different caregiver.

Without question, I needed to do something to manage the flow of information between me and what were now several caregivers. Regularly scheduled phone calls were out. These conversations invaded everyone's personal time and invariably led to a gossipy way of talking about Dorothy and dementia.

In the place of phone calls, I decided to try daily notes as a way to transmit and record information. I developed a short questionnaire so that caregivers could comment on what Dorothy ate, her sleeping habits, problems with toileting, her moods, and any ongoing changes in Dorothy's behavior or daily skills. I also included an "other comments" section so caregivers could mention things not covered by the other questions.

Keeping daily notes helped create a library of need-to-know information. In the short term, it seemed like nothing more than a repeated litany of Dorothy eating an open-faced ham and cheese sandwich for lunch, the expected mustard or mayonnaise argument, taking a morning and an afternoon nap, refusing to use the walker, repeated conversations, and another day without a shower. The "other comments" section gave the caregivers the ability to write about back pain, outings to the library or the local senior center, and anything else that seemed odd, wonderful, or unusual.

Looking at the daily notes over the span of one or several months revealed subtle changes in Dorothy's condition. Reviewing them helped me appreciate that toileting was becoming more of a problem, language was becoming more and more impoverished, and back pain and exhaustion—two things Dorothy would never admit to—were making trips away from home difficult.

The daily notes helped us make appropriate adjustments to Dorothy's care. And writing and presenting Dorothy's doctor with a quarterly summary helped guide his decisions as well. But most important, the daily notes made it easier to discuss her care in an efficient, productive, and professional manner.

MEDICAL CARE

Doctors and other health care professionals are foundation members of your "getting-the-help-you-need" team. These clinicians include primary care doctors, such as family doctors (general practitioners), internists, and geriatricians, who can provide your family member's day-to-day medical care. Your loved one may need to see other specialists such as a psychiatrist or a neurologist to evaluate and fine-tune the medications used to manage depression, anxiety, delusions, and hallucinations.

Because people who have dementia often have other medical conditions, they may see doctors who treat such things as heart disease, cancer, kidney failure, and diabetes. Oh, and remember to keep up with your family member's dental, hearing, and vision care. Foot care from a podiatrist is a good idea—especially if your loved one has diabetes or difficult-to-trim and ingrown toenails.

And don't forget that every doctor needs a copy of your family member's durable health POA. Having a health POA included in your loved one's medical files makes it possible for the doctor to discuss their medical care with you.

Taking Dorothy to her primary care doctor was always an ordeal. Her repeated questions about the date and time of her appointment made everyone nuts. Showing her the day and time on the calendar didn't help. The day before her appointment, after weeks without washing her hair or showering, she would demand to go the hair salon, and sometimes she would agree to take a shower. Her sudden attention to hygiene was her way of showing that she was okay—there was nothing wrong with her.

A few days before her appointment, I would e-mail a brief descriptive summary of any changes in Dorothy's behavior or daily living skills to her doctor. I also included any questions or concerns that I and the caregivers might have about Dorothy's care or treatment.

If your loved one's doctor does not use e-mail or a patient portal to communicate with patients or their family caregiver, consider sending your summary and questions to the office in a stamped envelope. Other alternatives include giving the summary to the office secretary or the doctor's nurse when you arrive at the office, or simply using it as a reference to guide conversation during the appointment. Because Dorothy did not allow me to join her in the examination room, it was important that her doctor read the summary beforehand.

After Dorothy's medical exam, her doctor and I met privately in another room. What Dorothy's doctor told me in our private discussions didn't change much over the years. "Your mother claims she is healthy and can take care of herself. She pays her own bills, does her own shopping, and feels she doesn't need caregivers. She says her back doesn't hurt, that she never falls, and there is no reason why she cannot drive."

As part of our back-room meeting, the doctor explained the results of Dorothy's lab work, which included blood tests for anemia, kidney and liver function, and blood lipids. While it's hard to say what is normal for a woman in her late nineties, the blood work did reveal anemia and kidneys that were beginning to fail. He also said that because Dorothy would not permit him to do a physical exam, he could not do much more than chat, test her balance, and sometimes give her a mini mental status exam.

Then her doctor and I, often in the company of a nurse case manager and a medical social worker, met with Dorothy to discuss his findings and our mutual concerns. Her appointment concluded with the paperwork associated with prescription refills, a next appointment, and the accompanying lab work.

Once home, her sullen mood often erupted into anger. Her doctor was crazy and too young, and he did not have enough experience. In efforts to find herself a new doctor, Dorothy frantically punched random phone numbers. Anyone who answered the phone got an earful before hanging up on what was certainly a deranged caller. Eventually, Dorothy would give up and go to bed for the rest of the day. With time, her anger subsided, and we were back to hearing her repeated questions about her next doctor appointment.

Obviously, things were not working out as well as they should. Perhaps we needed a different doctor. Dorothy's primary care doctor thought this was worth a try and suggested I take her to a geriatrician—a physician who specializes in caring for older people. As it turned out, the idea of changing doctors was more disturbing to her than remaining with the doctor who wouldn't give her permission to drive.

PALLIATIVE CARE

It's never too soon to think about palliative care. Many people have heard about palliative care; however, only a few people know what it is. Some assume palliative care is only for people who have cancer. Many feel that palliative care begins when death is imminent. Others believe palliative care is the same as "pull the plug."

Throughout the progression of a life-threatening disease like dementia, palliative care always takes into consideration patient comfort and dignity. Palliative care provides relief from physical pain, manages distressing symptoms, and addresses the fear and anger people experience when confronting a life-threatening illness. Palliative care is comfort care.

Research shows that people who begin palliative care shortly after receiving a diagnosis of a life-altering or life-threatening disease experience less depression and anxiety and, overall, have a higher quality of life. Palliative care, when started early, often extends life by several months.

In the most general sense, palliative care is a philosophical approach that focuses on maintaining the quality of life of patients who face a serious illness. Cancer is certainly one of those serious illnesses. But other illnesses, such as rheumatoid arthritis, multiple sclerosis, congestive heart failure, kidney disease, Parkinson's disease, and dementia, are just as serious.

Palliative care exists alongside standard treatment; however, the overall emphasis of the two types of care changes as people transition from early to advanced stages of their illness. At first, people primarily receive standard treatment. For a person who has dementia, this may include medication to slow memory loss, participation in engaging and stimulating activities, and receiving care for any other conditions or illnesses they may have, such as high blood pressure or diabetes. During the early stages of dementia, the palliative component includes such things as addressing psychological well-being and helping the patient and family plan for future needs.

As dementia progresses and cognitive function deteriorates further, such things as safety, nutrition, bodily functions, and symptom management become more important. The patient still receives treatments for any ongoing conditions they may have, as well as for episodic illnesses like pneumonia. Comfort care and managing symptoms become more important than having the patient undergo difficult testing procedures. At this point, family begins to play a bigger decision-making role.

Advanced dementia brings comfort care to the forefront. The family, often with the guidance of the patient's doctor, medical social worker, or chaplain, makes decisions that reflect the patient's advance directives (see chapter 13). The doctor may begin to eliminate certain medications, such as those used to control cholesterol blood levels. As events such as aspirated food and infections become more frequent, patient dignity and quality of life become defining factors for palliative care.

HOME MEDICAL ALERT SYSTEMS

For some of us, the words *medical alert* immediately brings to mind the campy 1980s television commercial where Mrs. Fletcher cries out, "Help, I've fallen and I can't get up." Her line, now trite with overuse, is a grim reminder that, according to the Centers for Disease Control and Prevention, falls are the leading cause of injury-related deaths among people sixty-five years or older.

Elderly people fall when they lose their footing, trip on rugs, or miss a stair. Changes in balance, vision, and muscle tone, in addition to the side effects of the many medications elderly people take, are other risk factors.

Dementia adds another layer of risk when your family member can no longer connect something like a wet floor with the need to walk more carefully.

Even if your family member receives twenty-four-hour care, purchasing or leasing a medical alert system is something worth considering. Today, unlike the days of Mrs. Fletcher, there are many medical alert devices to choose from. Use the internet and the keywords "medical alert systems" and "medical alert system reviews" to begin researching for the products that best meet your budget and your loved one's capabilities.

We installed a medical alert system in Dorothy's home. Not unexpectedly, Dorothy refused to wear the necklace. She said she didn't need it because she didn't ever fall. Reminding her that she had already fallen resulted in a quizzical look or denial. Rephrasing and explaining that wearing the necklace would keep her safe should she happen to trip on something didn't work. Dorothy was simply incapable of understanding "in case something might happen."

It took a few more falls before she was willing to wear her necklace; however, by that time she couldn't understand how to push the button for help and soon she wasn't even aware of "that thing" around her neck. Fortunately, I or one of the caregivers was there to pick her up off the floor. Basically, the medical alert system was a good emergency backup for her caregivers.

EMERGENCIES

It is important to create emergency plans and discuss those plans with the caregivers and any other people, such as immediate family and neighbors, who might be involved in your family member's care. Some emergencies include the any number of reasons why caregivers cannot come to work. But for the most part, emergencies involve sudden changes in your loved one's health.

Caregivers who work for agencies must follow company rules about administering first aid or doing things that go beyond housekeeping, companionship, and activities of daily living. Rules about administering first aid or making clinical decisions vary from one home care agency to another. Concerns about lawsuits, rather than common sense, often determine what an agency caregiver can or cannot do. In our case, the agency caregivers were required to call 911 for just about everything.

I didn't discuss my first aid expectations in any great detail with Dorothy's independent caregivers; however, they did know to call me if they had any questions or concerns. They also knew to first call 911 if Dorothy should do something like break a bone, get burned, or have symptoms that might indicate a stroke or heart attack. You know—use common sense.

Sometimes the emergency is simply one where your family member's behavior is more than you or the caregiver can handle. When this happens, calling the Crisis Intervention Team, rather than 911, may be the best option. The Crisis Intervention Team, or CIT, refers to the police officers in your community who have special training in how to manage a variety of behavioral, drug-related, and mental health crises. Be sure to include the phone number of your local CIT in your list of emergency phone numbers.

THE BIG "WHAT IF"

Dorothy's headaches, stomach aches, falls, and back pain were all things we were used to handling. But the caregivers wanted to know what they should do if they found Dorothy dying or dead. This scary question was one that the independent caregivers and I discussed at length. For all of us, this part of life was an unknown; it was something that was outside of our experience.

The agency caregivers were considerably more matter-of-fact about the eventuality of Dorothy's death. In fact, the agency administrator left a "Do Not Resuscitate" sign and told me to tape it to Dorothy's refrigerator door. Yikes!

I certainly wouldn't want to have that thing staring me in the face. And what about Dorothy? I told the agency administrator that I would tape the sign to the hot water heater located in the garage.

But "What if?" The question haunted me for a long time. Gradually, I began to understand that advanced age, in combination with dementia and congestive heart failure, were events and conditions that mark the end of a life. With time, I began to feel comfortable with the idea that my job was to provide the kind of home care that would support Dorothy's dignity and comfort.

RESPITE

Respite. Just a few moments free from interruptions, emergency phone calls, and impossible demands. Relief from the overwhelming stress that comes from years of doing more than our abilities, circumstances, and resources would normally withstand. An intermission from the topsy-turvy world that dementia imposes on our lives. Respite.

A study by researchers at the University of Utah and the California State University at San Bernardino shows that respite services enhance the quality of daily life for family caregivers and the family member in their care. Yet, in their national survey involving more than nine hundred family caregivers, these same researchers found that access to respite was the most desired and needed kind of assistance.

Without question, home care, adult day care, and organizations that provide overnight or multiple days of respite can be a lifesaver. Home care is a resource many family caregivers forget to consider as a short-term option. Affordability, in combination with the feeling that you must shoulder the entire caregiving responsibility, is an issue for many people; however, hiring a paid caregiver, even for a few hours per week, can give you the time you need to decompress, relax, or participate in a favorite activity. These few scheduled hours will seem inexpensive when compared to the toll long-term dementia care can take on your family and on your own physical and mental health.

There are many community and faith-based organizations that provide affordable respite care. The Alzheimer's Association and the Office on Aging are examples of two community resources. The Catholic Charities and Jewish Family Service are examples of faith-based, nonprofit organizations that help people, regardless of ethnicity or religion, stay in their homes for as long as possible. Some agencies offer respite reimbursement to help make respite care more affordable.

The internet is another search strategy. In addition to using the name of the community where your family member lives, use key phrases like "senior companions," "faith-based eldercare," and "dementia home care" to find organizations that provide paid or volunteer assistance. Many organizations use a sliding fee scale so cost does not become a deterrent.

Adult day care is another possibility. Located in community senior centers, nursing homes, churches, synagogues, hospitals, or schools, adult day care provides stimulation and companionship for seniors who need medical assistance and other kinds of supervision during the day. Usually open during business hours, adult day care centers give the family caregiver time to go to work, to attend to personal business, or to relax while knowing their loved one is safe.

The cost of adult day care depends on the kinds of services offered, available reimbursements, and geographic location. Medicare and insurance usually do not cover adult day care costs; however, you may find financial assistance through Medicaid, the Older Americans Act, and the Veterans Administration (see Helpful Resources).

Not every state regulates or licenses adult day care centers; therefore, it is important to visit nearby care centers before enrolling your loved one in a program. Be sure to talk to staff and to the other families who use the center. You want to make sure your loved one is in a healthful environment that meets their medical, emotional, and social needs.

Your friends, family, and neighbors are another source of short-term respite. These people may actually mean it when they say, "Please be sure to call if you need any help." Some people are naturally generous, and others, because of their own experiences, understand the difference a little extra help can make.

And think about this: your loved one may also enjoy having respite from your hovering presence.

When a friend, neighbor, or another family member comes to visit, your family member can enjoy the companionship of a person who has the time, energy, and patience to hear their stories (again), take a walk, or maybe enjoy a cup of tea.

Make sure your respite angels have the information they need to make their visit pleasant and safe. Give them suggestions about activities or snack foods your loved one might enjoy, explain how to prevent or manage difficult behaviors, show them the emergency contact list, and, most importantly, tell them how they can contact you.

Your family could use a break as well. After months of having to live with a preoccupied and emotionally fragile person (you!), your family might like to spend some time with a more relaxed you. A weekend at a wonderful bed and breakfast or maybe a nice dinner and a movie can help give some sparkle to your family life.

Some of the home care services mentioned earlier in this chapter may offer short-term overnight assistance. Try to schedule an overnight respite with a caregiver who is familiar with your family member and the place where they live.

Many assisted living and dementia care facilities offer weekend or week-long stays. In addition to giving you a much-needed break, a few days at a residential care facility could be a nice change of scenery for your loved one; however, be sure to tell your loved one that you promise to bring them home in a few days. Write the dates of your loved one's "vacation" on a calendar and mark in red the day they will return home. Your loved one may no longer remember their daily and personal details, but something like a breach of trust has a way of sticking.

Family caregivers use respite time in different ways. Some sleep, while others go shopping, spend time with friends, read, walk, or take time to participate in a favorite hobby or sport.

Respite can range from a few hours to several days. Make an effort to schedule respite breaks for the same time each week. Plan ahead so you will know how you will spend your precious time. That way, even on a difficult day, you will always have something to look forward to doing. But whatever you decide, make respite a priority before feelings of exhaustion, isolation, and resentment take over.

Do not use respite time, as one person suggested, to do something like getting your knee fixed. Surgery is not respite. Like any job, taking time off for surgery is well-earned medical leave.

DISTANCE CARE

Perhaps you get the news from your loved one's neighbor, or maybe it's a phone call from a relative. In either case, what they say makes you worry. Unlike what your loved one says during your Sunday morning chats, the neighbor's report makes you feel that maybe things really aren't just fine.

Your loved one's younger brother takes a more blunt approach. He tells you to come home—now! He says your mother gets lost going to the grocery store and sometimes cannot find her way to his house.

Yes, you think to yourself, Mom does repeat herself, but maybe it's because she lives alone. And sometimes when I call, she does get me mixed up with other people. But aren't all older people forgetful? But it does seem strange that she gets lost going to the grocery store. How could that be? She has lived in that neighborhood for more than fifty years.

Many family members find themselves in the situation where they live far away from a loved one who needs their help. Managing their care, either alone or with the help of other people, is a considerable undertaking.

As a first step, consider writing a list of the things that you and other relatives need to do; however, be prepared to continually revise your outlined care plans as you learn more about your loved one's condition and eligibility for local medical and community services.

Determining the skills where you loved one needs assistance is a good place to start. A visit to their home is the best way to assess their daily living skills (chapter 4, worksheets 4.1 and 4.2). During this same visit, take the time to establish contacts with people and organizations that can help you coordinate your loved one's care from a distance. In addition to neighbors, friends, and other family members, contacts may also include community organizations that offer eldercare services, home care agencies, and your loved one's doctor. Contacting a local lawyer is especially important if your parent has not already established a power of attorney.

Make an appointment to speak with a bank officer at your family member's financial institution. Doing so may help you find a person who can manage or monitor your loved one's banking transactions. An accountant, one who lives near you or your family member, can make the financial management aspects of distance care easier.

Some families opt to engage the services of a geriatric care manager when, for any number of reasons, they cannot provide sufficient supervision themselves. These health and human services professionals plan and coordinate your loved one's care. The geriatric care manager can find appropriate housing and home care, coordinate medical care and socialization services, and oversee your loved one's financial and legal planning. Their goals are to improve quality of life, maintain independence for as long as possible, and assure cost-effective continuity in the services your loved one receives.

You can learn more about geriatric care managers on the National Association of Professional Geriatric Care Managers website. Costs for services depend on the geographic location. Many geriatric care managers charge a flat fee for the initial consultation and bill by the hour for services that can range from referral placements and crisis intervention to guardianships and conservatorships.

In addition to private geriatric care management practices, you can often find similar—and less expensive—"case management" services through various city, county, and nonprofit organizations, such as the Agency on Aging (see Helpful Resources).

In the event that distance care is no longer sufficient, you may need to consider moving your loved one into assisted living or to a dementia care facility. The next question is where. It could be a facility in your parent's hometown or a place closer to you or another family member. Another option is moving your loved one into your own home. The biggest consideration with respect to "here or there" is the agitation and confusion he or she may experience. You also need to consider how well you and your family can adapt to living close to or with your parent or other family member.

WAYS TO PAY FOR CARE

Finances are probably the biggest reason why family caregivers donate nearly $244 billion per year of unpaid family care.

How to pay for care is a challenge many family caregivers face. In addition to your loved one's savings, property, and insurance policies, funding can come from such federal programs Medicare and various state programs, such as Medicaid. Some family caregivers discover they must make personal contributions to their loved one's care.

Many family caregivers are either unaware of their family member's financial situation or do not have access to their accounts. A diagnosis of early-stage dementia may be the only opportunity you will have to discuss income, assets, and long-term financial arrangements with your loved one and the other family members involved in their care.

With a durable POA on file, you have access to your family member's bank accounts and have the ability to sign checks. Joint tenancy, or joint ownership, makes you a co-owner of the account. Although joint tenancy can simplify probate and some aspects of settling the estate, it does come with an element of risk. A joint ownership can expose your loved one's money to litigation should you, as the joint owner, become involved in a lawsuit or divorce proceedings.

If having enough money is the primary stumbling block, a reverse mortgage may provide sufficient income. A reverse mortgage, also called a home equity conversion mortgage, is a loan option that allows people to convert home equity into a monthly cash payment while they continue to live in their home. Having additional income is not a consideration when applying for a reverse mortgage; however, there are eligibility requirements. The homeowner must be sixty-two years of age or older, and if they haven't already paid off the mortgage, they must be close to doing so. The property can be a single-family home, a home consisting of one to four units, a Housing and Urban Development (HUD)–approved condominium, or a manufactured home that meets Federal Housing Administration (FHA) standards (see Helpful Resources).

Renting your family member's home is another way to generate income. Of course, this assumes your family member will move to your home or to an assisted living facility. Speak with an eldercare or estate lawyer to make sure you have the legal authority to rent and to manage your family member's property if they are incapable of doing so.

Selling your family member's assets, such as stock, fine art, or land, is another way to raise money for their care; however, unless you are a co-owner, you must be their court-appointed conservator in order to sell their personal assets.

Many family caregivers use their own funds to pay for their parent's care. When possible, divide the expenses equally among your siblings. But be sure to take into consideration circumstances that may make it difficult for your family to make equal monetary contributions. Your brother may have one or more children in college. Your sister may have a mother-in-law who also requires assistance and she or her husband may be unemployed.

When family finances are at issue, take into consideration the value of time. Perhaps your brother can take care of your mother's yard or keep her car in running order. Maybe your sister can be responsible for keeping track of finances or agree to spend two afternoons a week with your mother. When it comes to asking siblings for contributions, be flexible and creative.

LONG-TERM CARE INSURANCE

Many people have special insurance policies to cover their long-term care. Dorothy often told me about her insurance policy that paid for a skilled nurse to come to her home. Between her durable general POA, a paid-off house, and having thoughtfully included me as a co-owner on her savings accounts, she was certain that she could live out her days in her own home.

When I finally found a copy of her nursing care policy buried among a bunch of random papers, I was horrified to read that it paid $10 a day for a registered nurse to come to her home and nothing more.

I called the insurance company and found the bad news was just that. The premiums Dorothy had paid for more than thirty years would not cover similar care today.

I am grateful that Dorothy had only one useless insurance policy. Many elderly people, out of fear and the desire to make things as easy as possible for their families, are duped into buying numerous and useless insurance policies; however, it can be very helpful if your family member planned ahead and bought a long-term care (LTC) insurance policy.

People who can take advantage of their LTC insurance may not be ill as we usually define illness. Instead of something like cancer or Parkinson's disease, they may have poor balance, be frail, or be unable to dress, bathe, get in and out of bed, walk, or use the toilet without assistance.

Long-term care insurance provides those services not usually included in health insurance policies and Medicare. A long-term care insurance policy will pay, up to a certain daily limit, for all of the expenses associated with home care, assisted living, adult day care, and nursing home and dementia facility care. It will also pay for a live-in caregiver, companion, housekeeper, therapist, or private duty nurse up to seven days a week and twenty-four hours a day. The only catch is one must buy a policy before a change in health necessitates service.

MEDICARE, MEDICAID, AND RELATED PROGRAMS

There are many government agencies that offer services and funding to help families provide care for loved ones who have chronic and debilitating diseases and conditions. Information on many of these programs is challenging to find and complex to comprehend when you do find it.

Medicare

If your family member is sixty-five years of age or older they are entitled to Medicare benefits. Basically, Medicare is a national insurance program funded through paycheck withholdings. Even at its most basic level, Medicare is a complex topic. Just remember Part A is hospital insurance and Part B covers medical expenses. Medicare Part C is a combination of Parts A and B; however, Medicare Part C, unlike Parts A and B, requires using only certain doctors and hospitals. Medicare Part C also covers prescriptions. Medicare Part D covers prescriptions for those people who prefer the Parts A and B option.

A geriatric case manager, eldercare lawyer, or your local Office on Aging are some of the people and organizations who can help you sort out the Medicare puzzle.

Medicaid

Medicaid is a federal program that allocates funds to states. Therefore, the number, type, and program requirements vary from state to state.

The purpose of Medicaid is to help very low income people get the health care they need. For elderly people, eligibility requirements for Medicaid benefits are grim. In most states, the person in your care, excluding the house and car, can have only a few thousand dollars in a bank account. Each state stipulates the maximum monthly income your family member can receive and still be eligible for Medicaid benefits. Spend-down of personal funds for home care and assisted living care is how many elderly people become eligible for Medicaid.

If your loved one is eligible for Medicaid, they must contribute all but a small portion of their monthly income to pay for assisted living or nursing home care. Your loved one may use the remaining dollars to buy any personal items they may want or need. Medicaid picks up the difference between your loved one's contribution and the cost of care. Not every care facility accepts Medicaid patients, and most limit the number of Medicaid patients they will have at any one time.

Medicaid and Related Programs

Under certain circumstances, Medicaid will contract with private home care agencies and pay them to provide in-home care and personal care, such as assistance with bathing, dressing, and cooking.

Some states participate in Medicaid-funded Cash and Counseling programs. Under the Cash and Counseling program, the family member who provides the care receives payment for their work; however, as is true for all Medicaid programs, your loved one must have limited financial assets to meet eligibility requirements.

Some people become eligible for Medicaid assistance by hiding their money and other assets in certain types of trusts. If your loved one owns a home or has diverted money into a trust, the state Medicaid Estate Recovery Program, upon your loved one's death, may require reimbursement. The estate or the trust returns a portion of the public funds used to pay for their care to Medicaid. Often the money comes from selling the house.

Program of All-Inclusive Care for the Elderly (PACE)

In addition to Medicaid, each state has an Aging Service Division that administers programs to help frail elderly people stay in their homes for as long as possible. One such program is the Program of All-Inclusive Care for the Elderly (PACE). To be eligible for PACE services, people must be age fifty-five or older, live in a PACE state, and be unable to perform at least two activities of daily living (e.g., dressing and personal hygiene) but otherwise able to live safely at home (see Helpful Resources).

FOR VETERANS AND THEIR CAREGIVERS

The U.S. Veterans Administration (VA) offers a broad range of services to help veterans who have dementia. In addition to medical care, the VA offers access to home and community-based care, VA and community nursing homes, and State Veteran homes. Veterans, who have the financial means, pay a co-payment for services (see Helpful Resources).

To take advantage of the various VA programs and services, the veteran must be enrolled in the VA health care system. While the veteran does not have to have a service-related injury to receive dementia care, the veteran must have an honorable or a general discharge.

Examples of VA services and programs include the Caregiver Support Line; the VA REACH program (Resources for Enhancing Any Caregivers Health); VA community living centers; VA-contracted community residential care facilities; and adult day care centers. The VA Caregiver Support Services website is a good starting point (see Helpful Resources).

FREQUENTLY ASKED QUESTIONS

1. The caregiver I have hired to care for my mother comes from another country and insists I pay her in cash. Is this legal?

This is an important question that is beyond the scope of this book. To legally work in the United States, your caregiver must have a work permit or be a permanent resident. It's not illegal to pay for services in cash, and you must keep a record of payments to your caregiver that includes all state and federal deductions. This is especially important if you are deducting home care as medical expense on your parent's state and federal taxes. How to pay an independent caregiver is a topic every family caregiver should discuss with an accountant or an eldercare lawyer.

2. My mother is in late-stage dementia. She also has congestive heart failure and severe osteoporosis. I am her durable health power of attorney. Her advance directives state that she wants all artificial life-sustaining measures and resuscitation. The nurses tell me her ribs and other bones are too thin and weak to withstand resuscitation. What can I do to avoid going to court to become her guardian?

This is a difficult situation, and one that caused me considerable worry and lost sleep. In the end, Dorothy's doctor reminded me that I was my mother's health power of attorney. That meant she had given me her permission to make decisions on her behalf. While this situation opens obvious opportunities for doing wrong, her doctor was confident that my motivations were honorable. So in the end, we let nature take its course.

3. My father designated me as his durable general power of attorney. He never signed a durable health power of attorney, and now that he is in mid-stage dementia, he is not competent to sign one. I am in the process of becoming his guardian; however, the lawyer wants me to file conservatorship papers, too. Is this necessary? Why isn't the durable general power of attorney enough?

You are correct; your father's durable general power of attorney does give you the right to manage his financial affairs; however, there are several reasons why it is a good idea to become your father's conservator. First of all, your father can terminate his durable general power of attorney with you. If this should happen, you will have to go back to the lawyer and start the process all over again. Therefore, it is best to obtain guardianship and conservancy at the same time.

Having extended capabilities is another reason for becoming your father's conservator. Acting as his general power of attorney allows you to act in his place. You can write checks and make deposits and withdrawals from his bank accounts; however, conservatorship gives you the right to buy or sell stock, open or close accounts, move money from one bank to another, and sell property. This flexibility is especially helpful if you need to find funds to pay for his care. Conversely, you must keep his estate separate from yours.

Talk to your lawyer or accountant for further clarification if you are a joint owner on any of your father's financial holdings. And remember, to protect your father's estate from mismanagement, you must keep detailed records and report your financial transactions to the court and to other family members.

4. I recently discovered that my much older sister designated me as her power of attorney. She never asked me, and I never signed anything. While I am happy to help her, it might have been nice if she had asked first.

Yes, this is the kind of surprise most people do not appreciate. Nonetheless, in many states the power of attorney document does not require your signature. If you find you are unable or unwilling to take on this responsibility you can ask your sister to name another person as her POA. If she has dementia or some other debilitating illness, perhaps another previously named designee can take over your role. If not, talk to a lawyer who can start proceedings to make her a ward of the state.

5. When I discuss caregiving or financial matters with my mother, I feel like I am speaking to a raging adolescent, or maybe to an angry two-year-old. I am trying as much as possible to include my mother in the decisions that affect her life. What can I do to make this situation less volatile?

First of all, I want to compliment you on trying to include your mother in these discussions; however, what you say about a raging adolescent is a good description of the situation. Think back a few years. Did you always give into your children's demands? Hopefully, you listened and, if appropriate, modified your thoughts based on what they said. But then, as the adult, you were the one who made the decision. It's tough to think of your mother or father as a child. But, discussing caregiving and finances with a person who no longer has adult reasoning capabilities just doesn't work.

6. The other day I called Medicare to get information about my father's hospital bill. The Medicare representative said they could not give me that information. In fact, they told me the government does not recognize the POA. What's that all about?

Yes, I had a similar experience, and it's one of those situations that can make a difficult day even worse. I have since learned from an eldercare lawyer that government offices do not accept the POA because the legislative statutes are state specific.

WORKSHEET 7.1:
Communication Form

Making a check-off list of regularly scheduled housekeeping chores will make it easier for you and the caregivers to organize the day and, if there are two or three work shifts, know who did what.

Chore	Who Did It	Date
Wash laundry	_____	_____
Dry laundry	_____	_____
Put laundry away	_____	_____
Change bed sheets	_____	_____
Sweep floors	_____	_____
Fill pill box	_____	_____
Call pharmacy	_____	_____
Pharmacy pick-up	_____	_____
Clean bathroom	_____	_____
Clean refrigerator	_____	_____
Wash dishes	_____	_____
Put dishes away	_____	_____
Water house plants	_____	_____
Take out trash	_____	_____
Take trash to curb	_____	_____
Take in mail	_____	_____
Feed pets	_____	_____
Clean cat box	_____	_____

WORKSHEET 7.2:
Template Caregiver Directory
(Electronic or Hard Copy)

Use the templates below to write a directory of important information. Some information should only be available on a need-to-know basis. For example, only certain family members should have access to bank account numbers.

Important People and Their Contact Information

Family phone numbers and other contact information:

Name and relationship: _____

Home phone number: _____   Cell phone number: _____

E-mail address: _____

Caregivers:

Name: _____

Home phone number: _____   Cell phone number: _____

E-mail address: _____

Address: _____

Doctors:

Name and specialty: _____

Office phone number: _____   On-call number: _____

E-mail address: _____

Address: _____

Other health professionals (dentist, medical social worker, etc.):

Name and profession: _____

Office phone number: _____   On-call number: _____

E-mail address: _____

Address: _____

(continued)

WORKSHEET 7.2:
Continued

House Information:

Door code: _____   Alarm code: _____

Garage code: _____   Location of spare key: _____

_____

Trash day instructions: _____

_____

Neighbor's name and contact: _____

_____

Need to Know Only

Insurance Company Information

Name of company: _____

Phone number: _____

Agent name: _____

Policy number: _____

Other benefits (Social Security, Medicare, Veteran, etc.)

Name as written on card: _____

Identification number: _____

Name as written on card: _____

Policy number: _____

Banks

Name of bank: _____

Phone number: _____

Name of manager: _____

Account number: _____

Address: _____

Safety deposit box (must be a cosigner)

Location: _____

Location of key: _____

Financial Advisor

Name of company: _____

Phone number: _____

Agent name: _____

Address: _____

Accountant

Name of company: _____

Address: _____

Accountant's name: _____

E-mail address: _____

Phone number: _____

Lawyer

Name of company: _____

Address: _____

Lawyer's name: _____

E-mail address: _____

Phone number: _____

Stockbroker

Name of company: _____

Address: _____

Stockbroker's name: _____

E-mail address: _____

Phone number: _____

Account number(s): _____

8

WHEN THE LITTLE THINGS ARE REALLY THE BIG THINGS

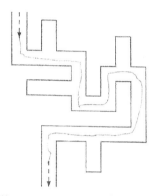

Woman, age seventy-nine, maze.

The words *house* and *home* aren't the same. For most people, the word *house* produces a mental image of a building. It may be the house where you now live or it may be a generic house with a pointed roof and brick chimney.

The word *home* stimulates an array of complex feelings. *Home* may cause you to remember the smell of your mother's cooking, the view from a childhood tree house, the sound of your children playing, or the feel of your loved one's kiss. Home is more than four walls and a roof. Home is memory, personal history, and a bountiful source of comfort.

The decision to care for a family member in their home or yours can be a difficult one. If your loved one remains in their own home, you may have added travel time, plus the expense of caregivers, and the responsibility of managing a second home. Giving work and your own family the attention they deserve presents additional challenges.

If moving your family member into your home seems like the best option, you have sacrificed your privacy and personal space, and you have unwittingly involved your whole family in your loved one's care. On the other hand, a multigenerational home can be an enriching experience when you open your home, and not your house, to your loved one.

Either way, there are many pluses and minuses to consider.

Other reasons are purely emotional—a promise to your loved one to never move them from their home. Or the promises that you made to yourself.

It's hard to say if a person who has dementia can always tell the difference between house and home. Yet, it is clear that food, music, and art can help people who have dementia make connections to their past. You can see it in their eyes and on their faces. For a moment they may smile, sing, or become unusually animated. Because of that, I am sure, somewhere in your loved one's heart they know when they are home.

DEMENTIA AND THE CREATIVE SPIRIT

Family caregivers tend to focus their effort on providing the basics. The goals are to get through the day and to see that the person in our care has food, clothing, and a safe place to live. It's difficult to think about, much less provide, our loved one with meaningful and creative activities, too.

Researchers and art educators are beginning to see the positive role art, music, poetry, dance, and theater can play in improving the quality of life for people who have dementia. As Bruce Miller, MD, says in a presentation to the Mind Science Foundation, art gives people who have dementia the ability to "express what they can with what they have." Miller also states that participation in the arts can tell us "from the inside" what it feels like to have dementia.

Art

Making and finding art opportunities for your loved one may not be as difficult as it may appear. Set up some watercolors, paper, and brushes at the kitchen table, and you are good to go.

The Museum of Modern Art (MoMA), located in New York City, set the standard for making art accessible to people who have Alzheimer's disease and other dementias. With the guidance of specially trained museum docents, visitors explore selected museum collections where they can see and, when appropriate, touch wall art and sculpture. Interactive installations may invite viewers to experience sight, touch, and sound. Conversation is another facet of the MoMA program Do keep in mind that feelings and memory—not art history—are the inspirations for meaningful interactions and conversation.

Museums throughout the world use MoMA publications to start similar programs in their community. Use your search engine and the keywords "dementia" and "creative," as well as various combinations of such key words as "arts," "writing," "poetry," "dance," and "activities," to find other local resources. The Alzheimer's Association publications *Memories in the Making Revised Program Manual*, by Selly Jenny, and *I'm Still Here*, by La Doris "Sam" Heinly, are two references you can use to develop meaningful and creative activities for your whole family.

To find nearby programs, do an online search using the keywords "museum," "Alzheimer's," "dementia," and "outreach," plus the state where your family member resides.

The Thursday Art Project

The year after Dorothy's death, I made the decision to volunteer some of my newly realized free time to the dementia community. After speaking with my local Alzheimer's Association, I developed a curriculum that I hoped people who have dementia would enjoy.

My brief presentation to a local support group captured the interest of four eager participants. The three men and one woman had various types of dementia. One man had dementia with Lewy bodies, another had early-onset dementia, and the remaining people had a diagnosis of Alzheimer's disease.

Throughout the course of the year, the artists learned basic design principles, made relief prints, painted self-portraits, and designed and printed T-shirts for themselves and family members. Donations covered the cost of supplies.

I expected that the spouses would use class time to run errands. But as it turned out, they spent the two hours in a nearby coffee shop. Soon, "just coffee" morphed into family dinners.

One of my most precious moments was when one man, a retired aeronautical engineer, said the Thursday Art Program made him feel that he was "becoming" something rather than losing what he had once been.

Music

Music connects people to their life history and culture. Music transports people back to happy and sad places, such as the memory of a concert with friends or a reminder of a long-deceased relative.

People have positive reactions to the popular music of their youth or the kinds of music that reflect their taste and preferences; therefore, don't assume the person in your care will want to hear Glenn Miller or Bing Crosby. Baby boomers may prefer Elvis, Janis Joplin, the Beatles, or the Rolling Stones. Some people may favor classical music, jazz, or opera.

There are many simple ways to bring music into your loved one's life. At home you can download music from the internet and watch or listen to broadcast performances. Together, you can sing, play a musical instrument, or use bells, sticks, and homemade drums to create a home-style rhythm band. Consider inviting family members, friends, and other caregivers and their loved ones to participate in a jam session. Serve coffee and cookies, and you have an event!

Choral groups are another option. The Giving Voice Initiative, located in Bloomington, Minnesota, can help you locate or organize a choral group in your community. See Helpful Resources at the end of this book for more information.

It's always a nice break to take excursions outside of the home. Combining an early afternoon concert with lunch or an early supper is another way to enjoy a day and enrich a relationship. Senior centers are another place where you can find performances and music classes your loved one might enjoy. Many nonprofit organizations, such as the YMCA, sponsor music programs designed especially for people who have dementia and other disabilities.

The Poetry Project

Gary Glazner, the founder of the Alzheimer's Poetry Project, returns the joy of the spoken word to those quieted by Alzheimer's disease. It's amazing to see the transformation. Familiar poetry, all spoken in a cadence reminiscent of inborn body rhythms, reveals smiles. Silly poems make the whole room break out in laughter.

Creating and performing a collaborative poem is another aspect of Glazner's program. To encourage engagement, he asks a difficult question: "What does spring taste like?" "Manure," says one woman. "My grandfather's farm," says another. And from a woman, in a voice just above a whisper, "Spring tastes like tomorrow."

GARDENING AND THE GOOD EARTH

Similar to art and poetry, gardening makes for creative and soothing moments. The aroma of freshly overturned earth truly does "taste like tomorrow" and reminds us of new beginnings. Soon there will be flowers, birds, and the possibility of fresh fruits and vegetables. A garden is a place to relax, observe, discover, imagine, socialize, reminisce, meditate, and exercise. Gardening is purposeful work, and even something as simple as watering potted houseplants can make your loved one feel useful and needed.

There are many ways to bring the garden to your loved one. Cut flowers and houseplants can bring a bit of cheer to a dreary winter day. A window herb garden can make a high-rise apartment seem like a forty-acre farm. And a backyard garden is a place everyone can enjoy.

Dorothy loved her yard. She liked to sit on her porch, listen to the birds, watch the sky, and tell us about World War II victory gardens. Eventually, Dorothy's storytelling would lead to reminiscing about an old family friend who only grew onions in his World War II garden patch. Dorothy always wondered what anyone would do with so many onions.

In some communities, adult day care programs sponsor garden clubs for people who have early- and mid-stage dementia. Some clubs have monthly meetings. In addition to socializing, participants pot easy-to-grow plants that they bring home. Geraniums, coleus, pansies, rosemary, and mint are examples of colorful and fragrant plants your family member may enjoy.

Other clubs meet on a weekly basis and, similar to Dorothy's victory garden, work a small patch of land. Members tend to be those who are still physically active and enjoy social contact, exercise, and the sense of achievement that gardening can bring.

The internet is a resource where you can learn more about the benefits of gardening for people who have dementia. The keywords "Alzheimer's," "green thumb," "dementia," and "gardening" will lead you to many interesting and informative websites.

VISITING WITH FAMILY AND FRIENDS

Most people find visiting a family member or a friend who has dementia difficult. Visitors have difficulty following stream of consciousness conversation and may become impatient when they hear the same question over and over again. Visitors find the invisible changes that make their family member or friend unrecognizable disturbing. "And what if that happens to me?" is the thought that crosses everyone's mind.

During the last three years of her life, Dorothy saw few people other than her immediate family and caregivers. That's not to say a full social life came to a screeching halt. Dorothy led a quiet life. She moved from her hometown to live closer to her family. Most of her long-time friends had died. She lost interest in community volunteer work although she did look forward to her monthly book club meeting. She had polite, rather than social, relationships with her neighbors. Reading, making stone sculpture, and spending time with her family made her happy.

One of her caregivers said that it was rare for dementia patients to have visitors. The caregiver said dementia makes it like you never existed.

This all sounds pretty dismal; however, it is important that your family member see and socialize with other people. It's also important that other people see and socialize with those who have dementia. Perhaps doing so will lessen fear and reduce stigma.

DRIVING

Driving. Remember how hard it was to convince your parents you were responsible enough to get a driver's license? And remember, once you got that license, you had to prove to your parents that you drove well enough to use the family car? Well, guess what? "It's déjà vu all over again." Only this time, you have to take the car keys away from a person who has been driving for the past half century or even longer.

But before we delve into ways to get your family member off the road, early-stage dementia does not instantly disqualify a person from driving; however, early-stage dementia is a very good time to establish criteria for when driving is no longer safe, as well as to discuss other transportation options.

If you are lucky, something will happen—a minor fender bender or getting lost going to or from a familiar place that scares your family member enough to stop driving on their own. Otherwise, you, or another person, must initiate next steps (see table 8.1).

Table 8.1.   Signs It Is Time for Your Parent to Give Up the Keys

Has received two or more traffic tickets or warnings within the past two years
Has been involved in two or more accidents or near-misses within the past two years
Confuses the gas pedal with the brake pedal
Ignores traffic signals
Fails to signal or signals inappropriately
Has difficulty seeing pedestrians or other vehicles
Has difficulty making turns or changing lanes
Weaves across the road
Straddles lanes
Gets lost going to or from familiar places
Gets honked at
Drives too fast or too slow
Asks for copilot help going to familiar places
Lacks good judgment
Has poor parking skills or parks in inappropriate places

Note: Adapted from "Know When to Be Concerned," SeniorDrivingAAA, accessed June 6, 2020, https://seniordriving.aaa.com/resources-family-friends/know-when-be-concerned/.

Your family member's doctor can be a wonderful ally. Sometimes their voice of authority is enough and the parent agrees to give up the keys. If the doctor is unsuccessful in convincing your family member that driving is no longer appropriate, you or the doctor can write a letter to the registry of motor vehicles, stating driving safety concerns.

The American Automobile Association (AAA) offers a range of senior driver services. Their "Resources for Family and Friends" is especially helpful. Nevertheless, do keep in mind that people who have dementia may not have sufficient self-awareness to accept the suggestions the AAA, or anyone else, may make.

Obviously, it is important to protect your loved one's safety as well as the safety of other drivers and pedestrians. It is also important to do so in a way that respects your loved one's dignity. One family told me their approach was to demand their father, like a naughty child, hand over his driver's license and car keys to them. The same family expressed surprise at how angry their father became.

My husband and I did things a little differently. Dorothy kept her driver's license—she just didn't drive. And the car keys? Dorothy wasn't aware I had removed them from her keychain.

The driving regulations for senior citizens vary from state to state. Some states require annual written and road tests; others just require a written exam and a vision test. A few states do not have special rules for older drivers. The age when one becomes a senior driver also varies (see Helpful Resources).

I discussed my driving safety concerns with Dorothy's doctor several months after dementia became part of Dorothy's official medical history. He asked her a few questions, she claimed a perfect driving record, and he mumbled something about "anyone in this state who has a gun rack and can open a six-pack" can drive.

Hmm, this shouldn't be too hard. Dorothy didn't have a gun rack, and the trouble she had opening cereal boxes I was sure made opening a six-pack impossible.

Well, as it turned out, getting Dorothy off the road was far from easy. Rational discussion went nowhere. I hoped giving specific examples might work better. I told her that neighbors had mentioned their concern to me. I pointed out the dings on the garage door and the scrape marks on her car. I reminded her that a person who should not have been driving killed my father and her husband. I reminded her that, because her car was in the repair shop (really), it might be a good time to try senior citizen transportation services.

So she called a car rental company, and yep—you guessed right.

Once, just out of curiosity, my husband asked Dorothy when she thought she might stop driving. Without even a second's thought, she replied, "104." Just for the record, Dorothy didn't have a sense of humor.

As I have mentioned before, the weeks Dorothy spent in the hospital and the rehabilitation facility made her cognitive decline obvious; however, the reason for her hospitalizations gave us a new approach to the driving issue—driving will hurt your back. Dorothy, believing her back injury was a temporary condition, never stopped asking "when."

I hid the car keys in a spot where only the caregivers could have access to them. And when Dorothy told us she could do her own driving, the caregivers told her that, after all her years of hard work, she deserved to live like a princess. Saying that often made her smile (see table 8.2).

Table 8.2.   Examples of Alternative Transportation for Senior Drivers

Carpooling with a neighbor or friend
Escorted travel
Online ride request
Paratransit services provided by public transportation systems
Social service agencies and ride-pools or vans
Social service agencies and volunteer drivers
Taxi

Later, when Dorothy no longer had the strength or the coordination to open the car door, I no longer worried about her taking the keys and escaping. For us, the oft-repeated refrain, "when your doctor says it's okay," worked well. It wasn't "no," it did give her hope, and by passing blame on to her doctor, it prevented her from becoming angry with me. Eventually, Dorothy said she had forgotten how to drive and wanted driving lessons.

My approach doesn't work if your family member can find and reach the keys and, in addition, have the physical strength to open the door. In these situations, it is important to hide keys in a very safe place. Some families disconnect or remove the car battery. Other families park the car away from the house or arrange to have the car "stolen."

DAILY MONEY MATTERS

Money management, like driving, is a statement of independence. And again, similar to driving, early-stage dementia does not instantly make your family member unable to manage their own financial affairs; however, the early-stage dementia period is a good time to learn about your family member's finances and, if you are the POA, get your name on their bank accounts and credit cards. Over time, your role will gradually change from oversight to becoming the person responsible for such things as paying bills and taxes and managing investments.

But just because you and your loved one discussed finances earlier doesn't guarantee they will agree with those decisions now. Your family member may want to maintain control, and that feeling often overrides earlier agreements.

What to do! Some families ignore the protests and simply remove checkbooks and credit cards. Rather than taking Dorothy's checkbook away from her, the bank made a separate set of checkbooks for me to use. I also got a credit card with my name on it.

There were occasions when Dorothy insisted on writing a check to pay for services. That was okay. It helped her feel in charge and independent; however, what Dorothy didn't know is that I told people (such as the neighborhood kid who cut her lawn) to take the check and give it to me in exchange for one the bank would accept.

Dorothy did like having her own spending money. When asked, the caregiver took Dorothy to the bank, and with the teller's help, she withdrew the money she used to pay for her twice-a-month wash and set. I did put a limit on the amount of money Dorothy could withdraw at any one time, and I kept track of her account balance online.

The credit card never became an issue. Dorothy rarely went into stores and did not shop online or order things over the phone; however, the caregiver did use the credit card to buy gas for Dorothy's car, pay for prescriptions, and, on rare occasions, buy a few things at the grocery store.

This arrangement worked fairly well, and it was only right that Dorothy have access to her own money. Having Dorothy feel that she was still in control also avoided what would have been a terrible and never-ending argument.

NOT A LITTLE THING: FRAUD AND SCAMS

Many people of Dorothy's generation couldn't understand why anyone would want a computer in their home, much less use one. It was much easier to brag about their genius grandchildren than admit computers are a total mystery. That was pretty much the case for Dorothy—until the day when she announced she wanted to write to Bessie. Somehow, we managed to connect the two lifelong friends.

Dorothy sat at my desk, and, with some help, she slowly typed, "Bessie, I had soup for dinner." And shortly afterward came the response, "I did, too."

Dorothy was so proud of herself; she used a computer! Although, as far as she was concerned, once was enough.

Unfamiliarity with computers protected Dorothy and others of her generation from an onslaught of fraudulent e-mail and other online scams. Now, more people are computer competent.

Today, all of us are inundated with phone calls, door-to-door sales, and online (phishing) scams. Caregivers, tired and stressed, also may fall victim to these predatory tactics; however, elderly people and people who are in the early stages of dementia are easy targets.

Scammers pursue elderly people who are media naïve or who are lonely. These predators know to capitalize on the fear of losing Medicare and Social Security benefits. Scammers know that many older people are easily duped into sweepstake and lottery schemes. Seemingly friendly and empathetic scammers can trick seniors, especially those with mild cognitive impairment, into revealing personal information. Scammers read obituary notices to find people who are emotionally fragile and overwhelmed.

According to the U.S. Senate Special Committee on Aging, Social Security impersonation is the one most frequently reported to the scam and fraud hotline. Here, people claiming to represent the Social Security Administration (SSA) tell elderly people they face arrest or other legal action. Sometimes the scammers switch tactics and say that they want to help activate a suspended Social Security number. It's important that your family member understands that the SSA *never* initiates contact by phone, *never* makes threats, and *never* asks for credit card information. Report SSA and identify theft scams to the Federal Trade Commission (see Helpful Resources).

There are several things you can do to protect your family member from fraud and scams. Perhaps the most important is vigilance. Listen to your loved one—do they mention having made new friends? Do they sound worried about the person who calls every day and asks too many questions? Check the incoming phone call numbers as well as any voice mail messages.

GROOMING AND OUTWARD APPEARANCES

In part, who we are is how we present ourselves to others. Our clothing and grooming, more than merely an outward appearance, reveals what is happening inside.

Dementia is a disease that robs people of their sense of self. Who they are fades until the person we once knew is unrecognizable. Eventually, the disease creates a "near-stranger" dressed in an easy-wash jogging suit, baggy knee-high stockings, and Velcro sneakers.

Clothing

Often people who have dementia refuse to change their clothes. They want to wear the same shirt, pants, or dress every day. The accumulation of food stains and body odor makes it unpleasant and somewhat depressing for everyone.

Dorothy, who was once very self-conscious about her appearance, insisted on wearing the same beige blouse and brown pants for days at a time. Maybe wearing different clothing made it hard for her to recognize herself. Maybe making decisions about what to wear was too difficult. Our solution was to wash and dry her clothes after she went to bed at night.

Of course, the frequent washing was hard on the fabric, and pretty soon Dorothy's underwear and clothes were falling apart. Thinking she might enjoy having a present delivered to her house, I ordered some new outfits from an online store. What a disaster! "I can buy my own clothes!" And taking her out to shop didn't work any better. Dorothy, unable to focus on shopping, made loud and inappropriate comments about the people she saw in the store. That experience was trying and exhausting for everyone.

Shopping without Dorothy was the best solution. And so she wouldn't notice my purchases, I bought items of the same color and style as her worn-out clothes and put them in her closet and drawers without telling her.

For the most part, I was able to avoid the jogging suit and Velcro look. I bought button-down blouses as arthritis made getting in and out of pullover tops painful. Slacks made with an elastic waist fit better than those with buttons and reduced toileting accidents. Clothing made from natural materials, such as cotton, didn't seem to get as smelly as those made from synthetic fabrics. Nonetheless, Dorothy did like knee-high stockings, and, sadly, they did sag and bag.

Occasionally, I would find something on sale that I felt Dorothy might like. Realizing that her inability to shop on her own often led to arguments, I gave those purchases to the caregivers who, in turn, gave them to Dorothy as a present.

This roundabout way to give Dorothy a pretty blouse might seem like too much trouble. But it is amazing how much good came from making the extra effort. Receiving a present from "her girls" was a great mood booster and that, of course, made the day easier for everyone. It was also nice to see Dorothy wear something more colorful than her beige and brown uniform.

Finding clothes that fit was another challenge. Bone loss caused Dorothy to shrink from a height of five feet tall to as short as four foot ten inches or maybe even shorter. Loss of height translated into a curved back, a protruding midsection, and needing clothing larger than expected. I found that petite-sized capri slacks with an elastic waist fit Dorothy like full-length pants. The sleeves of petite-sized blouses were close to the right length, and a size medium or large fit around her chest and abdomen.

Finding shoes was perhaps the most difficult. What worked best was a call to a local shoe store and, after describing the situation, arranging for a time to meet with a salesperson likely to have the understanding and patience to fit Dorothy with a pair of shoes.

Dressing

For a person who has dementia, getting dressed can be a frustrating experience. Deciding what to wear, in combination with the difficulty of putting clothes on, can be too much. To maintain your family member's independence for as long as possible, it is helpful to offer no more than two choices. Lay out clothing in the order of use—underwear first and slacks last.

You may need to hand your family member one item at a time and give simple and step-wise instructions, for example, "Put on your socks." Stating "get dressed" isn't helpful if your family member no longer understands dressing is a series of orderly steps.

Dorothy wanted to dress herself; however, left to her own devices, she couldn't get much further than taking her pajamas off. Laying out washed clothing the night before reduced the anxiety of deciding what to wear. She almost always refused our offer to help her get dressed; however, she almost always needed assistance. Our usual ritual was to stand outside her door and wait for her call.

For Dorothy, having the option to ask for assistance was more acceptable than having help offered. Sometimes, getting dressed would take close to an hour. It was for this reason we avoided early morning doctor appointments.

Grooming

Your loved one may forget to brush their hair and not remember how to shave. Your loved one may no longer remember the purpose of a toothbrush or how to use nail clippers. The loss of cognitive and executive functions, in combination with other medical problems (such as poor vision and arthritis), can make it hard for your family member to attend to their own grooming.

There are many ways to encourage independent grooming. At first, a gentle reminder may be all that your loved one needs; however, as dementia progresses, they may need assistance. Sometimes, brushing your own hair or teeth alongside your loved one will help them copy your motions. You can also place your hands over theirs to guide the necessary motions. Some people who have dementia will not accept your assistance.

Another option is taking your loved one to a beauty salon, barber shop, or manicure salon. Make an appointment, rather than going "walk-in," to avoid long waits. Also be sure to ask for a beautician or barber who either knows your family member or who has the patience to work with a person who has dementia. Consider getting a haircut or a manicure at the same time as your loved one. It's an efficient use of your time and a pleasant activity to do together.

Many beauticians, barbers, and manicurists make home visits. It is especially nice if a grooming professional your loved one knows comes to the house.

If cost is a concern, many beauty and barber schools offer reduced-price services. Use your search engine and the keywords "student training salon," plus the name of the city or town where your family member lives, to find a more affordable haircuts and manicures.

In chapter 9, you will learn that agency caregivers have strict limitations on what they may do. Nail care is often one of them. Many home care agencies feel that filing and cutting fingernails and toenails is similar to providing medical treatment and, therefore, is beyond their employee's scope of work. While it's hard to think of red nail polish in the same context as glucose monitoring, many elderly patients do have foot problems associated with diabetes, poor circulation, ingrown toenails, and thickened toenails.

Mouth care is another sensitive issue. During the early stages of dementia, most people can do an adequate job of maintaining their oral hygiene; however, as dementia progresses, you may need to remind your loved one to brush their teeth or clean their dentures. Eventually, your loved one may need help with their oral hygiene.

A FEW WORDS FROM THE DENTAL OFFICE

It's easy to overlook your family member's dental care when you are already overwhelmed with other doctor appointments, house maintenance, and the challenges of difficult behavior. Nevertheless, poor dental health, especially in combination with diabetes, can cause pain and eating difficulties, and it can increase the risk for cardiovascular disease. In addition, a side effect of many medications used to manage behavior causes dry mouth—a condition that is uncomfortable and promotes gum disease and tooth decay.

Helping a person manage their oral health at home takes sensitivity and creativity. Having someone poking around in your mouth is invasive, unnatural, and uncomfortable. These feelings must be especially so for a person who has dementia.

Many dental hygienists and dentists suggest that you brush and floss together. Mimicking your motions makes it easier for your family member to follow direction and makes you seem less bossy. Over time, you may need to take a more active role in your loved one's at-home dental care.

Dental appointments create another set of challenges. Apprehension or refusal will probably be your first hurdle. Again, dental professionals suggest making the appointment seem more social than a "hav'ta do." Perhaps mentioning your hygienist misses seeing you and your pretty smile will reduce their resistance. Another strategy is to promise an enjoyable activity afterward.

Be sure to communicate your concerns to the hygienist and dentist so they are aware of your loved one's special needs. A phone call to the front office should suffice. It's also important that you, another family member, or a paid caregiver stay with your loved one in the examination room. The presence of a trusted person will reduce stress and need for sedation, and it will make the appointment go as smoothly as possible.

Hopefully, good preventative care will spare your loved one from having to undergo procedures to treat gum disease or remove decayed teeth. Otherwise, the dentist will discuss treatment options with you or another person able to represent the patient. Some dentists, under these circumstances, will suggest palliative procedures, rather than extensive repairs, to reduce pain, treat infections, and improve the ability to eat.

Many older people wear dentures or partial bridges to replace all or some of their teeth. Both kinds of dental appliances require care and maintenance. Your loved one's dental hygienist can explain and demonstrate the best way to clean the dentures or removable bridges, as well as how to identify problems that may require attention.

CAREGIVER HYGIENE

It's worrisome when doctors, nurses, and other caregivers do not wash their hands or use protective gloves. When we see this lapse in expected health care standards, we worry about getting sick.

It's hard to think that caring for your loved one can make you ill. After all, your family member isn't a stranger, and you feel confident of your own health. What many people do not realize is that everyone has bacteria and other microbes in and on their body. Most are harmless, but many microbes, when they get into an open wound or contaminate food, can cause illness.

The other concern is transporting disease-causing microbes back and forth between your loved one's home and your own family.

Just like people who work in a hospital, washing and gloving is a simple way to lower the risk of giving or getting an infection at home. Keeping soap—regular or antibacterial—by the kitchen and bathroom sinks, or a waterless antiseptic hand wash in convenient locations throughout the house, are good ways to remind yourself to wash your hands. Washing is especially important before handling food and after contact with body fluids like blood, mucus, urine, feces, or vomit.

It might sound silly, but in addition to washing your hands, it is sometimes important to also wear disposable gloves. For example, wear disposable medical gloves when helping your loved one with their personal hygiene. Afterward, remove and dispose of the gloves, and then wash your hands with a bactericidal soap or an antiseptic hand wash.

You can buy bactericidal soaps, waterless antiseptic hand wash products, and disposable gloves at most grocery stores and pharmacies. It is often more economical to buy gloves in larger quantities at such big-box stores as Walmart, Costco, Sam's Club, or Target. Online suppliers are another option. If you are allergic to latex, buy gloves made from nitrile or vinyl.

FREQUENTLY ASKED QUESTIONS

1. My husband misses his friends. Suggestions?

The easiest way is to create an event. It doesn't have to be fancy—coffee and dessert at home or in a local coffee shop, an easy hike, or an invitation to a sporting event, an art exhibit, or to a concert. But do limit the number of guests and schedule at a time when your family member is least likely to become confused and overwhelmed.

2. For as long as I can remember, my mother hoped that someday, when she had the time, she could join a choral group. Is this a possibility for her, and if so, how do I find a choral group?

The answer to the first part of your question is easy—yes! The second half is also easy. There are choral programs especially for people who have dementia. The same can be said for theater, dance, and art programs. Your web browser and the keywords "choral," "chorus," "dementia," and "Alzheimer's," plus the location where your mother lives, will give you the information you need.

There are many other "someday" opportunities for people who have dementia. The keywords "dementia," "Alzheimer's," "groups," "programs," plus the name of the activity of interest (such as hiking, ceramics, music, and dancing), will direct you to many helpful sites. And should skydiving be on your loved one's "someday" list, check out this link: https://togetherinthis. com/alive-alzheimers-skydiving-adventure/.

3. You give many examples of ways to work around various caregiving problems. What if I cannot think of ways to reduce the difficulties specific to my family member's care?

Well, first of all, don't be too hard on yourself. It's difficult to think of creative or even simple solutions when the challenge of being your family member's caregiver leaves you stressed and exhausted. The important thing is recognizing that you need the help and input of others. Your local Alzheimer's Association is always a good source of information. Another is the Dementia Society of America. Support group members are another wonderful resource. You can often find support group listings in your local newspaper. Or you can use the keywords "dementia," "Alzheimer's disease," and "support groups," plus the location where you or your family member lives, to find internet links and telephone contact information to local support groups.

9

HOME CARE AND CAREGIVERS

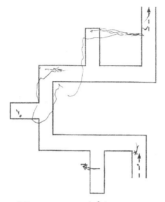

Woman, age eighty, maze.

A few days before Dorothy's anticipated discharge from the hospital, I met with the doctor responsible for her rehabilitation care. For some reason, it never occurred to me Dorothy would need more assistance than I could provide in her home or mine. Suddenly, I had to find caregivers, install bathroom railings, and arrange for the delivery of a wheelchair, walker, and hospital bed. I also had to figure out a way to adjust my day to meet her needs.

Her house wasn't ready, my house wasn't ready, and I wasn't ready.

My stopgap solution was to place her in a continuum of care facility where she would receive additional physical and occupational therapy. In the meantime, her back problems eased enough to transition from the nursing home wing to an assisted living area that included people in mid-stage dementia.

I will admit I hoped she would be willing to call this very luxurious care center home. I showed her the library, the beautiful gardens, the elegant dining area, and the arts and crafts room. After a total of nearly two months in a hospital and rehabilitation care facility, Dorothy wanted to go home. I can't blame her for that. I'm sure I'd want the same for myself.

At some point, we received a home safety evaluation from the hospital social service department. The improvements were minimal—safety rails in the shower and toilet area, a shower chair, and "child-proof" latches on cabinets containing cleaning supplies and other potentially dangerous substances. The safety consultant suggested Dorothy should have a hospital bed, a wheelchair, and a walker. In addition, she gave me a list of Medicare-approved hospital supply stores.

We returned the hospital bed a few days after its arrival. The bed was too high for Dorothy, as well as uncomfortable. It took a phone call and too much paperwork to get rid of the bed. The wheelchair and walker we stored out of sight. Dorothy made it perfectly clear she was never going to need or use them. For the record, the opposite was true.

CHALLENGES

Many families eventually resort to employing paid caregivers when dementia progresses to the point when they can no longer do it alone. There are other reasons why having paid caregivers may become a necessity. Distance is certainly an important one. Family and work responsibilities comprise many of the other reasons why adult children cannot devote several years to a parent's full-time care. Emotional distance is another.

Spouses, for similar reasons, may need outside help. When dementia disrupts a long-standing relationship, it impacts how two people share their home, it reduces the ability to enjoy time spent together or with friends, and it reduces much-needed "me time."

Older couples may not want to impose or become a bother to their adult children who are already juggling the responsibilities of children, home, and work. Emotional distance is another factor.

ADULT CHILDREN

Unlike a spouse, many adult children are no longer accustomed to spending extended time with their parents. As independent adults, they maintain the relationship with short visits, phone calls, e-mail, and face-to-face social media. If they live far away, holiday gatherings and life cycle events like births, weddings, and funerals may be the only times they get together. In many ways, time and distance weaken already fragile relationships.

In either situation—physical distance or overwhelming responsibilities—daily interactions with a parent who is becoming progressively more disabled becomes increasingly difficult. And you know what? Parents may find their children's presence or daily inquiries both intrusive and unwanted.

Emotional distance is another challenge many adult children have to overcome when dementia forces a change in the relationship. Memories of cruel words, indifference, and, in some cases, a history of alcoholism and drug abuse may emerge.

Some adult children can overcome past difficulties. Conversely, the reverse is also true—sometimes the past is too painful to forget. And you know what? That is okay. It is better and healthier for everyone when there is a realistic understanding of the situation.

Counseling or therapy may help you understand and overcome these difficult emotions. Or quite possibly, using paid caregivers to limit time spent with your mother or father is truly the best answer. In any case, it's important that you understand your physical and emotional limits. If other people question your actions, simply tell them, "I am doing the best I can under the circumstances." There is no need to explain the situation further.

SPOUSES

Dementia can put considerable strain between spouses. Particularly for retired couples, dementia often means household tasks they once shared, such as grocery shopping and yardwork, suddenly falls on the shoulders of one of them.

More than likely, one or both of them have other health problems to contend with. The caregiving spouse may have diabetes, or the spouse who has Alzheimer's disease may also have severe arthritis.

To compound matters, it's becoming increasingly common for grandparents to be raising their grandchildren.

Distance, both physical and emotional, may make it difficult for parents to accept help from their children. It may also be true that the longtime marriage may not have been a happy one.

CAREGIVER AGENCIES

Home care agencies may be small, locally owned businesses or large regional or national franchises. Most agencies offer an assortment of services that may include companionship, light housekeeping and cooking, transportation, and bathing and personal hygiene, as well as medication reminders. The agency, in addition to certified nursing assistants (CNA), may also have licensed practical and registered nurses on staff who can provide more medically complex skills, such as insulin injections or wound care.

Finding the right agency is a time-consuming process. As always, your friends and neighbors can tell you about their experiences with various agencies. Your loved one's doctor, medical social worker, or nurse case manager may have suggestions.

An internet search is another approach. The keywords "home care," "dementia," "eldercare," and "Alzheimer's" will link you to a spectrum of local and franchised home health care agencies. Adding the keyword "review" will uncover opinions from current or former clients.

Agency web pages often contain extensive and detailed information. The "Who We Are" or "About Us" sections present their philosophy and business history. Many agency websites contain tabs that link to such things as dementia information, the services they provide, and contact phone numbers and e-mail addresses.

Often the website will have a tab or link for people looking for job opportunities. Reading this section is a good way to learn about the people the agency employs. It is interesting to note that having been a caregiver for a family member, rather than education and training, is a quality many agencies look for.

Home care agencies are usually nothing more than an office. Therefore, after making contact, an agency representative will ask to meet you where your family member lives or will live. There are some practical reasons for meeting away from the office. The agency wants to know as much as possible about their client and family. They also want to evaluate the caregiver's work environment. You might want to think of this "sizing up" as an interview or even as a first date.

Your meeting with the agency representative is a time to ask questions; however, before the interview, research the kinds of amenities this and other agencies provide. Friends who have used agency caregivers are a good place to start. Websites are another. Often, the information posted on the website doesn't reveal the services they do *not* provide or the tasks their caregivers *cannot* do. Table 9.1 contains examples of the questions you may want to ask the agency representative.

I made the habit of asking questions that would reveal more than expected information. "Why do you work in the home care industry?" "What do you find interesting, satisfying, or exciting about your job?" "What do you tell your family or friends about your workday?"

First of all, I wonder about the effectiveness and motivation of an administrator who responds by saying "I don't know," "I never thought about that," or "It paid enough." Sometimes their answers reveal a difficult workplace with

Table 9.1. Examples of Questions to Ask a Home Health Care Representative

What is the minimum and maximum number of hours a caregiver can work each day or week?

May the caregiver drive my family member's car?

Who makes and keeps track of doctor appointments?

May the home caregiver call in prescription refills, go to the pharmacy, or dispense medication?

Does the caregiver cook meals or use prepared and packaged foods?

Can your caregivers help my family member make or count change or use their credit card?

What is the holiday rate?

What is included in "light housekeeping"?

Are there extra charges if my family member needs help during the night?

Do your caregivers wash and style hair?

May your caregivers cut and file fingernails and toenails?

What is the protocol if a caregiver cannot come to work?

What is the protocol if my family member needs to go to the emergency room?

Do caregivers provide their own meals?

What kinds of cognitive and social stimulation do your caregivers provide?

How do your caregivers communicate with me and each other?

How do we coordinate care so that all caregivers know what to do?

Do you provide respite care?

Who should I contact if I have a question? Phone, text, or e-mail? Typical response time?

frequent employee turnover. Your response to this uncensored and candid information is simply a friendly, "Thank-you." There is no need to pry further.

The agency representative will have many questions for you. He or she will want to learn about your loved one's personality and behavior, as well as their favorite activities and foods. Refer back to worksheets 4.1 and 4.2 in chapter 4 to help organize your thoughts about the kinds and amounts of services your loved one may need.

The representative may also ask to see the kitchen, bathroom, and bedroom. They will want to see staircases that lead to the basement, upper levels of the house, and the backyard or patio. In part, they are looking for potential safety issues. In addition, they want to choose a caregiver physically able to help your family member navigate a potentially challenging living space. The administrator may suggest how to improve bathroom or kitchen safety and request that you install handrails, remove throw rugs, or add locks to doors leading to the basement or the backyard.

Be sure to ask the representative for local references. Some agency representatives will bring with them the names and numbers of former or current clients. Other times, the agency representative will provide reference information in a follow-up phone call.

My conversations with former agency clients often revealed two problems: (1) difficulty in communicating with the agency office, and (2) the time it took for the agency to find the right caregivers. I suspect these are problems common to most home care agencies.

The agency I selected gave me a special phone number and e-mail address to use when I needed information, had a problem to report, or needed to reschedule caregiver hours. There were many times when I had to leave a phone message on their twenty-four-hour phone service, and sometimes it took longer than expected to get a response. I quickly discovered that e-mail was frequently ignored, never made it to the right person, or the right person had left the agency.

Consistent care was an ongoing difficulty. Sometimes the agency, without much warning, would transfer caregivers to another home. Other times, the caregiver—citing such things as Dorothy's behavior or a long commute, would ask for another assignment. And for the first few months, Dorothy, not understanding her situation, would frequently announce, "I don't need your help. You're fired!"

Even though Dorothy was usually happy to see the caregiver the next day, I was careful to take into consideration other reasons that might cause Dorothy to dislike certain caregivers. Once, when it was obvious that a poor match was the problem, I requested that the agency send a different caregiver.

The biggest obstacle was the number of hours an agency caregiver could work each week. Even when we limited care to thirteen hours per day, it meant more people were in and out of Dorothy's house over the course of the week than she could tolerate. Dorothy couldn't remember one caregiver from another, and having all those strangers in her home made her feel confused and unsafe. It was primarily for this reason that I switched from an agency to privately hired or independent caregivers. The other reason was expense. Dorothy's dwindling bank account was making it hard for me to sleep at night.

Agencies are more expensive. But despite the added cost, there are some advantages to using an agency. One of them is the company is responsible for the weekly payroll.

Paying the agency is similar to paying rent on an apartment. Some agencies ask for an upfront deposit to cover the last weeks of the caregiver's salary. Then, once service begins, you receive a detailed monthly bill. Considering there may be a rotating cast of caregivers in and out of your loved one's home, it is very helpful that the agency is responsible for monitoring hours worked and money earned. The agency's monthly bill also makes it easier for you to keep track of your family member's medical tax deductions.

In addition to payroll, there are other benefits. First of all, the people they send to your loved one's home have successfully completed a home care training program. Second, agency home caregivers are insured and bonded. The assurances that come with a background check remove some of the concerns and worries associated with a stranger having access to your loved one's home. And finally, many agencies provide their employees with health insurance and workers' compensation.

WHO ARE AGENCY CAREGIVERS?

Agency caregivers are people who work for a business or an organization that provide various kinds of home care services. Monitoring, certification, and employee standards differ from state to state.

Agency employers may require their caregivers have nursing assistant (CNA) certification or proof of having received training from another home care agency. Some agencies will train otherwise promising employees. In addition, agencies often require additional in-house training and participation in continuing education classes.

A clean background check is another requirement for employment. Some states require having passed a TB (tuberculosis) screening test as a condition for employment.

THE ROLE OF AN AGENCY CAREGIVER

The caregiver's role is difficult to define. In the most general sense, the agency caregiver provides homemaking, companionship, and personal care services. Agency caregivers, sensitive to the amount of assistance their client needs, can bathe and dress your loved one, as well as wash and comb hair, brush teeth, and clean dentures. Most agency caregivers can take your family member to doctor appointments, out to lunch, or to group activities. Making the doctor appointments is your responsibility (see table 9.2).

Grocery shopping and meal preparation are gray areas. With the availability of prepaid online shopping as well as home delivery options, the caregiver has little reason to go to the grocery store.

Meal preparation is *the* gray area issue. Does the agency limit the caregiver to prepackaged foods? Are there caregivers who can accommodate vegetarian, vegan, and kosher diets? Ditto for lactose- and gluten-free diets.

If the caregiver drives your family member's car, make sure the car is in good working order and that the caregiver has a way to pay for gasoline. Even though the insurance is on the car, and not on the driver, you may want to notify the insurance company that another person will be the primary driver.

Table 9.2. Caregiver Interview Questions

What would you like me to know about you?
What makes you happy or proud?
What do you like to do for relaxation?
Tell me what you like about working with people who have dementia.
Tell me what you know about dementia.
Describe other caregiving experiences you have had.
My father repeats himself to the extent that it becomes annoying. How will you handle that kind of situation?
My mother often cannot get to the toilet in time. How would you handle toileting accidents?
Sometimes my father sees things that aren't there. What would you do to lessen his fear?
What will you do if you cannot come to work because of illness, weather, or personal reasons?
Dementia behaviors are difficult for everyone. How might you lessen the effects of a difficult day on your behavior?
Define abuse. Give some examples.

If the caregiver uses his or her own car, make sure they carry adequate insurance. It is a good idea to investigate the caregiver's driving record. Call the State Department of Motor Vehicles office to get access to the caregiver's driving record.

Most agency caregivers may not change bandages, clean wounds, dispense medication, cut toenails, or help with home dialysis. If your family member requires this kind of assistance, the agency can send employees who do have the necessary training and qualifications.

Laundry and light housekeeping are other tasks agency caregivers do; however, most do not wash floors or windows or clean bathrooms and refrigerators. You may find these same people, working off the clock, will do these chores with a cash payment from you.

Agency employees do not do yardwork or make house repairs. If you have neither the time nor the inclination to cut the lawn, replace light bulbs, repair the roof, or change furnace filters, you need to find people or services to maintain your family member's home.

I made the decision to pay Dorothy's longtime housekeeper Becky to do the heavy cleaning. There were several reasons for having what might seem like an unnecessary expense. First of all, it would help Dorothy feel she was in charge of her home. It made her angry when I or one of the caregivers cleaned her house. On the other hand, Becky and Dorothy had a more than twenty-year relationship. I am quite certain Dorothy felt having Becky in her house made things seem normal and familiar. And paying the housekeeper was an "I can do" opportunity; however, Dorothy could no longer write a check or count money. To get around this difficulty, I paid the housekeeper who returned Dorothy's miswritten check or miscounted money to me.

Yes, as I have stated many times, trust and finding creative ways to work around problems is an important aspect of caregiving, especially if doing so helps maintain dignity and a sense of self-sufficiency.

Independent caregivers may be willing and able to do certain "clinical" tasks. Dorothy's independent caregivers called in pharmacy refills and, under my direction, dispensed her medications into a weekly medication box. They also gave Dorothy the nasal drops she took to slow bone loss. We all took turns at getting Dorothy's medications at the pharmacy.

Using mail-order pharmacies can simplify this aspect of your loved one's care; however, mail-order pharmacies usually fill prescriptions in three-month allotments. Using mail-order pharmacies, then, is not a good idea for new medications your family member may not tolerate or for prescriptions likely to change within three months.

INDEPENDENT CAREGIVERS

Independent caregivers are people you hire. In other words, you are now a business owner and employer—a topic I will discuss at length in the "Business Owner and Family Caregiver" section of this chapter.

Finding caregivers that are both affordable and a good fit with your loved one's needs and personality is a time-intensive process. As always, friends and neighbors are often a good resource; however, be aware that your friends and their acquaintances are not likely to give up a wonderful caregiver currently in their employment. But it's still worth asking. Their caregiver may have a friend or relative who would like to work for you.

Dorothy's first independent caregiver was a woman who had worked for us through the home care agency; however, to hire her, I had to pay the agency a finder's fee to release her from the contract I had signed. Getting out of the contracted agreement was expensive, but the advantages outweighed the expense.

Reduced cost is an important benefit of using independent caregivers. Even though I paid the caregiver more than she received from the agency, it was still about 50 percent less than what the agency charged per hour. It took only a few weeks to earn back the finder's fee.

Now, rather than four different caregivers, Dorothy only had two—one who worked Monday through Friday, and an agency caregiver who stayed with her all day on Saturday and until dinner time on Sunday when Dorothy had dinner and spent the evening with my husband and me.

I was pleased to discover that the weekend agency contract still gave me coverage for any extra or substitute help I might need during the week.

Having two caregivers made it easier for Dorothy to understand her day and to accept the presence of caregivers in her home. But even with just two new people in her life, she was unable to remember their names. Dorothy often used "she" and "the girl" when speaking about them. The caregivers said they responded to any name Dorothy used.

Eventually, the weekday situation fell apart. Although the caregiver said she preferred working with a single client, she could not handle the long hours with a person who was often verbally abusive. As a result, I had become an intermediary and mediator. It was a particularly difficult phone conversation with the caregiver that made me realize the situation wouldn't improve.

My strategy in getting new caregivers was to ask the remaining ones if they knew anyone who would be a good fit for our situation. Often it was a friend or another member of their extended family who became a next caregiver.

It took a while, but eventually I got the perfect combination when a mother-in-law/daughter-in-law team came into our lives. Unlike many other caregivers, these two women thrived in the open-ended work environment I expected. Basically, I wanted Dorothy to have someone with her from 8 a.m. to 9 p.m. every day. How they split their hours was up to them.

Flexible hours helped both women attend to their own families and get the breaks they needed to prevent burnout. Eventually, they added the weekend hours to their schedule. Occasionally, another person in their family, such as a sister or a niece, would take over when both caregivers had schedule conflicts. Yes, it did require a considerable amount of trust on my part—but in this case, it worked.

Not having to work with and around the constraints of the agency contract is one of the benefits of using independent caregivers. Nevertheless, that freedom also comes with the concerns of having people in your parent's home who may be neither insured nor bonded. You might get yourself into a workers' compensation situation if the caregiver hurts themselves in helping your loved one in or out of the bathtub. In addition, you are opening their home to a person whose honesty is based on the words of other people. Although I did not do this, it might be worth the expense to pay for a background check. In hindsight, I could have created a disastrous situation. In any case, the reality of theft, plus your family member's delusions of stealing, means it is important to maintain a presence in your family member's home.

Dorothy was quite certain that "her girls" were taking things from her house. She also believed that the girls had changed the bathroom tile. It didn't take long for me to discover Dorothy was hiding jewelry, family pictures, and favorite knickknacks in strange places throughout the house. Then, when she couldn't find her necklace or her favorite sweater, she was certain one of the girls was a thief.

The independent caregiver's education and training is another unknown. Those independent caregivers who once worked for an agency often do have the expected skills. Some caregivers come with a wealth of self-learned experiences, and with others, you hope they are people who have common sense and unending patience.

The mother-in-law/daughter-in-law team I mentioned earlier was candid, and told me that while they did not have dementia care experience, they felt they could do the job. The mother-in-law had once worked for an agency that provided care for developmentally disabled people. Her daughter-in-law was a part-time caterer and substitute teacher. They seemed willing to learn and right for the job, and I am glad I took the chance and hired them.

The Job Interview

It's a big step to give a stranger the keys to your parent's home and all that it contains. You hope this stranger is as trustworthy, patient, and kind as they made themselves appear in their interview. You want to believe that the people who offered glowing recommendations were truthful. To overcome some of these worries, I opted for a formal interview conducted at a local coffee shop.

As part of the interview, I asked questions that would help me understand their motivation to spend so many hours with an elderly woman who was often unpleasant, manipulative, and uncooperative. Many cited the satisfaction of having provided care for a member of their family or other clients. Others said their mother or father did not receive appropriate care. By helping others, they felt they were righting a wrong.

Their experience with dementia was another topic of discussion. Some did describe their experiences with other dementia patients; however, most stated such things as remembering their grandmother's behavior or described other work experiences. In the end, I found that dementia experience was not as important as the ability to give reasonable answers to "what would you do if" questions.

The personality characteristics I looked for, irrespective of dementia experience, were a high tolerance for difficult behavior, flexibility, and a desire to learn more about health and health care (see table 9.2).

Our best caregivers were those who had experience caring for people who were both physically and mentally disabled. Those caregivers understood the importance of maintaining a daily schedule. They were also skillful at managing the difficult behaviors that come from a changed brain.

I learned that it was important to stress my expectation for teamwork. I wanted caregivers who were considerate of each other and did not purposely leave all the hard or unpleasant tasks for the next shift. Teamwork also included coordinating work hours with their colleagues and writing daily notes so the next shift would know what had happened earlier. I wanted them to know that I, too, was an active member of Dorothy's caregiving team (see worksheet 7.1 in chapter 7).

The interview was also a time for the candidate to ask questions and to discuss any concerns or special requirements they may have. While pay is certainly a relevant topic, I hoped to hear other kinds of inquiries. I wanted to hire people whose first concern was Dorothy and the kind of help she needed.

Overtime and holiday pay is something you need to discuss during the interview. Many caregivers expect and truly deserve overtime and holiday pay. Be sure to define which holidays are special enough to warrant extra compensation. I had one caregiver who wanted extra pay for nearly every holiday on the calendar.

My usual way of handling major holidays like Thanksgiving and Christmas was to give a full day's pay for a half day's work—thus giving the caregiver time to spend with their family without having to sacrifice their paycheck. Dorothy spent the hours without coverage in our home.

The next step was having the newly hired caregiver sign my homemade Agreement for Services form. My form stated such things as the expected daily responsibilities, specific household and caregiving tasks, and what to do in case of emergencies. The contract also stated my responsibilities, such as prompt payment. I don't know if my Agreement for Services carried the authority of a legal document, but I do feel that having one made for a business-like relationship.

Business Owner and Family Caregiver

I never wanted to be a business owner, and becoming one was definitely one of the "unintendeds" the title of this book describes.

Employing an independent caregiver is more than providing a set of keys and a paycheck. As an employer, there are legal requirements, such as getting an Employer Identification Number (EIN). You need the EIN to file a new-hire report with federal and state agencies. The EIN is the same as the FEIN, or a Federal Employer Identification Number. Many states have additional new-hire requirements.

The EIN identifies businesses; therefore, you, in the role of your family member's power of attorney, are now in the caregiving business! There are important reasons for getting an EIN. First of all, it is a first step in making the expenditure a tax deductible medical expense. This alone makes the hassle of getting the EIN well worth the effort. In addition, the EIN makes it possible for the business to contribute to the caregiver's Social Security and unemployment benefits.

Your new employee must sign a W-4 form, the Employee's Withholding Certificate, so they can pay state and federal income taxes and eventually receive their Social Security payment. Together, the EIN number and W-4 link the caregiver to the pay they receive from the business. Some states require an additional W-4 form.

Often, independent caregivers are immigrants. Foreign nationals must have the legal ability to work in the United States. To prove work eligibility, the caregiver must complete an I-9 form, titled "Employment Eligibility Verification," from the Department of Homeland Security's U.S. Citizenship and Immigration Services.

Unlike the EIN, you keep the completed form on file, along with copies of other required documentation of work eligibility like a Green Card, a U.S.-delivered work permit, or a U.S. ID card.

In the bibliography's listings for this chapter, you will find online resources that will point you to the various federal, state, and foreign work permission forms.

As the employer, it is important to establish and maintain business-like habits. In addition to creating a professional and mutually respectful relationship, keeping detailed records is necessary for tax purposes.

With respect to bookkeeping, I developed a time sheet where caregivers recorded their hours each day and a spreadsheet where I recorded hours worked, gross pay, the various state and federal withholdings, net pay, and a running year-to-date tabulation of each payroll category. I also developed a payroll form so caregivers would have a detailed record of their earnings.

The Federal Insurance Contributions Act (FICA) is the money that goes into the employee's Social Security and Medicare withholdings. Currently, the rate for wage or salaried employees is 12.4 percent, split evenly between the employer and the employee. Medicare, at 1.45 percent, is another evenly shared withholding.

Federal and state withholdings are additional payroll deduction categories. Unlike FICA and Medicare, the federal and state deductions depend on the number of dependents and exemptions the employee claims on their W-2 Wage and Tax Statement form. Employees must receive their W-2 by January 31 of the following year. The W-2 form is the official Wage and Tax Statement that reports an employee's annual wages, no matter how small, and the amount of taxes withheld from their paycheck. The employer must file a copy of the employee's W-2 with the Internal Revenue Service (IRS). Since these rates may change, call your local Internal Revenue Service or State Office of Taxation to get the most up-to-date information.

I know all of this is considerably worse than horrible and so much so that you may be tempted to pay your caregivers in cash. Sometimes caregivers request payment in cash or ask that you do not file their employment information with state and federal employment and taxation offices.

For so many reasons, taking the under-the-table route is not a good idea. As you read earlier, you lose the medical tax deduction. In addition, the caregiver does not accrue Social Security, Medicare, and unemployment benefits. Plus, should the IRS notice, you will be responsible for paying back taxes and penalties.

Try to remember, the tax deduction alone makes the hassle of getting the EIN well worth the effort.

In addition to keeping track of payroll, it is important to develop a payroll schedule. I collected time sheets on Tuesday evening and distributed paychecks on Wednesday afternoon when I delivered groceries.

Why mid-week? Wednesday is double discount day at the grocery store, and combining grocery shopping with the caregiver's payday was an efficient use of my time. Perhaps, collecting time sheets on Thursdays and delivering paychecks on Friday would work better for you. But whatever you decide, pay your family member's caregivers the same day each week, as many caregivers live under very tight economic circumstances.

NOT-FOR-PROFIT ELDERCARE SERVICES

I wish I had known about the variety of not-for-profit eldercare services in my community. Having their help would have reduced some of the difficulty I experienced with managing Dorothy's home, finances, and medical care.

While most not-for-profits do not provide the level of care that people who have dementia require, many do offer other helpful services. Assistance can range from "honey-do" workers who do simple household repairs and yard maintenance to elder day care programs and caregiver respite grants.

While many not-for-profits are faith-based organizations, all assist people of all religions and ethnicities. Sliding-scale payment is another feature many not-for-profits have in common; therefore, your loved one will have to meet criteria, such as a specific monthly income, to receive a reduced rate. Overall, not-for-profits charge less than what you might expect to pay an agency or independent workers. Still, similar to agency caregivers, these workers are insured and bonded. Most not-for-profits depend on community fund-raising events, donations, and grants to make up the difference between the charged fee and what their employees earn.

Perhaps the biggest benefit of finding a local not-for-profit organization is relief from some of the smaller, and never-ending, tasks that take up so much of the family caregiver's time and energy. Looking back, having their help would have made things so much better for me and my family. And maybe Dorothy would have enjoyed having a home companion come to the house to chat or read to her.

Finding a local not-for-profit organization is not as easy as locating a home care agency. Limited budgets mean that you don't often see newspaper or other advertisements. Your friends and neighbors, especially those who have church and synagogue connections or who work or volunteer for social service organizations, are often a good place to start. The internet is another. Using phrases like "not-for-profit caregiver," "caregiver respite," "not-for-profit eldercare," "not-for-profit dementia care," and "not-for-profit senior care" will bring up a variety of organizations and services. These search engine phrases will also uncover not-for-profit community and faith-based dementia residential care facilities. Even though your current focus is getting the help you need to keep your family member at home, it is always good to collect information that may come in handy at a later time.

LAST AND NOT LEAST

Dorothy's hospital evaluations made it obvious she no longer had the daily skills to stay at home without assistance. Friends and neighbors told me I had lots to do to get Dorothy's home in shape for her arrival.

In addition to finding a home care agency, I had to make Dorothy's home safe for both her and the caregivers. Some of these tasks included the installation of properly placed and anchored grab bars and a handheld shower attachment in the bathroom. Other safety items were a shower chair, toilet handrails, and a toilet seat riser. With the exception of the handheld shower attachment, I bought those items at a local hospital supply store. Shower attachments are available at most hardware stores.

Getting her kitchen ready was an interesting window into Dorothy's history—and as it turns out, mine as well. In addition to replacing burned-out pots and pans and beyond-dull knives, I discovered that it had been at least forty years since Dorothy bought any kitchen gadgets. I suspected the can opener that required using a hammer or a hand-powered egg beater would mystify many younger caregivers.

The can opener brought me back to memories of a can of Puss 'n Boots cat food and a couple of Band-Aids. I have to admit it was fun to find my set of ancient copper-colored gelatin dessert molds that I "purchased" with carefully saved Green Stamps.

Although kitchen archeology was fun, it was time to focus my energy on preparing her house and finding caregivers. Another concern was my university teaching responsibilities.

FREQUENTLY ASKED QUESTIONS

1. My father's caregiver has finally received subsidized rent; however, she discovered that the amount she earns as his caregiver makes her ineligible for reduced rent. She asked if I would pay her in cash. This seems a little shady, but I would like to make things easier for her.

Cash payment means your parent loses his medical deduction on his taxes. In addition, the caregiver is no longer entitled to her earned unemployment, workers' compensation, or Social Security benefits. In addition, her government subsidy increases the likelihood that cash payment will get her into trouble—and, as a consequence, you as well.

2. I simply don't have the head for running a business. On the other hand, I cannot afford the cost of an agency caregiver. Suggestions?

If, for any number of reasons, you do not want to use agency caregivers, working with an accountant or a bookkeeper is an affordable alternative to running the business on your own. He or she can take care of the EIN and other forms. Nevertheless, you will need to keep detailed payroll records so the accountant or bookkeeper can file the required monthly state and federal contributions.

10

IT'S DINNERTIME!

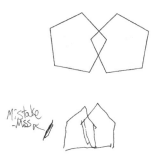

Man, age seventy-four, pentagon.

Dorothy always liked it when I did the grocery shopping and made dinner—and I don't mean during the dementia years. I was ten or eleven years old when I first began to do the grocery shopping and cook the family dinner. To me, Saturday morning at the grocery store was an adventure. With $25 in hand, I purchased our groceries for the week. It never occurred to me that everyone else pushing a shopping cart was much older.

Making dinner for my parents, and a few years later just for my mother and me, was fun. Dorothy's repertoire was pretty much limited to boiled, broiled, and baked. On my own, I figured out how to make spaghetti sauce, chicken soup, and, a few years later, bread—something I continue to do today.

Now, nearly fifty years later, I was again shopping for her groceries. I have to admit that despite my complex day, I liked going to the store for her. It was relaxing. It was a break from the pace of the day. Maybe shopping for her groceries gave me a moment to indulge in pleasant memories.

Grocery shopping did present challenges. At first, when she thought her situation was temporary, Dorothy looked forward to finding surprises in the grocery bags. She liked the interesting crackers and said the hard candies helped her dry throat. Oh, and ice cream, too! But it didn't take long until shopping and independence became one and the same.

Dorothy insisted she didn't need my help. To prove it, she had the caregiver drive her to the grocery store. Exhausted by the trip, Dorothy stayed in the car while the caregiver went inside and bought a chicken. It was a little thing, but it gave Dorothy the ammunition to announce, "I don't want you running around for me, and *she* can leave at the end of the week. I can drive myself to the store."

Dorothy didn't have the stamina to walk from handicapped parking to the store entrance. She didn't have the skills to do something as complex as buying groceries, use a self-service checkout counter, and then make payment. Dorothy no longer remembered how to write a check, and she didn't understand how to use her credit or debit cards. Even if she would allow us to help her, there were so many other reasons why grocery shopping was one of the many things she could no longer do.

It took a while to figure out the best way to sidestep the grocery issue. My solution was to deliver groceries when Dorothy took her afternoon nap or when she had gone to bed for the night. In addition to circumventing a trigger for difficult behavior, these odd delivery times had other advantages. The caregivers could discuss their observations and concerns, and we had a few moments where we could schmooze, laugh, and just get to know each other better.

I don't know if Dorothy ever wondered why she never ran out of milk and eggs. She never said anything. But once in a while, "I want my own chicken" would resurface. And what is wrong with that? It's just a little thing, and it made a big difference to her.

FOOD IS A SENSORY EXPERIENCE

Smell, taste, texture, and appearance are what make food appealing and appetizing. Research shows that our sensitivity to the five taste sensations—sweet, sour, bitter, salty, and umami—diminish as we age. *Merriam-Webster* defines the term *umami*, a taste category unfamiliar to most of us, as a type of savory that imparts a taste sensation we associate with cheese, cooked meat, mushrooms, soy, and ripe tomatoes.

In addition to age-related physical changes (e.g., kidney failure, Parkinson's disease, and dementia), some medications, as well as smoking and chemotherapy, can make marked changes in taste and smell. The combination of diminished and altered ability to taste and smell may cause people who have dementia to lose or gain weight, or consume nonedible substances.

Dementia caused some obvious changes in Dorothy's ability to taste and in the kinds of foods she wanted to eat. Fresh fruit, something she had always enjoyed, became unbearably sour. The strawberries that my husband and I found quite sweet would make her grimace and shiver. Dorothy became un-characteristically interested in snack foods. Suddenly, after a lifetime of criti-cizing anyone who ate junk food, she craved potato chips and candy. Because she ate well at mealtimes, we didn't make a big deal about her salty and sweet snacks. Besides, eating them gave her pleasure.

In addition to changes in taste and food choices, some people who have dementia lose the ability to distinguish fresh from spoiled food or even food from inedible substances like cosmetics and soap. It is important, therefore, to frequently clean the refrigerator and to make sure the person in your care does not eat nonfood items. Eventually, as dementia progresses, you may need to put safety locks on kitchen cabinets or store nonedible substances in a locked cabinet.

In consideration of your loved one's dignity, make part of the kitchen easily and safely accessible. Just the ability to independently make a sandwich or get a snack is one of those little things that can make a big difference in helping your loved one feel independent.

FOOD WARS

Food wars consumed a lot of my energy. Dorothy had her standards. She, with a few exceptions, wouldn't eat prepared or frozen foods. One exception was pizza. As far as she was concerned, pizza always came frozen and in a box.

Her dislike of frozen foods focused mostly on the fresh meat and fish that I or the caregiver divided into small portions and froze for later use. Vegetables and bread did not present the same problem. Those we bought and used be-fore they spoiled. It was quite infuriating that Dorothy demanded that she do her own shopping and, at the same time, expected that I make daily trips to the grocery store. But over the years, I gradually learned to accept that, with respect to logic, Dorothy lived in a different world.

Taking the time to consider Dorothy's difficult behavior in the context of her history made it easier to understand—although not necessarily easier to manage. Frozen foods and home freezers large enough to store more than a single box of green peas weren't widely available until the early 1960s. Before that time, women did shop for food every day. For some women, having a home freezer was the innovation that liberated them from the kitchen. But for women like Dorothy, frozen food was the symbol of the unfit wife and mother. She was proud that, unlike the other mothers, her meals did not come straight out of the freezer. And TV dinners—oh, how I wished for one.

Sad to say, lying was the strategy that kept the frozen food war from escalating. If Dorothy asked, we told her the fish she was eating had never been frozen. We just had to be careful to thaw her daily portion out of view.

The food wars included more than the frozen food battle. If Dorothy didn't like the caregiver, she wouldn't eat anything the caregiver prepared. To quiet the situation, the caregiver quickly learned to tell Dorothy I was the one who made dinner.

Dorothy's short-term memory loss was another contributing factor. The time it took to make a sandwich was too long for her to remember that she had asked for mustard and not mayonnaise. To prevent an argument, the caregiver learned to put a spoonful of each condiment on Dorothy's lunch plate. That way, Dorothy got to choose and spread whatever she wanted on her sandwich; having the choice made her feel in control.

Forgetting that she had already eaten was another difficulty. Sometimes reminding Dorothy that she ate breakfast less than an hour ago was sufficient. But when a reminder didn't work, it was better to give her an early morning breakfast-like snack than argue.

NUTRITION

You may wonder why your loved one's nutrition is such an important topic. After all, people who have dementia are usually elderly *and* suffer from a terminal illness. One would think this is the perfect time to eat a pint of ice cream. To a limited extent this is true. Nonetheless, good nutrition still plays an important role in maintaining overall health, independence, and well-being.

Everyone, regardless of age, needs to eat foods from the five basic food groups each day. The five basic food groups are carbohydrates (bread, pasta, and grains), vegetables and fruits, dairy products, meat and meat alternatives (fish, eggs, beans, tofu, and nuts) and fats.

Older people, because of inactivity and a slower metabolism, need fewer calories per day than younger people; however, changes in the ability to absorb or use the nutrients means that older people have higher requirements than younger people for iron, calcium, vitamin D, and the B vitamins, as well as for several other nutrients. The combination of fewer calories consumed and higher nutrient requirements can make healthful eating a challenge.

The Alzheimer's Disease Education and Referral (ADEAR) Center is an excellent resource where you can find many helpful hints regarding healthy eating and related topics. Some hints include the following:

Buy healthy foods that include vegetables, fruits, and whole grain products.
Be sure to buy foods the person likes and can eat.
Give choices—although not so many as to create confusion.
Provide nutritious snacks, such as fresh fruit, raw vegetables, and cheese.

EATING IS MORE THAN FOOD

Your family member, especially an elderly parent, may have been living alone for a long time, and they may have developed eating habits that reflect a solitary life. Instead of cooking a meal, they eat packaged meals or perhaps just have cheese and crackers for dinner. Eating in the company of a family member or a caregiver may be a welcomed change.

When you or the caregiver joins your family member during mealtimes, use this occasion to engage in pleasant conversation rather than commenting on what they are or are not eating. While background music can create a pleasant ambience, television is an unwanted distraction.

Many older people, and especially those who have dementia, are overwhelmed by large amounts of food. It's too much food for a small appetite, and if they have trouble chewing, swallowing, or using a fork and knife, it's too much work.

Using a smaller plate, rather than a dinner plate, can make meals more appealing and approachable. Colorful dinnerware and a cheerful tablecloth or placemat are other little things that help make eating enjoyable and mealtimes pleasant. Buying holiday dishes off-season or discontinued dishes and tableware is an inexpensive way to set a welcoming table.

Changes can be difficult for a person who has Alzheimer's disease or other kinds of dementia; therefore, in addition to creating an uncluttered and pleasant environment, it is also important to maintain accustomed routines and serve familiar and favorite foods. Be sure to inform a home health aide, or other person responsible for making meals, of your family member's preferences. Doing so will make things easier for everyone.

I REMEMBER WHEN!

We all have had the experience when the aroma, taste, or crunch of a certain food transports us back in time. Maybe the aroma of homemade tomato sauce reminds you of your grandmother. Or perhaps biting into "ants on a log" (a celery stick filled with peanut butter and topped with a couple raisins) reminds you of your mother and after-school snacks.

My fondest food memory is making potato latkes with my father. And much to my amazement, this one sentence transports me back to a small mid-century modern kitchen table and wonderfully intimate moments with my father.

If you are at a loss as to how to discover memory foods, ask family members or similarly aged friends what they enjoyed eating during their childhood.

But do be prepared to listen to stories about how they once lived and played together. Talking about food is an amazing way to learn about your family genealogy as well as everyday history. When possible, include younger family members in this adventure.

Just for fun, check out the nostalgia websites! There you will find links to the most memorable recipes of the decade, jingles to remind listeners to buy processed cheese and irresistible potato chips, and recordings of all sorts of radio and television shows. I guarantee the whole family will enjoy many laughful moments (see Helpful Resources).

Old cookbooks and internet searches are wonderful resources. According to *Betty Crocker's Cooky Book*, French lace cookies were the best cookie of the mid-1960s. Along with the recipe, Betty Crocker notes two historical highlights: the launch of the Echo I communications satellite (1960) and, in 1962, Colonel John Glenn's orbit of the earth in a rocket-boosted spaceship.

I still have my copy of *Betty Crocker's Cooky Book*. I bought it with my own money in 1963.

The bottom line is that food and cooking gives you, and your entire family, the opportunity to indulge in a little fun.

On the other hand, the smell, taste, or appearance of certain foods may transport people back to horrific events they endured many years ago. Food can trigger terrifying flashbacks to a childhood in World War II concentration camps or years of confinement in a Vietnam-era prisoner-of-war internment encampment.

BE A LITTLE EASY ON YOURSELF

It's perfectly okay to take some shortcuts. While it's all good and wonderful to use mealtime as an occasional side trip into family history, you do need to give yourself a little "me time." Do consider taking advantage of various grocery store and restaurant home delivery options. Boxed dinner subscriptions, containing all the ingredients you (or another caregiver) need to prepare dinner, are another possibility. And finally, purchasing a share in a CSA (community-supported agriculture) is an easy way to buy seasonal and locally grown fresh produce. Many CSAs make home deliveries.

Online shopping can be a more cost-effective way to buy groceries and assorted dry goods. Many grocery chains and big-box stores will do the shopping for you. All you have to do is go to their website, create a grocery list, and, at an arranged time, go to the drive-up window. Some stores make home deliveries.

Gee—I sure wish some of those services were available when I was my mother's primary caregiver. I did, however, take advantage of the Meals on Wheels program.

IN-PERSON SHOPPING

Keeping a home stocked with sufficient groceries, paper goods, and cleaning supplies takes a little planning. Make a list and, as much as possible, try to avoid making extra trips to the store. To save time, buy groceries and household supplies for your loved one at the same time you buy your own.

Find a grocery store where you can purchase perishables in amounts a single person can consume in a week and have a selection of healthy and, not so healthy, snacks.

A big-box store is often the best place to stock up on economy-sized household supplies, such as detergent, soap, napkins, toilet paper, absorbency products, and paper towels. You will find that dementia care entails using surprisingly large amounts of cleaning supplies.

MEALS ON WHEELS

Meals on Wheels is a nationwide program whose mission is to "drive away senior hunger in America." Some programs serve meals at senior centers, others deliver meals to homebound people, and some programs do both. The cost is income based and even full price is quite reasonable.

Meals on Wheels volunteers do more than just deliver a hot meal to a homebound person. Recognizing that loneliness is another kind of hunger, volunteers take the time to socialize. In addition to bringing a few moments of companionship, volunteers can alert appropriate medical services and community organizations if their client appears unwell or needs assistance.

A few moments of midday conversation with a friendly volunteer can be a welcomed source of caregiver respite, too. And, if food wars are one of your challenges, Meals on Wheels puts a big distance between the caregiver and the food on the table.

STAGES OF DEMENTIA AND EATING

You may notice changes in your family member's relationship with food as they progress from early- to late-stage dementia. During the first stage, your loved one may limit herself to a few easy-to-prepare foods, such as cereal, canned soup, toast, and tea. They may forget to eat or forget they have already eaten. Consuming spoiled food and eating from dirty dishes are other common problems. Forgetfulness may cause your family member to either undercook or burn food. When asked, they may not give realistic information about the food they ate over the course of a day.

Forgetting to eat and difficulty in using a fork and knife are common problems associated with mid-stage dementia. Hoarding and hiding food and eating nonfood items are other behaviors associated with mid-stage dementia. People in mid-stage dementia cannot reliably report what they have eaten.

During the last stage of dementia, your loved one may neither recognize food nor know what to do with it. During this last phase, your loved one may lose the ability to chew and swallow food. Your loved one may refuse to wear their dentures. When this happens, you or the caregiver will need to learn feeding techniques so your loved one can receive safe mealtime assistance.

PREPARING MEALS

Cooking for a person who has dementia is different than preparing family meals. In addition to catering to old habits and fluctuating likes and dislikes, one also needs to take into consideration the ability to chew, swallow, and use a knife and fork. Many people who have dementia prefer small portions of easily identified and familiar foods.

Breakfast was easy. Dorothy was happy with the tea, orange juice, and toast or English muffin that she had eaten every morning for most of her adult life. Sometimes, Dorothy's caregiver would surprise her and make scrambled eggs or give her a single pancake and freeze the rest for another time.

Lunch presented small challenges. In addition to the mustard or mayonnaise problem mentioned earlier, Dorothy was stuck in the "single slice of bread with one slice of reduced-fat mozzarella cheese" habit. Sometimes, Dorothy accepted the caregiver's suggestion and had a small piece of pizza or a bowl of soup for lunch.

Dinner was the problem meal. Defining the caregiver's job was one of the difficulties. The contract I signed with the home care agency clearly stated their employees assemble meals from prepared foods. In other words, agency caregivers were happy to open boxes, bags, and cans, and they were quite adept at using the microwave. Oh—I forgot to mention that as far as Dorothy was concerned, the microwave was just as evil as the freezer.

In the beginning, I did not realize how strongly Dorothy would react to people whose sense of food was different than hers. Was Dorothy's behavior an attempt to take control of her situation? Unquestionably, yes! But nonetheless, I couldn't ignore it. She was using their inability to cook, contractual and real, as an excuse to be verbally abusive to me and to them. Basically, Dorothy was in "survival mode" and would do whatever it took to get these strangers out of her house.

Although Dorothy's attempts to control the situation were obvious, she did not suffer caregiver cooking every night. Once a week, Dorothy had dinner with my husband and me. In the beginning, we brought her to our home. But as she became weaker, and less able to get around, we brought dinner to her. I always made extra food, so at the most she had caregiver dinners three or four times a week.

Cooking for Dorothy required that I transport hot meals to her house. Eventually, after several messy mishaps with plastic- and foil-covered dishes, I discovered rectangular Pyrex containers—the ones sold with tight-fitting plastic lids. These containers keep cooked foods hot, microwave well (remember to loosen the lid), and stack well, and best of all, they don't leak.

Collapsible silicone food containers are a relatively new product. They don't leak, are microwave safe, and collapse into a space-saving shape.

Eventually, I replaced agency caregivers with ones I hired. Among other benefits, I hoped this change might reduce food war tensions. The first independent caregiver was quite willing to cook meals. Unfortunately, it didn't occur to me to probe further. I assumed cooking meals meant cutting, mixing, boiling, and baking with fresh ingredients.

The first independent caregiver assumed cooking meals meant opening a box or can, microwaving, and for a treat, fast food carry out. She really didn't know anything different, and that was how her family ate. After several months of trying to work with her, we parted ways over her inability to make a baked potato. The next caregivers, the ones who stayed with us to the end, were both willing and able to cook in the old-fashioned meaning of the word.

FINGER FOODS

Finger foods are the next step when poor coordination makes it difficult for your family member to use a fork and knife. Although taking this step may seem a little sad, finger foods are one of those little things that help maintain your family member's sense of independence and dignity. They can pick the items they want to eat and be in control of the amount of time it takes to eat their meals. Finger foods allow your loved one to eat without assistance.

It takes a little imagination to prepare well-balanced meals that don't require using a knife and fork. As before, your parent will enjoy an array of colorful and familiar foods.

Make a mini buffet containing an assortment of sliced fruits, vegetables, cheese, quartered hard boiled eggs, and small sandwiches. Sandwich fillings like sliced meats, tuna salad, egg salad, hummus, or peanut butter are easy to prepare. For variety, use breads made from different grains and mini-sandwiches made using tortillas and rolls.

For hot meals, your loved one may enjoy eating baked potatoes or sweet potato slices, small pieces of deboned fish or chicken, and an assortment of cooked or raw vegetables. Pizza, quiche, and vegetable tarts, all cut in small portions, are other finger food options. You can find these in the frozen food section of your grocery store.

If you run out of ideas, look at the cooking magazines and internet sites that specialize in appetizers and other party food recipes; however, you may need to adjust the recipe to accommodate any dietary requirements your family member may have. Appetizers tend to be high in fat and salt, and they often are very spicy. Because some people who have dementia cannot tell the difference between edible and inedible things, avoid appetizers held together with toothpicks.

If your family member can still use a spoon, consider serving chunky or thick soups, puddings, or baked custard. In addition to offering a variety of tastes and textures, soup, pudding, and baked custard are nostalgia foods. Your mother may remember making split pea soup for her family, and your father may reminisce about the baked custard his mother once made for him.

PUREED FOODS

Pureed foods are the next step when your loved one can no longer chew food, move it to the back of the mouth, and swallow. Rather than using jarred baby food, you can puree adult foods using a food mill, an electric blender, or food processor. Add enough liquid to give the food the consistency of yogurt. Placing a small spoonful of food toward the back of the mouth can make it easier to swallow. If you are having difficulty finding the right spot, ask to speak with a palliative care nurse.

FREQUENTLY ASKED QUESTIONS

1. Are there dietary supplements or foods that can slow the progression of Alzheimer's disease?

The combination of eating nutrient-rich foods and a healthy lifestyle may reduce risk for developing dementia; however, there is no conclusive evidence showing that taking certain nutrient supplements or eating specific foods can reduce the risk of developing dementia, improve cognitive function, or slow the progression of the disease.

2. Are there dietary supplements or foods that people who have dementia should avoid?

Taking certain dietary supplements and eating certain foods can alter how well the body absorbs medications. For example, if the person in your care takes an antiseizure medication as an off-label mood stabilizer, eating grapefruit may lower the amount of medication circulating in blood and put them at risk for having a seizure. It is important, then, to ask their doctor about known interactions between specific dietary supplements, foods, and any medications that may be prescribed to manage dementia symptoms.

3. Am I required to provide meals for my family member's caregiver?

As is true for many things—it depends. If you are working with an agency, they will stipulate the requirement in the contract; however, when hiring independent caregivers, the issue of providing meals is something you can discuss with them. Many will prefer to bring their own food. As a matter of courtesy, it is a nice gesture to provide beverages and snacks.

4. Although preparing or talking about memory foods is a lovely idea, it seems like just one more thing I have to do. I don't have the time—and besides, I make efforts to spend as little time as possible in the kitchen. Suggestions?

Preparing and talking about memory foods is just one way to stimulate pleasant and interesting conversation. Other topics can include talking about childhood games, seeing a television for the first time, favorite movies or radio shows, or memorable teachers. For an eye-opener, ask your baby boomer family member about air raid drills and "duck and cover." Watching online videos can make conversation even livelier.

WORKSHEET 10.1:
Reflective Writing

Talking about food can help your family member connect with their past. Listening to their stories is a wonderful opportunity for you and other family members to learn about your personal history.

Their stories can help you understand some of your family member's behavioral quirks. For example, discovering that cooking in the 1950s was all about experimenting with frozen foods, cake mixes, and other convenience foods helped put Dorothy's difficult behavior in the context of her history of refusing to go along with what is popular.

As suggested in earlier chapters, reflective writing is a good way to sort out the day, learn from past mistakes, and consider better ways of approaching caregiving challenges. Use the following ideas to start your reflective writing adventure. Who knows, your responses might eventually lead to writing your family's history.

List or describe your family member's behaviors that may come from their experiences as a younger person.

List things you can do to encourage your loved one to talk about how their family coped with such things as World War II, the polio epidemic, or having spent their childhood living away from their parents.

What does your family member say or do when they eat foods they may have enjoyed fifty or more years ago? And once you get your loved one talking, what did you learn, and how does that information change your feelings and approach to their behavior?

WORKSHEET 10.2:
A Family Project

Write a mini-cookbook that contains family recipes and memories. If you want to get fancy, find an online company that can assemble your family recipes into a bound book. The cookbook will be a lasting memento that your whole family will enjoy. To get you started, here is Dorothy's gingerbread recipe.

Dorothy's Maryland Gingerbread

I remember watching Dorothy make Maryland gingerbread when we lived in Chevy Chase, Maryland. Because the kitchen was very small, my mother did all of the measuring and mixing on the kitchen table. I don't remember having any counter space. I thought adding hot water to the cake batter was strange, but I later discovered that many gingerbread recipes include this step. By the way, substituting the black coffee for the hot water is a nice addition, as coffee and molasses are a particularly flavorful combination.

Ingredients

2	eggs
¾	cup melted shortening or vegetable oil
2¼	cups flour
¾	cup brown sugar
2½	teaspoons baking powder
¾	teaspoon baking soda
2	teaspoons ginger
1½	teaspoons cinnamon
1	teaspoon cloves
½	teaspoon nutmeg
¾	cup molasses
1	cup boiling water (or black coffee)

Method

1. Add beaten eggs to sugar, molasses, and melted shortening (vegetable oil).
2. Add sifted flour and other dry ingredients to the egg mixture.
3. Carefully mix in the hot water or coffee.
4. Pour into an oiled and floured 9 × 9 pan or a prepared cupcake tin.
5. Bake at 350 degrees for about 40 minutes, less time if cupcakes.
6. The gingerbread is done when it pulls away from the sides of the pan.

11

FINDING THE
RIGHT CARE FACILITY

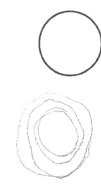

Woman, age seventy-nine, circle.

I started to research residential care options long before it became necessary to move Dorothy from her home. My community offered several choices that ranged from private homes to continuum of care facilities.

A phone call to the facility director often resulted in an invitation to visit. Some I declined because of the cost or location. And in one case, even though they gave me a blueberry pie to take home, the complicated floor plan told me it was the wrong place. The pie wasn't any good either.

The visits were eye-openers. Some seemed more like warehouses than places that offered compassionate care for people whose health will never improve. Others, while they looked clean and orderly, smelled like urine. And the memory care units were filled with ghosts and expressionless faces but no meaningful activity.

Caring for Dorothy was a challenge, but seeing these other elderly people told me the time wasn't right. Without question she had dementia and required assistance, but compared to the ghosts, Dorothy was doing pretty well.

Visiting facilities and meeting their residents helped me understand dementia as a progressive and terminal disease. Basically, dementia care comes down to creating an illusion of independence, maintaining quality of life and dignity, and doing what you can to avoid problems. The caregivers and I could certainly provide that level of care for a while longer. After a lengthy discussion with my immediate family, we committed ourselves to helping Dorothy stay home until it was no longer safe for her or for us.

Within a year, we could see obvious changes. Dorothy's vocabulary became limited. Rather than using nouns and adjectives, she relied on words like "it" and "they" to express ideas and needs. The short walk from her bedroom to the kitchen left her breathless. Dorothy rarely left the house, and conversation repeated on what seemed like a ten-second cycle. Her short-term memory was pretty much on the same schedule. The situation was still manageable, but I knew that rather than having the luxury of time, I might have to "turn on a dime" to find more appropriate care.

More phone calls and more visits. Eventually, I found a dementia care facility that was different from the others. First of all, they used the phrase "memory care unit" and not the "lock down wing." And rather than a multistory building with decorative bars on the windows, this place looked more like a ranch-style home with a walled garden and walking paths. I saw the groundskeeper helping a resident plant spring flowers. The fragrance of freshly baked muffins welcomed me at the entrance. I have to admit, that alone sold me on the place.

Yes, the ghosts lived there, too. Yet you could sometimes see inklings of former lives. The music professor, although he no longer talked, did play the piano. Residents, with supervision, could go to the kitchen and make a sandwich or cookies. It seemed this memory care unit was as good as it was going to get.

I had a long conversation with the director. I explained our situation and told her "not yet, but probably within the year." She was honest and said they could not guarantee a space, but they would help us as best they could. There was no pressure, and there were no requests to sign a contract or make a deposit. She did ask if she could call once in a while to hear how we were doing.

The feeling of relief was immediate. I had a path to follow and the help I needed to guide me through the next steps.

ANTICIPATE AND PLAN AHEAD

Most family caregivers will see themselves in one or more of the following scenarios. On the whole, things are going well. Your family member is receiving the care they need, and you are managing well enough. Moving your loved one from the comfort of their home or yours just doesn't seem like anything you need to consider at this time.

It may also be true that things aren't going as well as you might hope. Your loved one is difficult to manage, you are getting behind at work, and your family is concerned about your health. Still, you made a promise you intend to keep.

Your loved one's declining health is becoming obvious. Behavior is more difficult to manage, and safety—yours and theirs—is of increasing concern. You wonder, how much longer? You aren't sure what event will make an assisted facility necessary—but you figure you will know when the time is right.

As with all progressive illnesses, time reveals worsening signs and symptoms. After months of smooth sailing, health and behavior issues may suddenly make home care impossible. For these and other reasons, you have reached the invisible line where you know you cannot do more.

People enter residential care facilities for a variety of reasons. It's very unusual, but on occasion, one finds an early-stage resident living in a dementia care facility. Some of these residents, committed to making things as easy as possible for their family, made the decision to move. Others, because they do not have family, understand the importance of planning ahead.

For the most part, the people who live in residential care facilities have mid- to late-stage Alzheimer's disease. And nearly all do not enter voluntarily. Unmanageable behavior and incontinence are the two last-straw reasons that cause many family caregivers to move their loved one into a residential care. Use worksheet 11.1 to help organize your thoughts about this very big decision.

Even if you never intend to move your loved one from their home, it's important to survey facilities close to where you live. You might have reason to change your mind, or you may want to take advantage of the short-term respite care some facilities offer.

When declining health and safety issues let you know the time is right, making the decision about "where" is much easier if you have already done the research. Rather than a mad scramble, one or two phone calls are all you have to do. And because you have already seen the good, bad, and horrible, you can feel comfortable the choice you made is the right one.

Placing a loved one into a care facility doesn't just happen. To begin with, you have to overcome two difficulties: First, more than likely, your loved one does not want to move, and second, they are not competent enough to make this decision for themselves. Like everything else, discuss this next step with other family members. Their understanding and support are important elements in making the move as easy as possible.

It is also necessary to get an approval for placement from your loved one's doctor. The doctor's consent, far from busywork, is a step that protects older people from unscrupulous relatives. Some states require a second, independent evaluation from another doctor.

Paying for care is another aspect of planning ahead. If you are very fortunate, there is sufficient money so that all you have to do is use a credit card to cover the deposit and the monthly fees. Long-term care insurance is another way some people finance their residential care; however, for many families, finding a way to pay their loved one's assisted living fees takes time, resourcefulness, and patience.

Discussing money is always a difficult subject. You feel uncomfortable about prying into your family member's financial life. You are concerned they, or other family members, may believe you are greedy and thinking only of yourself. Despite these natural concerns, it's never too soon to learn about your loved one's finances. To help make these first discussions with your loved one go as smoothly as possible, consider a group meeting with an eldercare lawyer, a financial advisor, or a geriatric care manager present.

Your local Alzheimer's Association office can help you navigate the financial aspects of dementia care (see Helpful Resources).

HOW TO PAY FOR CARE

There are many options to consider when there are insufficient funds. Some involve converting assets like real estate, stocks, and bonds into cash; however, consult a lawyer to make sure you have the legal authority to sell your family member's property. Others include the following:

Converting a life insurance policy into a long-term care policy
Securing a reverse mortgage, where house equity becomes income
Renting your family member's home
Spending down to Medicaid eligibility

Be sure to do some careful research to make sure these options meet your needs and are truly as good as they appear.

Often, families must make monetary contributions when there are insufficient assets. For many adult children, a difficult economy plus the expenses of college tuition and a mortgage can make contributing to their parent's care difficult or impossible. Family harmony often suffers when some siblings cannot meet the financial expectations of their better-off brothers and sisters.

When differences in income become an issue, it is important to find other ways family members can contribute. Examples include overseeing the sale of your loved one's home or making sure they have sufficient clothing and toiletries.

There are occasions when the caregiving spouse does not have access to their husband's or wife's bank accounts, investments, annuities, or property. It is of utmost importance to make their financial relationship equitable before there is need to do so—especially before competence becomes an issue.

The process in making these modifications differs from state to state. Speaking with a lawyer, accountant, bank manager, or financial advisor can help you navigate the relatively easy steps to creating financial fairness.

Medicare may pay all costs associated with facility care if, in addition to dementia, your family member has another medical problem, such as a broken hip or severe depression. Another Medicare requirement is that nursing home care must follow within thirty days of a three-day-or-more hospitalization. This Medicare benefit applies to rehabilitation hospitals, transitional care hospitals, nursing homes, and continuum of care facilities.

As you may recall, Dorothy did spend a few weeks in the nursing home section of a continuum of care facility. Her hospitalization for back pain followed by weeks spent in the rehabilitation hospital met the "within thirty days of a three-day-or-more hospitalization" requirement. Surprisingly, it was a bladder infection, and not her original reason for hospitalization, that made her Medicare eligible. Medicare did not pay for her residential care once the bladder infection cleared up.

Medicaid, a federal program administered at the state level, may cover all or some of the cost of nursing home care. Eligibility requirements vary from state to state, but in general, Medicaid helps very low income people who have few assets. Under certain circumstances, the Program of All-Inclusive Care for the Elderly (PACE) described in chapter 7 may pay for residential care; however, most assisted living facilities cannot or will not accept Medicaid or PACE patients. Affordability makes finding good-quality residential care particularly challenging (see Helpful Resources).

A final option for long-term residential care is the U.S. Department of Veterans Affairs (VA). Although combat duty is not a requirement, your veteran family member must be registered in the VA medical care system to receive VA assistance (see Helpful Resources).

TYPES OF CARE FACILITIES

Residential care is a place where patients receive twenty-four-hour care in a location other than their or another family member's home. That person may receive residential care in an assisted living facility, a nursing home, or in a continuum of care facility. Assisted living facilities may include private

Table 11.1. Types of Care Facilities

Type of Care Facility	Description
Assisted living facility	An assisted living facility is one where residents receive "assistance" with their daily living skills. Assisted living facility employees do not have the licensure to give injections, administer pain control medications, or perform medical procedures. Many facilities have on-call nurses and physicians.
Continuum of care facility	A continuum of care facility covers the entire spectrum of need—from independent living to memory care.
Nursing home	A nursing home is for people who don't require hospitalization but can't be cared for at home. Nursing homes have registered nurses onsite twenty-four hours a day and on-call physicians.
Rehabilitation hospital	A rehabilitation hospital is one that gives physical and occupational therapy treatments, as well as speech therapy to help patients regain function.
Transitional care hospital	A transitional care hospital is one for patients, otherwise stable, who will have long recoveries. Examples include wound care, stroke and brain injuries, and pulmonary support.

(and certified) homes that serve one or several residents as well as large locally owned and franchised businesses. These last two options may range from relatively small facilities to community-like buildings that may house several hundred residents (see table 11.1).

Unlike assisted living facilities, nursing homes provide skilled nursing care. Nursing homes have staff trained and licensed to start and manage intravenous lines, give injections, provide wound care, and administer dialysis or respiratory therapy.

Continuum of care facilities are a relatively new option in the caregiving business. These facilities provide a range of residences that range from independent housing, assisted living, and nursing home care. Often relatively healthy individuals or couples opt to move from their homes into independent living quarters.

These independent living apartments look just like any other apartment. Many independent living residents have cars, participate in activities elsewhere, and travel. Residents can elect to have some of their meals in a communal dining area, and should they become ill, medical care is available on the premises.

Independent living is a good choice for single people who do not have other family living nearby or when a healthy spouse is the caregiver for the less healthy one. When health and other needs dictate, residents move from independent living apartments to assisted living quarters.

LEARNING ABOUT ASSISTED LIVING FACILITIES

I was surprised to find that states, and not the federal government, regulate assisted living facilities. That means each state has different rules that determine every aspect of assisted living licensure—from meals and activities provided to staffing requirements and fire safety. The National Center for Assisted Living publishes an Assisted Living Regulatory review.

The term *assistance* describes the kinds of services assisted living facilities provide. The people who live there may require help taking medication, preparing food, and feeding or dressing themselves. Residents receive assistance when balance and physical strength difficulties affect walking and the ability to safely get in or out of bed. In other words, people living in an assisted living facility receive assistance with the daily living skills they can no longer reliably or safely perform.

Assisted living is how many people who have dementia first enter into residential care. Transition into a dementia care unit within the assisted living facility occurs when dementia progresses and the resident needs continuous supervision.

It's important to know that assisted living facilities do not take patients who already require skilled nursing care; therefore, if your family member requires dialysis, specialized wound care, or respiratory therapy, a nursing home or the special care unit of a continuum of care facility is a more appropriate option.

The assisted living facility I chose for Dorothy only accepted residents who have dementia but are otherwise fairly healthy. They called themselves a "memory care facility" to distinguish themselves from those assisted living facilities that take residents who need assistance for other reasons. A *special care unit* is another term used to describe facilities that provide care for people who have Alzheimer's disease and other types of dementia.

Memory care facilities have a higher staff-to-resident ratio, and the people who work in memory care facilities receive more training than those who work in other kinds of assisted living facilities. Activities and meals are tailored to meet the needs of residents who have dementia. To prevent residents from leaving the premises on their own, memory care facilities are lock-down units. You may hear the phrase "to prevent elopement." It's just a friendlier way to say "locked-down facility."

Some assisted living facilities state they embrace a philosophy of person-centered or personalized assisted living. In a person-centered facility, care providers know the names and the backgrounds of each resident. Person-centered caregivers understand that people who have dementia are individuals who have unique interests and desires.

A range of health care providers work in assisted living facilities. Certified nursing assistants (CNAs) and people trained by the assisted living facility provide most of the day-to-day care. Similar to what you would look for in the individuals you may have hired as home caregivers, attributes like patience and a warm and nonjudgmental personality, rather than advanced degrees, are some of the most important qualifications for staff.

Assisted living facilities, although they do not provide skilled nursing care, do recognize that residents must have access to medical care. Some assisted living facilities have a medical director. Most often the medical director is a registered nurse (RN). The nurse may be on the premises for only a few scheduled hours per week; however, the medical director should be available for phone consultations and to make "house calls." Some assisted living facilities arrange for a local medical group to care for their residents. A podiatrist is another medical professional who may make regularly scheduled visits. Foot and nail care is especially important for residents who have diabetes.

Many assisted living facilities employ licensed practical nurses (LPNs) who, with the supervision of an RN, dispense medications from the medicine closet and perform other simple medically related services. In some states, LPNs do not have the training and licensure to do such things as give insulin shots. Some assisted living facilities provide the training required to allow other staff to hand already measured amounts of medication to residents.

Assisted living facilities may have a staff psychologist, medical social worker, or an art therapist to help residents and their families cope with the ongoing challenges of dementia. Another important staff member is the recreation director. He or she provides meaningful activities that emphasize resident participation and pleasure rather than a specific outcome, such as making a holiday card or completing a puzzle. Housekeeping and grounds personnel maintain the building and the garden areas.

Many assisted living facilities have either a small hair salon or arrange for a hairdresser to cut, wash, and style hair. Physical and occupational therapy, to help maintain resident independence, is another service available at some assisted living facilities.

Many states require assisted living facilities employees complete a certain number of continuing education (CME) credits each year. Staff members, through classes, reading materials, online resources, and conferences learn about dementia, aging, and new approaches to successful dementia care.

ACCESS TO MEDICAL CARE

Facility residents can receive medical care from an independent medical practitioner who makes assisted living facility "house calls" or from their family doctor. In either case, the doctor will bill the resident and Medicare for payment. Should your family member choose to stay with their primary care physician, you are responsible for scheduling appointments and arranging transportation. Scheduling dental and eye care appointments are also your responsibility.

The availability of in-house medical care was an important factor in choosing the assisted living facility that would best meet Dorothy's needs. The care Dorothy received from her family doctor, although excellent, was an ongoing source of stress. Getting her dressed and ready for a scheduled appointment was difficult. Dorothy, a dedicated back seat driver, made the trip to his office an exhausting experience. And, as described in an earlier chapter, her behavior before, during, and after the appointment made the rest of the day difficult for me and her caregivers. Unscheduled medical problems often meant a long wait in the emergency room. Having "in-house" care, we hoped, would make things easier for everyone, as well as eliminate trips to the emergency room.

Dorothy responded very well to her new doctor. In part, the "new face" factor may have made it easier for the new doctor to interact with her. And without question, his old-world European charm made Dorothy as cooperative as possible; however, another reason for improved cooperation was that Dorothy believed the doctor was her ticket out of there.

Relocating her medical care to the assisted living facility, although needed, was not an easy decision for me. I respected her family doctor and wasn't sure I had the energy to go through the process of working with a new one. Much to my relief, an introductory consultation with the physician assigned to her quickly revealed his passion for eldercare. Geriatrics and dementia care were his chosen specialty.

CHOOSING AN ASSISTED LIVING FACILITY

Finding the assisted living facility that is affordable, meets your loved one's needs, and provides an acceptable standard of care is far from an exact science. You can get recommendations from friends, review state or county inspection reports, make scheduled and impromptu site visits, and—as always—ask lots of questions. But in the end, your gut feelings are often your most valuable guide.

Talking to friends is a good place to start. Your friends can tell you why they chose to use, or not use, a particular facility. They can also tell you if their initial impressions matched the service their family member received. While too many opinions can hinder the decision-making process, having input from two, maybe three, other people can be helpful.

INSPECTIONS AND INSPECTION REPORTS

It can be surprisingly difficult to find unbiased assisted living facility online reviews. Accessibility to impartial information would make it considerably easier to choose the assisted living facilities that seem worth visiting.

In some states, one can find information on the Department of Health website. In other states, information is available on county or city Department of Health websites. A good starting point in your internet search is to use keywords like "assisted living facility," "evaluations," "inspections," and "reports," along with the city, county, or state location where your family member will live.

Blogs and other types of interactive media are sources of helpful information. But just like restaurant or product reviews, people who post opinions tend to be those who are angry or disappointed; however, reading several posts that describe similar deficiencies may be good cause for caution.

A phone call to the state, county, or city Department of Health is another option. Simply ask the health department operator to connect you to the office responsible for assisted living inspections. The inspection office can give you information about specific assisted living facilities and point you to online information sources.

The kinds of information available vary. In general, most reports include a description of the facility, the date of the most recent inspection, the number of residents, the staff-to-resident ratio, and information concerning the types of payment accepted. Building safety, kitchen cleanliness, food quality, pre-employment background checks, staff training, and drug dispensing procedures are some of the other things that inspectors evaluate. Inspectors also look for signs of resident abuse.

Electrical problems, fire hazards, improper food storage, insect and rodent infestations, inadequate pre-employment background checks, and insufficient employee training are frequently reported problems. Inspection reports can make all facilities seem like bad news. Sometimes, by combining information from earlier and recent reports, you can get a broader sense of how well a facility conforms to local regulations. Based on what you have read, does it appear that the facility corrects deficiencies and that recent inspection reports show improvement over earlier ones? Are there reports of abuse? Are there records of fines or legal action brought against the facility? Reviewing inspection reports with an eye toward finding evidence of good business and caregiving practices can help weed out those assisted living facilities that aren't worth visiting.

Group, or congregate, homes must conform to local inspection standards. Located in neighborhoods, group homes must follow local zoning laws and neighborhood covenants.

COMMUNICABLE ILLNESSES IN RESIDENTIAL CARE FACILITIES

As I am writing, people living in the United States and elsewhere are living under mandated social-distancing, shelter-at-home, and quarantine rulings. The reason for this immense change in our everyday life is COVID-19, or Coronavirus Infectious Disease 2019. The fact that this virus is a new and naturally occurring microbe means our immune system cannot protect us from this virus.

Younger people, and people in otherwise good health, are less likely to die of COVID-19; however, this is not the case for elderly people and especially those who have other underlying conditions (e.g., diabetes) or are immunocompromised. People living in assisted living, nursing home, and other kinds of long-term care facilities are particularly vulnerable to COVID-19.

The Centers for Disease Control and Prevention (CDC) recently published safety guidelines for health care providers, residents, and visitors; it's important to be aware that safety guidelines change in response to the most recent research findings. Currently, the CDC recommends hand washing, in combination with social distancing and wearing a mask, as the best way to reduce infection rates.

There are many reasons why it is important that residents receive vaccinations prior to moving into a communal living situation. Perhaps the most important one is the difference between living at home versus living in close proximity to other residents, visitors, and facility employees.

At the time of this writing, assisted living facilities do not require that residents and employees receive vaccination for vaccine-preventable diseases, for example, influenza, shingles, and hepatitis. Be sure to discuss this aspect of your loved one's transition to communal living with their doctor or other health professional. In table 11.2, you will see a list of the recommended vaccinations.

Table 11.2.   Suggested Vaccinations for Vaccine-Preventable Diseases

Name of Vaccine	Purpose
Shingles	Prevents shingles, a viral infection that causes a painful rash. This infection puts elderly people at higher risk for ongoing pain and hearing and vison loss. The virus can infect the brain, too.
Pneumococcal	Protection from getting bacterial pneumonia. Elderly people are at high risk for getting and dying of this lung infection.
Influenza	Prevents flu or influenza. Elderly people are at high risk for getting and dying of this lung infection.
Tetanus, diphtheria, and pertussis (Tdap)	Prevents three potentially lethal infectious diseases: tetanus, diphtheria, and whooping cough, or pertussis. Everyone should receive a Tdap booster every ten years.
Hepatitis A	Prevents hepatitis A, a liver disease, caused by eating contaminated food or water.
Hepatitis B	Prevents hepatitis B caused by exposure to contaminated blood and other body fluids. In addition, the vaccine prevents the kind of liver cancer the hepatitis B virus may cause.
TB (tuberculosis) skin test	Screens for exposure to tuberculosis.

PREPARING FOR YOUR SITE VISIT

Planning ahead can make your site visits as productive as possible. If you haven't already, review the websites of the facilities you plan to see. Doing so will give you a sense of the services you and your family member need, as well as help you come up with questions to ask (see worksheet 11.2).

Some facilities charge a flat monthly fee. Others, in addition to the costs of room, board, and basic care charge by the number of times your family member calls for assistance. Some facilities charge separately for laundry and similar services.

As mentioned earlier, Dorothy lived for several weeks in a rehabilitation hospital. Because patients spent time away from their room working with physical and occupational therapists, many, including Dorothy, choose to wear their own clothes. Those weeks of transporting urine-soaked clothing across town during the hottest part of the summer made it very clear that laundry service was a high-priority item on my list of needed services.

FIRST STEPS

Your evaluation begins with a phone call. How long did it take until someone answered the phone? Was that person courteous? Did that person, or any other people you spoke with, listen and make appropriate responses? Were they willing to make an appointment at a time most convenient for you?

Ask a family member or a friend to accompany you. Having another set of eyes and ears—and a nose, too—with you is a strategy that has many benefits. In addition to the emotional support, the backup may make it easier for other family members to accept the decision to move their loved one into residential care.

It's a good idea to take notes to record your sensory impressions, responses to questions, and any other pertinent information. Worksheet 11.3 can help organize your notetaking. Later, you can use your notes to refresh your memory.

Your next evaluation step begins when you approach the assisted living community. Is the street and neighborhood clean and quiet? Is there enough visitor parking? Is the building in good condition? Is the entryway inviting?

Once inside, your senses and your emotional radar system become your most important evaluation tools. What do you see, hear, and smell? Are people sincerely kind and friendly? And as for the overall ambience, is it welcoming or institutional?

Aromas and odors are often some of your first sensory clues. If the kitchen is near the administrative area, it is quite likely that the scent of lunch or dinner may greet you. It's easy to distinguish the greasy and salty aroma that brings back childhood memories of school cafeteria food (canned peas, steamed hot dogs, and fried fish sticks) from the scent of soup, fresh vegetables, and baked chicken. Either way, you can use this first sensory impression to introduce discussion about food, the weekly menu, and even the possibility of having lunch with the residents.

Body odor and urine may be another immediate sensory clue. As you well know, people who have dementia are often unwilling to take a bath or shower. A strong body odor smell in the building can indicate infrequent bathing, little attention given to personal hygiene, and inadequate ventilation. Be sure to ask about the bathing schedule and how they manage people who do not want to bathe. During your facility tour, ask to see the bath and shower rooms.

The unmistakable odor of urine is probably one of the most unwelcome clues. Immediately, you assume you are in one of those nightmare facilities where residents must suffer the indignity of wearing wet and soiled undergarments. Do remember that dehydration, bladder control problems, or urinary tract infections, rather than negligence, may be the source of this unmistakable and overwhelming odor.

People who do not drink enough water or other liquids make very concentrated and strong-smelling urine. A few drops of concentrated urine on clothing or chair covers produce an odor that, even with washing, can be difficult to remove.

Some facility residents may have bladder control problems caused either by an enlarged prostate (men) or stretched and weakened pelvic floor ligaments (women). Both of these medical conditions cause urine to leak from the bladder.

Urinary tract infections are a chronic problem for many older people. Bladder infections produce foul-smelling urine, a feeling of continuous urgency, and dribbling. Singly, or in combination with dehydration, physical changes to the urinary tract and bladder infections make odor control a challenge for even the best dementia care facilities.

If you do smell urine, be sure to politely mention this to the facility director. Give them a chance to explain the situation. Responses like "What do you expect from old people?" or "To prevent accidents we don't give them much to drink" are not acceptable. Replies that address some of the issues described earlier may help improve your impression.

Communicable diseases—influenza and COVID-19, in particular—are on everyone's radar. It's important, then, to ask about the infection control measures the facility takes to prevent the transmission of illness to and from residents and employees, as well as transmission to and from the community.

Ask the facility director if a tuberculosis (TB) screen and vaccinations against pneumonia, shingles, and hepatitis A and B are requirements for employment. Do employees receive infection control training? With the exception of TB screening and infection control education, you will discover that "no" is nearly always the answer. Hopefully, our tragic experience with so many assisted living residents becoming ill or dying of COVID-19 will turn many of the "nos" into "yeses."

THE SITE VISIT

The receptionist is usually the first person you meet. Undoubtedly, they will ask you to sit and wait until the executive director is available. The executive director's office is another assessment opportunity. Use your now well-honed evaluation radar to get a feeling of the person you are about to speak with and the facility he or she represents.

Does the office look like someone actually works there? Do you see any books, magazines, or professional journals? Does it appear that the executive director makes an effort to keep up with the latest eldercare developments? Has the director or the facility received any honors or awards from community groups or from the eldercare industry? Is there any evidence that the director is interested in meeting the needs of same-sex couples or accommodating various religious or ethnic traditions?

The interview begins—and yes, you are interviewing each other. Discussion might start with the director saying something like, "How can we help you?" or by simply picking up on something you mentioned in the introductory phone conversation. The idea is to get you talking. The facility director, and any other people present, should want to learn about your loved one and the family they hope to serve.

You, on the other hand, want to find out if their facility is one that meets your family member's physical and emotional needs and is safe, clean, and comfortable. You also want to know if moving your family member to their facility will give you respite from the unrelenting stresses dementia care creates. This is where doing your homework can make the difference between learning what you need to know and getting overwhelmed with too much well-polished talk. Be sure to bring a list of questions and your responses to worksheet 11.2 to help guide your discussion.

The facility director, and possibly the medical and marketing directors, too, will want to learn more about your loved one and their family. Some of the questions, such as inquiries about religious affiliation, their profession, important life cycle events, and your family dynamics, might seem too personal; however, these and other similar questions are important ones. The assisted living facility uses this kind of information to help new residents, and their families as well, feel comfortable and welcome.

The majority of the executive and marketing director's questions will be about everyday things, for example, your family member's food preferences, daily living skills, personality characteristics, sleep patterns, and interests. They should also ask if your family member has health problems that may go beyond their capabilities and licensure.

After the discussion, you should receive a facility tour. It can be upsetting to see the realities of residential dementia care units. The doors to the care units have keypad locks. It's hard to link kindness, respect, caring, and dignity to doors that your family member cannot open.

Some dementia care units look a little like a hospital with a central nursing station. Others look more like homes, or maybe a motel. Newer, or recently remodeled facilities may have a circular floor plan so that residents can walk without getting lost.

Dementia care facilities have other rooms where residents gather, eat, socialize, and participate in various activities. Walled gardens are often another feature. Gardens promote socialization and well-being, and they provide a little solitude and sunshine. One dementia facility I visited had areas where residents could grow flowers and vegetables in small, raised beds. Another facility garden was home to two goats, several chickens, a couple of peacocks, and three big rabbits.

I also visited a multistory facility that looked like an apartment building or maybe a hotel. Assisted living residents, some in early-stage dementia, spent most of the day in their room. Getting to the dining area and TV room required navigating a maze of similar-appearing hallways and an elevator. It was obvious that making one's way around this building would be confusing to anyone—and especially people who have cognitive impairments.

The mid-to-late-stage dementia residents lived in a below ground-level area. A cheerful and colorful décor was an honest attempt to compensate for the lack of windows and natural light. To reach the garden, caregivers had to escort residents through a locked door and then take an elevator up to the next floor. Entry to the garden was through another locked door. This dementia care facility, although clean and efficient, did not provide the kind of environment people who have dementia need.

Your tour should include meeting a few residents. Does the director speak in a demeaning or child-like voice? Does the director call the resident by their first or last name? Does the director recognize titles like doctor, professor, or reverend? Are there friendly introductions that indicate the director knows something about the person to whom they are speaking? Are there hugs or other indications of a warm relationship?

The seemingly normal appearance of some residents may make you wonder why they are living behind locked doors; however, once you hear the litany of repeated phrases and observe mindless meandering, the reasons why they are living in an assisted living facility become obvious. The director may mention that many of the residents were once doctors, professors, business executives, Girl Scout and Boy Scout leaders, or teachers.

Residents are usually pleased to speak with a visitor. Some may tell you how happy they are in their new home. Others may ask if you know where their husband is hiding or if you know why their daughter never visits. The weather is another frequent topic of conversation.

During your tour, you will see caregivers interacting with residents. Do they smile? Does their body language demonstrate that they are at ease? Do the caregivers connect with the residents in a friendly, yet respectful, manner?

If you haven't already, this would be a good time to ask the facility director about the resident-to-staff ratio during the day, over the weekend, and at night. Depending on the state requirements, resident-to-staff ratios can range anywhere from one staff member for every eight residents to one staff member for every fifteen residents. During the night, there may only be a few staff people present in the building. You should also ask about the availability of upper management personnel during the night and weekend hours.

Some assisted living facilities advertise twenty-four-hour medical coverage. Ask if a medical professional is in the building or available by phone. If your family member has diabetes, a disease that can sometimes require immediate attention, not having a person licensed to give insulin shots on the premises can be a dangerous situation. Inquire how the facility responds to medical emergencies, such as a heart attack or a stroke, during the day, at night, and on weekend hours.

Staff retention is another topic that can provide important clues about the working conditions and possibly the quality of care, too. On average, do their caregivers stay six months, one year, five years? Do take into consideration the difficulty of working with people who have dementia. Do facility caregivers rotate from dementia to nondementia care units? Does the care staff rotate shifts, and can your loved one expect to see a favorite caregiver the same time each day? You might also inquire about the average hourly wage that caregivers at that facility receive.

Ask the executive director, or other management-level personnel, about their background and interest in eldercare and how long they have worked at this particular facility.

MEDICATIONS REVISITED

The use of medication to reduce anxiety, depression, belligerence, and hallucinations is a touchy issue. Overmedicating makes people sleepy and disengaged from their surroundings. Some medications—sleeping pills, in particular—can cause balance difficulties and increase risk for falls and injuries. Conversely, under-medicating or withholding medication may cause undue pain and suffering.

Unfortunately, headline news decrying the inappropriate use of antipsychotics in nursing homes can give the impression that it is best to refrain from using behavior-modifying drugs.

As stated earlier, the decision to use antipsychotics is not an easy one. Studies show there are associated health risks for elderly people taking antipsychotics. In addition, it takes time and patience to tell if boredom, overstimulation, or dementia-related brain changes are the cause for difficult behavior.

One assisted living facility medical director I spoke with estimates that nearly half of all dementia residents receive medication to relieve behavioral symptoms. While 50 percent might seem extreme, one should take into consideration the following: (1) behavior is the primary reason why families opt to send a loved one to an assisted living facility, and (2) many residents first received behavior-modifying medication while still living at home.

It's hard to find information about medication practices in specific assisted living facilities; therefore, as a consumer, your best option is to ask the kind of questions that reveal if medication is used more for convenience than it is for the resident's benefit. Some of these questions include asking how they identify a resident's trigger points for difficult behavior and what they do to improve behavior without resorting to medication.

MEDICATING FOR OTHER CONDITIONS

Many older people take a variety of medications to treat or prevent illnesses; therefore, it is quite likely that your family member may take medications to control high blood pressure, reduce cholesterol blood levels, or prevent anemia. Some assisted living residents can manage their medication by themselves. Others, particularly those who have dementia, may need varying degrees of assistance.

Most people assume a nurse will manage their family member's medication. While a nurse or other licensed health professional administers (gives) medications to patients in hospitals or living in nursing homes, this is generally not the case in assisted living facilities. Many states assume assisted living facilities do not have a full-time registered nurse on staff and have developed laws to allow employees other than nurses to give residents their medication.

Medication aides are assisted living facility employees who have taken the state-mandated training that qualifies them to administer medication. Delegated authority, where a staff nurse trains facility aides to give patients medications, is another way that residents may receive help taking their medications. A third way uses unskilled facility employees who assist residents as they self-administer medication. "Assistance with self-administration" is a broadly defined term that includes opening a container, dispensing the medication, and if necessary, guiding a resident's hand to their mouth or placing medication on a resident's tongue.

During your interview and tour, make sure you ask questions that clarify the facility's medication management program. You need to learn about the education and training of the employees who dispense (prepare) and administer medication. You also need to find out if drugs are stored in a secure location and, when necessary, under refrigeration. Record keeping is another important aspect of medicine management. Ask who keeps drug-usage records and how often a registered nurse or pharmacist reviews them.

RELIGIOUS AND CULTURAL PRACTICES

For many people, religious beliefs and cultural heritage are fundamental aspects of their identity. Finding a dementia care facility that embraces particular religious beliefs or welcomes a diversity of cultural backgrounds can make a positive difference for you and your family.

Faith-based facilities can provide your loved one with the comfort that familiar rituals bring to life. In addition, faith-based assisted living facilities may be less expensive than privately owned facilities. Similar to finding other kinds of residential services, it is important that you do your homework and look at inspection records, speak to people familiar with the quality of services and care, and visit the facility.

Faith-based assisted living communities do take residents who practice other religions or who aren't religious. Nevertheless, it will still probably take some effort on your part to help the facility accommodate your loved one's beliefs and religious needs.

Non-faith-based care facilities tend to observe the holidays most people in the United States celebrate. Although willing to include other holidays (e.g., Chinese New Year, Greek Orthodox Easter, Kwanza, or Hanukkah) in their calendar of events, they may ask for your assistance. If you cannot help them, call a local clergy person who may be very happy to conduct religious services or contact local volunteers to help prepare a holiday meal that all residents can enjoy.

Our cultural or ethnic lives have a way of becoming more important as people age. Your foreign-born mother may suddenly speak in the language of her childhood, or your father, born in the United States, may suddenly identify with his father's and grandfather's stories. Dementia may return those who survived such things as the European Holocaust, the cultural cleansing of China, the Great Depression, or the hardships of the Dust Bowl years back to very frightening times. If part of your loved one's history includes trauma of this nature, finding an assisted living facility that understands the impact of these events can be very helpful.

RESIDENTIAL CARE AND THE LESBIAN, GAY, BISEXUAL, AND TRANSGENDER (LGBT) COMMUNITIES

The definition of family in the lesbian, gay, bisexual, and transgender (LGBT) community may not include blood relatives. Many times, family is a family of choice. Nevertheless, this is not to say that all blood-family members step aside. Many loved ones, siblings, and children do maintain long-standing and close relationships with their LGBT family member and their family member's spouse or partner.

It's important to remember a person of choice can be a designated caregiver. The Caregiver, Advise, Record, Enable (CARE) Act of 2016 states that once a caregiver is named, regardless of that person's relationship to the patient, the hospital is required to record the name of the caregiver in the patient's medical records, inform the caregiver when the patient is being discharged, and give the caregiver sufficient training to safely care for the patient at home.

The health care power of attorney (HCPOA) gives a designated person the ability to make decisions when the person in their care cannot. This document can give the POA the authority to demand health care providers respect their patient's gender identity. Together the CARE Act and the health care POA prevent blood relatives from imposing their demands on the person *not* in their care.

For many people, finding a welcoming assisted living facility or nursing home can be a challenge. There are many clues that can help identify LGBT-sensitive facilities. A rainbow decal on the front door, while not a guarantee, is a good indicator that the facility accepts diversity and believes in a philosophy of inclusiveness. Look over the brochures and other literature used to advertise services to the public. Do you see photographs showing people from a variety of ethnic groups and ways of life? Do you see words that imply an acceptance of different kinds of families? Do the brochures describe activities—an ice cream social or a holiday dinner, for example—in such a way that you or your family member's partner feels welcome?

It's sad to say, but in all likelihood, your responses to most of the aforementioned questions will be "no." But take heart, the long-term care industry is just beginning to become aware of the more than two million older adults who currently self-identify as lesbian, gay, bisexual, or transgender. According to "The Aging and Health Report," the numbers of self-identified LGBT older adults will more than double by 2030.

Your interview with the executive and medical directors is another way to evaluate the facility under consideration. Do these administrators use the words *partner* and *spouse* interchangeably? Do they assume that the older man who accompanied you to this meeting is your father's brother? Other lines of questioning become possible if the older man opts to identify his relationship to you. Ask if staff receives training on various LGBT issues. You can also ask about your options should you or the person in your care experience harassment, discrimination, or abuse. Unfortunately, cognitive impairment can make it less likely the care facility will take appropriate measures.

A collaborative study by several organizations, including the National Senior Citizens Law Center and the National Gay and Lesbian Task Force, shows that many LGBT older adults living in long-term care facilities often experience abuse and neglect. Study conclusions are based on the survey responses of nearly eight hundred people. Of these, roughly three hundred people identified themselves as LGBT older adults. The remainder included responses from family or friends, and from various legal, social, and medical service providers. Presumably, some of these people are speaking for those who have dementia.

The results are sobering. The majority of respondents felt they could not be open about their sexual orientation or gender identity. Refused admission or abrupt discharge from the long-term care facility was something nearly 25 percent of survey respondents said they had experienced. Other problems included verbal and physical harassment from other residents and facility staff, refusal to honor POA documents, restriction of visitors, staff refusal to address transgender residents by their preferred pronoun and name, and staff refusal to provide basic services, care, or medical treatment.

These conditions make it especially important that you get recommendations from those who know from experience which facilities are safe and welcoming. In addition to local recommendations, the Services and Advocacy for LGBT Elders (SAGE) organization can help you find assisted living communities whose employees receive cultural competency training.

AFTERWARD

Exhausted? Well, you should be! You just spent several hours doing some very intense research. Take a break. Relax.

While unwinding from your day, your mind might wander to the things you saw and heard earlier. Have a pad of paper and a pencil nearby so you can write those fleeting thoughts before you forget them. Or maybe you prefer to record your mind-wanderings on your smartphone or other recording device. These thoughts are often the important ones. They may be the ones that truly represent your uncensored thoughts and feelings about the assisted living facility you saw earlier.

It's also good to talk about your visit.

Be sure to speak with the person who accompanied you to the assisted living facility. It's important to discover their impressions and to discuss areas where you are not in agreement.

A verbal summary with friends or family over coffee or dinner is another way to organize your thoughts and, again, reveal points not otherwise obvious to you. Their responses are another source of valuable feedback. Use worksheet 11.3 to summarize your thoughts about each of the assisted living facilities you visited.

FREQUENTLY ASKED QUESTIONS

1. I am at the point where I can no longer care for my father in his home. Moving him to our home is out of the question. For him, and for us too, assisted living is the best solution. Nonetheless, I do want to make his adjustment as easy as possible. How do I respond to the questions assisted living facilities ask about the things he likes or might enjoy?

The best you can do is put yourself in his place and tell them about the foods or activities he likes. If you tell them he was once the family expert barbeque chef, they may make efforts to have outdoor meals. His passion for golf may morph into an indoor golf tournament.

Does he dislike spicy or difficult-to-cut and hard-to-chew foods? Does he hate listening to opera or being in noisy places? Based on what you tell them, and what they eventually learn for themselves, facility staff will do their best to respond to your father's individual preferences.

2. I know that assisted living facilities do not provide skilled nursing care. What happens if my father gets sick or goes into kidney failure while in an assisted living facility?

This very important question is one you must discuss with the director of each assisted living facility you visit. Most will say it depends on the circumstances.

Shortly after Dorothy's move to her assisted living residence, congestive heart failure became our primary medical concern. We were fortunate that the on-call physician could manage her symptoms with oral medication; however, had that not been true, she would have been sent to a facility, such as a nursing home, able to provide a higher level of care.

But should your father require dialysis to manage end-stage kidney disease and lives in a continuum of care facility, a temporary move to the nursing home section of the facility may be sufficient.

Something like kidney failure is more complicated. The combination of your loved one's medical directives, input from their doctor, and input from family members will define next steps. If kidney dialysis is the decision, then your loved one will need to move to a facility that can provide that level of care. If "let nature take its course" is the decision, then your family member— along with the help of hospice—can stay in the assisted living facility.

3. I would really appreciate it if my brother would help me select an assisted living facility for our mother. Each time I ask, he says he trusts my judgment or that he is too busy. I really would like him there with me.

Be sure to tell your brother that, even though he trusts your judgment, having him there would give you the emotional support you need. But do consider the possibility that he is seemingly passing the buck because he is afraid of what he will see. If that is the case, be truthful. Yes, it is difficult, but also mention the reasons why his presence will be helpful and appreciated.

It may also be true that he is busy and cannot join you at the times you arranged for site visits. If so, the easy solution is to first ask him to suggest days and times convenient for him. If your brother still finds ways to avoid making site visits, ask another relative, friend, or perhaps a family friend, to join you.

4. My mother, a retired biochemist and former chairperson of a university biochemistry department, is now living in a nearby dementia care facility. The director tells me my mother is often belligerent and seems to have a particular dislike for one of the caregivers. I noticed this caregiver calls my mother "Annie" rather than "Ann." Sometimes, she doesn't even bother using her name and calls her "Dearie." No one calls my mother "Annie." Even her grandchildren say "Grandma Ann." Do you think this might be part of the problem?

Your question reminds me of the importance of telling the facility director about the subtle things that can make assisted residential care less stressful. How caregivers address residents can make a big difference in a family member's behavior. Although some residents are perfectly happy with informality, others may find it insulting. Your loved one's behavior might improve if the caregiver addressed her as "Professor" or "Doctor" plus her last name. "Professor Ann" might be another alternative. Certainly, "Dearie" is a totally inappropriate way to address your mother, or any other resident for that matter.

5. Many years ago, I promised my mother that I would never put her in what she called an "institution." Now she has dementia. At this point, my family and I are able to care for her in our home; however, eventually that may become impossible. I am struggling with what to do. Just thinking about the possibility of breaking my promise to her makes me feel so guilty I cannot even look into other caregiving alternatives.

Guilt is a powerful emotion some people feel in response to the judgment of others. Because of its external source, psychologists often describe guilt as a "wasted or a useless emotion." "Emotional abuse" is another phrase some psychologists use. That being said, most people experience guilt at various times. It's a natural part of being human. It's part of being engaged with friends, family, and society. Guilt often prevents us from taking logical next steps.

By the same token, broken promises are also a part of life. Often the promises we make are something we say to make another person feel happy.

These promises we make are often more like fulfilling a wish than something we can say with guaranteed certainty—"I promise to love you to the end of time," "I promise we will take a vacation next year," "I promise I will never put you in a nursing home."

There are many things we can do to quiet feelings of guilt. First of all, objectively evaluate the situation. Think about the word *institution*. It is an emotionally charged word associated with unpleasant conditions. Who would want that for themselves or anyone in their care? Perhaps you and your loved one are unaware of the fine eldercare facilities we now have in nearly every community.

Perhaps your loved one equates residential eldercare with abandonment. Remember, you can maintain a comforting presence even when a loved one is living in an assisted living facility or a nursing home.

Become actively engaged in the process of overcoming guilt. Try to imagine what your loved one would say or do if, for a few moments, they could step out of dementia and see how the illness is affecting the family they love. Imagine what your healthy mother might say or do if she were in your situation. Think about how you might feel if your mother suffered because you could not provide sufficient or safe home care.

Consider what you might say to another person experiencing a situation similar to yours. Taking our own best advice can be difficult. But often, just recognizing the influence guilt plays in our decision-making process is helpful. And finally, remember there is no shame in asking others for guidance. The benefits of talking to a spiritual or professional advisor can give you the strength and insight you need to take your next steps with confidence.

WORKSHEET 11.1:
Organizing Your Thoughts about Residential Care

1. List three events or situations that would make you feel continued home care would be unsafe or too difficult.
2. For each of your responses, describe a solution that could potentially make home care manageable. "None" is an acceptable answer.
3. Do you believe the following statements?

   A. Home care is best.
   B. Home care is safer than residential care.
   C. Home care is a family obligation.
   D. Home care is less expensive.
   E. Home care makes you a better person.
   F. Residential care is a punishment.
   G. Residential care is safe.
   H. Residential care means an uncaring family.
   I. Residential care is the same as giving up.

4. What do your responses to the above statements say about your feelings about home care and residential care? Does it appear that you have a bias toward one kind of care over another? Are your feelings based on exploring local options, personal opinions, or what you have heard from media reports, family, and friends?

WORKSHEET 11.2:
Important Services

Use this worksheet to take inventory of the services you feel are important to your family member's care. The first table refers to assisted living communities. The second table focuses on the services often found in memory care or dementia care units.

Assisted Living

Service	Required	Willing to Pay Extra	Provide Yourself
Unlimited calls for assistance			N/A
Cost of assistance calls based on number per month			N/A
Personal laundry service			
In-house social activities			
In-house medical care			
In-house foot and nail care			
Transportation to medical care			
Transportation to restaurants, cultural events, social activities			
Access to outdoor areas			
In-house hair care			
Absorbency products			
Support group for residents			
Support group for family			
Special meals: kosher, vegetarian, gluten free, other			
Cultural and ethnic events			
Religious services			
Family events			
Family can join residents at meals			N/A

Memory Care Unit

Service	Yes	Not Available or No	Other Options
Medical staff on site 24/7			
24-hour emergency response system			
Periodic medical and social evaluations			
Absorbency products			
Personal laundry service			
Hair care			
Circular floor plan			
Foot and nail care			
Easy access to garden			
Therapy animals			
Art, music, and other creative activities			
Housekeeping			
Linen service			
Exercise program			
Entertainment			
Transportation			
Religious services			
Modified diets			
Kosher meals			
Vegetarian meals			
Health monitoring			
Snacks and beverages			
Assistance with daily living skills			
Life engagement program			
Support group for family members			
Family events			
End-of-life care			

WORKSHEET 11.3:
The Site Visit

Use this worksheet to summarize your notes about the various assisted living facilities and memory care units you visit.

Name of facility:

Facility address:

Phone number:

Names of contact persons:

Date and time of visit:

Name and contact information for any accompanying persons:

1. Write a few words to help remember the following about each facility:

   Street side appearance:

   Entry-way appearance:

   Reception area appearance:

   Odors and aromas:

   Sounds:

   Overall ambience:

   Personnel manners and body language:

   Staff manners and body language:

   Resident-to-staff ratio:

   Cleanliness:

   Facility floor plan:

   Outdoor features:

   Appearance of residents:

   Behavior management:

   Standout features of inspection reports:

2. Shortly after leaving the premises, write a few sentences that summarize your overall impressions. List a few standout features—good or bad.

12

IT ISN'T HOME

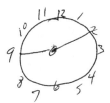

Man, age eighty, clock, 9:10 a.m.

Conversations with assisted living facility directors made it obvious to me that anyone would rather be home. It wasn't surprising, then, to hear that most residents had a difficult time adjusting to their new surroundings. One facility director assured me that most residents eventually acquiesce. And yes, they did use medication to ease the transition.

I suppose the look on my face revealed my thoughts. "Your mother needs to be here. It is the best thing for the both of you."

I wondered how long it would take Dorothy to adjust. Acquiescence, or giving in, was not part of her personality. And—what an awful word.

The staff was good about giving me daily updates. Dorothy was doing well. She seemed to enjoy listening to music, and believe it or not, she took a shower. Sometimes the news wasn't so great. Dorothy said mean things to the other residents. She refused to participate in group activities or to eat in the dining room. She told everyone that she needed to stay in her room so her daughter could find her.

Reports of Dorothy's behavior made me wonder if the care facility would send her back home. After one particularly trying day, I mentioned my concern to the facility director who laughed and said, "If good behavior was a requirement, we wouldn't be in business."

Visiting Dorothy wasn't as hard as I imagined. Much to my relief, Dorothy did not associate me with "this place." Still, the move had taken a toll. In a few weeks, she had changed from an elderly-looking woman into one who looked every bit of her ninety-nine and a half years. I also noticed a pile of unopened newspapers.

At her home, reading the newspaper was an all-day affair. We knew that she was doing little more than going through the motions—turning pages followed by a report of another slow news day. We thought that the familiarity, and even the normalcy, of turning pages must have been a source of comfort. It now appeared that, similar to her extended stay in the rehabilitation hospital a few years earlier, the move had disrupted the few remaining behaviors that linked her to her former self.

Her conversation was limited and repetitive. What kind of place is this? Why am I here? When can I go home? And unlike those other people, she insisted that she was healthy and would soon be driving again. Gratefully, the nursing staff would intervene and redirect Dorothy's attention.

Despite the difficulties, it was obvious that Dorothy enjoyed our visits. She was particularly happy to see her grown grandchildren.

I am certain that Dorothy did not acquiesce to this monumental change in her life. She did not have the capacity to understand that she needed help or that she was becoming increasingly frail. A familiar chair and a favorite crocheted blanket did not make this strange place home. But for us, it was a relief to know she was safe and receiving good care.

ADJUSTMENT

The memory care manager suggested that we not visit for two weeks or so. They said this would make it easier for Dorothy to make the adjustment. Their request seemed a little harsh—a little "cold turkey." I worried that Dorothy might feel abandoned and hopeless; however, I didn't question their judgment. The assisted living facility professionals must know what they are doing, and I understood the break was for my benefit as well.

Many years later, I wish I hadn't listened to them. A few days—that I can understand. A few weeks in a strange place—that is cruel.

Adjustment to assisted living takes time. For people who have dementia, it may be several months before they are comfortable in their new surroundings. The first days are the most difficult. Some new residents cry. Many refuse to eat, leave their rooms, or speak. Aggressive and destructive behaviors sometime occur. When behavioral methods, such as distraction and redirection, are not helpful, the medical practitioner responsible for your family member's care may use medication to help ease their transition.

Refusal to eat is short-lived. And it won't be long before your family member decides to watch the other residents from the security of a well-placed chair. Soon, she will join them in the various activities the facility offers.

The staff plays an important role in helping your loved one feel welcomed. Like any good neighbor, caregivers stop by to chat, introduce your loved one to other people, and accompany them to meals, as well as encourage participation in scheduled music, art, and exercise activities. Eventually, your loved one will begin to feel comfortable in these new surroundings.

Adjustment is not always a smooth process. More than likely, your loved one wonders how they got there. They may believe they were kidnapped. They may become depressed and anxious. When you think about it, these are normal responses to what must seem like a nightmare.

During the transition period, it is important to keep in close contact with the staff. Try to call during a relatively quiet time. If a staff member is unable to speak with you, leave a message containing specific questions. Be sure to leave your contact information. To avoid a telephone tag situation, mention the times when you are available to receive a phone call. Once you get a sense of the staffing schedule, you will know the best time to reach the person who has the most contact with your family member.

Your loved one isn't the only one who has to make a big adjustment. After many months or years, home care is no longer the focus of your day. In theory, you now have the time to concentrate on all those "I wish" things that you missed so much. But instead, you feel empty, adrift, and restless. You don't know what to do with yourself.

For many family caregivers, guilt becomes the overwhelming emotion (see worksheet 12.1). To compensate, you call or visit the care facility more often than necessary. In part, you want to dispel any thoughts—theirs or yours—that you are an uncaring, and totally awful, person. You wonder if you made a wise decision. Maybe you could have held on a little longer. Maybe your loved one really doesn't have dementia. Maybe your family member really wasn't that difficult. And oddly enough, you are also afraid the assisted living facility will send your family member home.

THROUGH THEIR EYES

Seeing the situation through your loved one's eyes may make it easier for you to understand their feelings. Your loved one, even if they had agreed to the move, probably does not remember ever saying so.

In many ways, your loved one is experiencing what must seem like a hallucination; however, unlike the bugs on the wall, you know the dementia care facility is real. As before, a kind and assuring tone will be more helpful than explaining why going home is not possible. Remind your loved one they are safe. Do and say things that show your love for them. Perhaps you can redirect conversation with a small present. But most of all, remember adjustment takes time, and your loved one needs to be there.

A NEW PLACE CALLED HOME

The nurses frequently talk about transition, adjustment, and acquiescence; however, I am quite sure "escape" is on the minds of many otherwise quiet and complacent residents. In one facility, a caregiver told me about a resident who threw his walker over the garden wall and then attempted to escape using a chair as a ladder. In another facility, the medical director described a situation where a resident managed to squeeze through a window. The resident proceeded to run (walker in tow) to the main road, where, at a stop light, she threw herself—headfirst—into an opened car window.

One day, while visiting Dorothy, I noticed a group of residents huddled around the door to the main lobby. The nurse told me I was witnessing the daily collaborative effort to break the door code. Today, like every other day, they were going to bust out of the joint!

Escape was in the forefront of Dorothy's thoughts, too. A friend, whose father was a facility resident, told me about the little lady she saw standing in the doorway to her bedroom. Pocketbook in hand, she looked like she was waiting for the bus. When my friend passed by the door, Dorothy asked my friend to take her home. Years later, that very sad image still stays with me.

MORE THAN AN ADJUSTMENT

The move to assisted living brings with it the problems of living in close proximity to people who truly are strangers. One of these challenges is exposure to infectious diseases, such as colds, flu, and various stomach bugs.

The other issue is the potential for elder abuse. Elder abuse is not an adjustment anyone should have to make. The bottom line is that elder abuse is unacceptable and should be reported.

It is important that family members be aware that elder abuse is something that can happen in any facility. Although far from an excuse, facility employees are often overworked. In some facilities, each caregiver may be responsible for as many as twelve to fifteen people.

Hearing about elder abuse is just plain awful. It can make anyone second-guess a decision to move a loved one from home into residential care. That being said, it is important to take into consideration that each community has a spectrum of assisted living facilities and nursing homes. Some provide consistently wonderful care, and some do not.

WHAT'S GOING ON?

It may seem like nearly every other phone call you receive from the assisted living facility informs you that your loved one has another "crud-bug." But don't worry, the caregiver says, your loved one is doing well and is on the road to recovery. You wonder what is going on. Aside from having dementia, your loved one is pretty healthy. You cannot remember the last time they had a cold. Upset stomachs and fevers were infrequent illnesses.

Your loved one's move from home into a communal living setting involves more than emotional acquiescence to a new environment. After years of living in relative isolation, your loved one is socializing, eating, and sleeping in close contact to many people. And unlike her home situation, she now sees many caregivers and other health care providers. Visitors are another source of exposure.

There are many reasons why older people are more susceptible than younger people to the various contagious diseases that circulate through the community. Some of these factors include an immune system that no longer works as well as it once did and presence of other underlying illnesses. In addition, the diminished ability to clear the throat and cough is a risk factor for pneumonia.

Another reason is the assisted living facility itself. Bladder infections and bladder and bowel incontinence are difficulties. Poor personal hygiene, specifically failure to wash hands and having feces and urine on clothing, makes it likely that doorknobs, chairs, or anything else residents touch are contaminated.

Gastrointestinal illnesses, ones that cause diarrhea, vomiting, and sometimes fever, are common within long-term care facilities. Hepatitis A, or foodborne hepatitis, is another problem in environments where fecal contamination is likely. Caregivers who forget to wash their hands after helping a resident use the toilet or before preparing a snack or a meal for residents play an important role in spreading intestinal diseases.

Respiratory infections are another assisted living facility concern. In addition to colds, living in close contact with other people increases the chances of getting influenza (flu) and certain kinds of pneumonia and meningitis. Here again, hand washing plays an important role in decreasing the spread of respiratory illnesses. In addition, it's important to cough and sneeze into your elbow, rather than your hands, and refrain from touching your face.

TB, or tuberculosis, is another concern for people living in close quarters or working in health care environments. Assisted living facilities do not require that new residents present evidence of a recent, and negative, TB test. In some states, a negative TB test is a requirement for employment in an assisted living facility.

For those residents who have diabetes, sugar monitoring can increase their risk for hepatitis B or blood-borne hepatitis. This can happen when poorly trained staff members use a glucose monitor without first cleaning and disinfecting the machine. Another cause is failure to wash hands between patients or failure to wear gloves when drawing blood. In some states, only licensed caregivers (nurses and doctors) may do these procedures. In other states, other staff members may perform glucose monitoring tests.

There are some simple things you can do so you do not become part of the infection transmission problem. Hand washing is number one! Wash your hands before entering your family member's room and again when you leave the facility. Wash your hands before handling food, after sneezing, or after helping your loved one use the bathroom. If soap and water aren't handy, be sure to bring a bottle of hand sanitizer gel or a box of sanitizing hand wipes with you.

An annual flu shot can protect you and your loved one from influenza. Even if you aren't sixty-five years old, having a family member living in an assisted living facility may make you eligible for the pneumococcal immunization. If you haven't already, get your hepatitis A and B vaccination series, too (see table 11.2 in chapter 11 for a list of recommended vaccinations). In truth, having those immunizations is a good idea for anyone who travels, eats in restaurants, or goes camping. And last, but not least, do not visit your family member when you have a cold or other illness. If there is a compelling reason why you must be there, wear a face mask.

ELDER ABUSE

The possibility of abuse is something you cannot ignore. According to a report by the Nursing Home Abuse Center, nearly 1 out of every 20 assisted living facility residents are subjected to some type of mistreatment. Stigma, the lack of nationally applied regulations, and infrequent facility inspections undoubtedly make this is a grossly underreported number.

In contrast, the Nursing Home Abuse Center reports that nearly 1 out of every 30 nursing home residents experience some form of abuse. The reason for this unexpected difference in findings between assisted living and nursing home data is hard to determine. Without question, stricter regulations and oversight makes it more likely that someone will notice and report incidents of abuse that take place in nursing homes.

Elder abuse includes at least five types of harm: physical abuse, neglect, sexual abuse, emotional abuse, and financial exploitation (see table 12.1). Signs of physical abuse include bruises, open wounds, burns, and abrasions. Sudden weight loss, soiling or the smell of urine and feces, infections, hair loss, and torn, stained, or bloodied clothing or bedding are all signs of neglect.

Table 12.1.   Types of Abuse

Physical mistreatment like hitting, burning, or using restraints
Verbal, emotional, or psychological abuse like teasing and insulting
Misuse of property or finances
Withholding food, water, and other daily living needs
Forced social isolation
Using fear and intimidation to control behavior
Enabling dangerous situations

Signs of sexual abuse, emotional abuse, and financial exploitation are not as obvious. You should be concerned if your parent suddenly displays infantile behaviors like thumb sucking, appears afraid of certain caregivers, or becomes listless and emotionally withdrawn. Sudden and unusual financial transactions may indicate financial exploitation. Other signs that may indicate abuse are caregivers who speak for the person in their care, ask you to wait before you may enter the room, and remain there during your visit.

Your loved one, thinking they will not be believed, may refuse to say anything against the abusive person. Your loved one may be unable to communicate with clarity or may feel that silence is the best way to prevent retaliation. Embarrassment is another possibility.

Many studies show that, in general, assisted living facilities that require a pre-employment background check and have a high staff-to-resident ratio tend to have fewer reported incidents of resident mistreatment.

A report issued by the National Center on Elder Abuse cites the primary factors leading to abuse in nursing homes as inadequate staff training, high staff turnover, and not enough caregivers for the number of residents. It seems reasonable to assume that their findings are applicable to assisted living facilities as well.

Your presence is probably the most important way to prevent abuse from occurring. Rather than predictable or scheduled visits, drop in at odd times. As one geriatric nurse specialist suggested, stay for a while. Sit on the couch, read the newspaper, and disappear into the background. Over the course of an hour or so, you will get a true sampling of how the staff treats the elders in their care.

Get to know your family member's caregivers. Keep in mind that, as your loved one's power of attorney or guardian, you have the right to read their medical chart. If you don't live nearby, designate a family friend, relative, eldercare consultant, or lawyer to take your place. The main idea is to make sure staff members do not get the impression that your loved one is alone and vulnerable.

There are many things you can do if you suspect abuse. Similar to workplace harassment, it is important to document incidents with the time, place, and duration. Be sure to photograph observable injuries (see worksheet 12.2). Review your loved one's medical chart to see if you can link incidents to a particular caregiver and report, in writing, your suspicions to the assisted living facility management. Be sure to keep a copy of your letter as well as any correspondences you receive from them.

If speaking with management does not clarify the situation, contact Adult Protective Services (APS). In most states, APS caseworkers are the first people who respond to reports of abuse, neglect, and exploitation of vulnerable adults. You can find your local APS office using your internet search engine and the keywords "Adult Protective Services," along with the state, city, and county where your family member resides.

The directory of state hotlines for reporting abuse in nursing homes, assisted living facilities, and board and care homes is another resource. You can find the link to the directory on the National Center for Elder Abuse web page. Another helpful organization is the National Long-Term Care Ombudsman Resource Center. This organization links long-term care residents to people who advocate in their behalf.

If you feel your loved one is in immediate danger, do not hesitate to call 911 or the local police and remove them from the premises.

Abuse, particularly financial exploitation, can extend to the resident's family. This happens when a facility caregiver, through seemingly innocent chatter, encourages conversation about the goings-on of the resident's grandchildren as well as other kinds of personal information. Now the predator has enough information to create a convincing story about a grandson in trouble and in need of money. Be sure to notify the family (and the grandson, too) of this troubling situation.

OTHER CHANGES

After years of living alone, your family member will find leaving the privacy and comfort of their home and transitioning to communal living extraordinarily difficult. The combination of having a roommate, sharing a bathroom, and having to deal with an imposed eating and sleeping schedule gives your family member many valid reasons to complain.

Most assisted living facilities can offer new residents the choice of a single or a double room. Single rooms are more expensive but do offer a little more privacy and respite from the constant presence of other people. Should you comment on the small space, the facility director is likely to mention that residents do not spend much time in their room. The director will say the small room encourages residents to socialize and participate in the activities the facility offers.

If you question the wisdom of having two strangers share a double room, the facility director will say that many residents enjoy the companionship and feel safer having another person nearby. And yes, you guessed right, the director will also mention that residents do not spend much time in their room.

A single room was the obvious choice for Dorothy. It wasn't that much more expensive, and her ability to share space and be polite was nil. For her, spending her last days with a roommate when she had her own house would be the biggest insult imaginable.

Her room did contain some of her home furnishings, books, artwork, and assorted sentimental items; however, Dorothy was upset to find *her* belongings in this strange place. She must have felt she was dropped into the Twilight Zone.

Although the facility encouraged socialization, Dorothy was a loner. And severe cognitive impairment did not lessen her disdain for what she considered frivolous activities. It didn't matter that she could no longer read, make art, discuss politics, or understand the National Public Radio news programs.

VISITING

It's hard to see your loved one in this different place. Suddenly, your parent has become one of those people you saw during your evaluation tours. Your loved one suddenly seems older, slower, and less able to engage with you and their surroundings.

You may wonder if medication is the cause for these changes. If you should ask, the facility medical director may say these changes are expected ones. The medical director may explain further and tell you your loved one can now relax—come out, so to speak. Your loved one is in a place where it is okay to have dementia.

Learning ways to make your visits a pleasurable and positive experience takes time and a little experimentation. Timing your visits, thinking carefully about the words you use, joining your family member in their world, and incorporating activities into your visit are all useful approaches. Schedule visits for mid-morning or early afternoon, a time when your family member is most likely to be in a good mood. Call ahead and arrange to have lunch with your family member. In addition to bringing a little normalcy into their life, your loved one will be proud to have a lunchtime guest.

Avoid going to see your loved one during late afternoon or evening, a time when they are more likely to be tired, agitated, or physically aggressive. The end of the day and evening is a time when many people who have dementia focus their thoughts on "get me out of here, I want to go home." Your presence during sundowning will be hard on everyone.

Orchestrating conversation with a person who has memory loss can be tricky. Avoid using trigger words that may make your loved one angry or agitated. Don't ask questions easily answered by a "yes or no" response, such as "Do you know who I am?" A response of "no" can be devastating to you and create a conversation dead-end.

Instead, you can say, "Hi, Dad. I am Mary, your youngest daughter." In return, he may say, "Yes, I know. Nice to see you." And if the opposite is true, he will enjoy visiting with this very friendly and charming person.

The phrase "do you remember?" may seem innocent enough to us. But to a person who has dementia, it can be an annoying question. Actually, most people find constant quizzing an annoyance! Your family member's response to, "Do you remember our house in Poughkeepsie?" may be nothing more than a confused look. Instead, you can try, "I was just thinking about our old house. The garden was so pretty." Converting questions into nonquestions may give your loved one the clues they need to say something in response. Even if your loved one doesn't remember, they will be happy to hear the rest of your story.

Connecting with your family member's world is another important visiting skill. In chapter 3, you learned about the "joining" strategy to prevent the behavior associated with hallucinations from escalating into something you cannot manage. Some people, when they enter a memory care facility, may become attached to a doll and treat it as though it were a real baby. Although your loved one's fixation on a doll may seem strange to you, try to remember that, in some way, it is a source of comfort. You loved one may use a toy telephone as though it is a real one, or they may believe they are in an airport waiting area. It's better to tell your mother, "The flight has been delayed, let's get a snack," than it is to convince her of your reality. As they say, there's no harm in pretending.

Visits tend to go better if you come prepared with an activity. Those that work best are activities that go to your loved one's strengths and interests. Looking through a family album, as long as you forgo the "do you remember?" phrase, can be a nice way to spend a morning together. Looking through a colorful coffee table book together is another, more neutral, alternative. Your loved one might enjoy looking at a book about English gardens or antique airplanes.

Many people who have Alzheimer's disease or another dementia enjoy making holiday cards; however, do keep in mind that it is the process and the time spent together, and not the product, that is most important.

A visit doesn't have to be all talk and chatter. Your family member may appreciate your quiet presence. Listening to music, taking a walk in the facility garden, reading poetry or short stories aloud, or watching an old movie are some other options.

It's easy to forget, but assisted living facilities aren't prisons. Once settled, your loved one may enjoy going out to lunch, visiting the zoo or a museum, or attending a local sports event. If your family member has a close friend, consider organizing an outing that includes them and their family, too.

Everyone has good days and bad days; however, for people who have dementia the difference between a good day and a bad one can be extreme. The situation can become even more volatile if your loved one feels tired or frustrated, or if he is in the early stages of coming down with a cold or another illness. Try your very best not to take what they say personally. Remember, it's the dementia, and not the person you once knew, who is talking.

Should you happen to stop by on a bad day, the best thing you can do is to cut your visit short. Do not respond in anger or reprimand your family member as though they are a misbehaving child. Instead, with a reassuring hug or a kiss, tell them you will come back another day. In all likelihood, the next time you visit, your loved one will be happy to see you.

VISITING WITH DOROTHY

At first, visiting with Dorothy was a scary prospect. No, it was more than scary. I expected her to punish me for the terrible thing I did. I also felt ashamed that I could no longer manage her care at home. Eventually, I realized I had misjudged her and the situation. Dorothy, rather than being angry with me, considered me a savior. Certainly, her trustworthy and capable daughter could find a way to get her out of there!

It goes without saying that Dorothy wanted to go home. And driving, that was another request. "When your doctor says it's okay." I was grateful that my small lie still worked. And by now, you know what comes next. It wasn't "no," it gave her hope, and it didn't create an impossible argument.

A FEW WORDS OF ENCOURAGEMENT

More than likely, your decision to move your family member into an assisted living facility was based on need. Something wasn't working. Your loved one requires more care than you can physically manage or afford. The commute and time away from work or your own family is becoming unmanageable. Your loved one's health is failing and needs more complex care than you or their current caregivers can provide. Because of unrelenting stress, your own health is suffering.

Assisted living facilities fill the gap between home care and a nursing home. Based on idealistic values of respect and dignity, assisted living facilities advertise that they give your loved one the assistance and supportive care they need. In all facilities, you will find some wonderful caregivers—people who are truly kind and compassionate.

Although your loved one's caregivers may not expect recognition, you can do your part by saying "thank-you" and perhaps mentioning their good work to their supervisor. A simple "thank-you" has an amazing way of making everyone feel good.

Many family caregivers, in describing the journey that eventually led to an assisted living facility, will say they wished they had moved their loved one much sooner. It was only then that they could appreciate how difficult the situation had become. Others, like me, will say they made the move just in time.

FREQUENTLY ASKED QUESTIONS

1. What do I say when various friends or family question my judgment in moving my mother into an assisted living facility?

Anyone who questions your judgment has never had to make a similar decision themselves. Don't get defensive or bother going into a prolonged explanation. Simply say, "Someday, if you should find yourself in a similar situation, you will understand I did the best I could under the circumstances."

2. Recently, I ran into one of my mother's casual friends at a social gathering. She seemed very concerned about my mother and was under the impression that I had "put my mother away" before making the effort to care for her at home. I have to admit, her comments surprised me. I have been my mother's primary caregiver for more than four years. While I know I am doing the best I can, it saddens me to think rumors are going around to the contrary.

It's easy to say what your mother's friend, or anyone else, believes doesn't matter. But in reality, we know rumors can be hurtful. What she and others may say does mean a lot to you. The best you can do is to assure her that your mother received good care at home for as long as it was possible. More than likely, your mother's friend is worried about herself.

3. The last time I visited my mother, she got very angry with me. She screamed and told me to leave and never come back. On the way out, she threw her shoe and hit me so hard it left a bruise. Needless to say, I was devastated. I don't know what I said or did that made her so angry.

First of all, I want to say that I am sorry this happened to you. As best you can, try to understand that dementia, and not your mother, is in control of her behavior. You were an innocent bystander who got caught in an unfortunate moment. Your mother cannot remember what she said and did to you; however, you should not ignore what happened and how you now feel.

Discuss the event with the facility caregivers; they may have some insightful suggestions. You may also learn that they, too, have to be very careful in her presence. Because the caregivers aren't your mother's daughter, they do not take what she says and does personally; however, they may be afraid of her. And that means your mother may not be getting the care and attention she needs.

Your mother's doctor may say that medication is the best way to reduce your mother's angry and violent outbursts.

But before you visit again, make sure you have a self-protection plan in place. Consider bringing another family member or a friend with you. Even when people have dementia they sometimes behave better in the presence of a different face. For example, Dorothy's caregivers and I quickly discovered that we could accomplish all kinds of things if my husband was there to lend a manly presence. He didn't have to do or say anything!

Another self-protection tactic is to ask a caregiver to stay nearby while your visit. That way, the caregiver can intervene in your behalf before the situation becomes unmanageable or unsafe.

Another kind of self-defense is the emotional backing you get from support group members. These people truly understand your situation and how you feel. What happened to you was hurtful in so many ways. So don't be afraid to seek professional help from a counselor, medical social worker, psychologist, or support group.

4. My father enjoys it when his roommate's daughter visits with her four children. One of them is a preschooler. Even when the child has a cough and a runny nose, he comes along with his brother and two sisters. Of course, all the kids give their grandpa and his roommate a hug and a kiss the moment they arrive and again when they are ready to go home. What should I do?

You are right to be concerned as you don't want your father or any of the other residents to get sick. Mention your concern to the medical director. Let her handle it. She can talk to the family, or better yet, the medical director can post a note so all visitors know to stay home when ill.

WORKSHEET 12.1:
Afterthoughts

Many people find that after moving their parent to an assisted living facility, feelings of guilt replace hoped-for relief. Use the questions and prompts below to organize your thoughts and reflect on the impact of this recent change.

1. Write three to five words that describe how you feel.
2. Suppose a friend, in a similar situation, used the same three to five words to describe themselves. What would you say to her? What advice would you give her? In what ways is your advice the same or different from what you expect of yourself?
3. What three to five words might a friend or family member use to describe their impression of you as a caregiver? Do you agree? Are you surprised?
4. List three to five ways that you, your family, or your place of employment benefits from your family member's assisted living placement.
5. List three to five ways that your family member benefits from assisted living services and care.

WORKSHEET 12.2:
Documenting Abuse

Documenting abuse provides the evidence you need to keep your loved one safe.

Date and Time of Incident:

Person Harmed:

Observations:

Name of Abuser:

Witness(es) and Contact Information:

Documentation:

People Informed, Date they were informed, and Contact Information:

Other Comments:

13

FAILING HEALTH

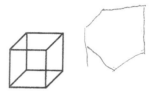

Man, age eighty-nine, cube.

On the whole, Dorothy was amazingly healthy for a person well into her nineties. But then again, she ate healthy, even before cholesterol and triglyceride blood levels were a mainstream concern. She took naps and, until the incident with the nameless lady, swam several times a week; however, Dorothy was not aware of the big changes osteoporosis had made in her height and posture. She believed that the medication she took for high blood pressure was a temporary situation. Dorothy often said that, unlike other people of her age, she didn't have any health problems. Those beliefs made medicating to manage her behavior and to treat osteoporosis and high blood pressure even more of a challenge when swallowing became difficult.

Dorothy did not remember the intestinal bleeding she experienced several years earlier. The results of the colonoscopy had revealed a mass in her intestines. A blood test showed low-grade anemia, but it was, as they say, "nothing to write home about." Even then, when her doctor explained the situation, her attention went elsewhere. She was fine. Everything was okay.

The colonoscopy took place before anyone had considered dementia a part of her medical history. The combination of age and the location of the growth made surgery too risky. Her doctors felt it was best to leave things alone. So we did. Dorothy, as usual, understood their decision as confirmation of her good health.

A few years later, with dementia as part of the picture, slight anemia became significant anemia. Her face was ashen. She tired easily and was often short of breath. Her doctor suggested another colonoscopy.

"No! Absolutely not!" was my instantaneous response. Toileting was already a struggle. The difficulty of preparing her for the test would be beyond horrible. I told her doctor if a colonoscopy was truly necessary, she must have the preparation in a hospital where experienced medical personnel, not people involved in her daily care, would be responsible.

A colonoscopy might provide answers—but would it lead to a solution? If the preparation and the procedure itself didn't kill her, the anesthesia needed to undergo the colonoscopy might worsen brain function. And surgery, with an even greater likelihood of a poor outcome, was not appropriate as long as she had a functioning bowel. Her doctor and I discussed other alternatives. The end result of our conversation was the decision to keep her comfortable and to manage symptoms.

To limit confusion and belligerent behavior, we didn't tell her about the blood transfusion to treat her anemia until the day before the appointment. As expected, she said that she didn't need one, that she was healthy, that her blood work was perfect, and that all of us, including her doctor, were crazy.

The next day, we did manage to get her dressed in time to get her to the hospital for a 10 a.m. appointment. It didn't take long to see the nearly immediate effects of the blood transfusion. Color returned to her face. And although she did find the experience exhausting, it was obvious that she felt better. By the time she finished lunch, all was forgotten. From that time on, we focused on care that managed symptoms or maintained or improved her comfort.

A DIFFERENT KIND OF PHONE CALL

I knew something different was going on when the assisted living nurse called to say that Dorothy's doctor needed to speak with me. In the few moments it took him to come to the phone, my mind had already wandered to the possibility of a fall and a broken hip, food aspiration, or maybe, as she sometimes threatened, a purposeful injury.

"Congestive heart failure," he said. "Your mother's heart can no longer efficiently pump blood through her body. Her legs are swollen. She is coughing and having difficulty breathing." He then explained that he had prescribed medication and supplemental oxygen to alleviate symptoms and to reduce discomfort.

I have to admit, this new twist to Dorothy's health did not surprise me. It explained why she so easily became breathless and exhausted. Even her recent falls could have been the result of feeling dizzy or lightheaded.

These latest events helped me understand the move to an assisted living facility happened just in time. She wouldn't use her walker, and getting her to take medication was a twice-a-day trial. The prospect of having to deal with supplemental oxygen and even more pills was one of several breaking points for me—and the caregivers, too. Without question, Dorothy's care had entered a new phase.

END-OF-LIFE CONSIDERATIONS

For many of us, end-of-life wishes are concerns that float somewhere in our consciousness. For some people, it's too scary to take next steps and compose a living will or an advance directive. Others feel an advance directive will bring them bad luck.

It's easier and healthier to consider your advance directive as a gift to your family. Your advance directive will prevent disagreements among family members. Your advance directive will ease the emotional burden of having to make some very difficult decisions for a person unable to speak for themselves. The living will informs others how you want to live and die.

The advance directive contains questions to guide your thoughts regarding such things as tube feeding or heroic measures to prolong life. Each question includes three choices: 1) I choose to, 2) I choose not to, or 3) I choose to let my agent (power of attorney or guardian) decide. Many people write a lengthy addendum where they expand upon the multiple-choice questions, including their wishes concerning tissue and organ donation, cremation, a green burial, and funeral details.

Health care providers will want to know if your parent has a DNR, or a "do not resuscitate" order. The DNR is a request not to have cardiopulmonary resuscitation (CPR) should the heart or breathing stop. Advance directives do not have to include a DNR order, and conversely, the DNR can be a stand-alone document.

You can find advance directive forms on the AARP (American Association of Retired Persons) website. The keywords "no-cost," living will," and "advance directive" will bring up many online options. Be sure to give a copy to a family member, friend, or your doctor. Another option is to inform others where they can find your advance directive papers.

WHAT SHOULD I DO?

It is a difficult situation when a loved one nearing the end of life does not have an advance directive in place. Particularly when dementia prevents people from stating their wishes, the power of attorney (POA) or guardian must make decisions based on what the person may have once said or what the POA or guardian believes that person would choose.

Even if you feel very settled about your own end-of-life wishes, making similar choices for another person is a tremendous emotional burden. Having the support and backing of your family can reduce your stress and feelings of self-doubt. The reverse may happen when family members express opinions opposite to yours.

Talking about end-of-life care, particularly when it's not theoretical, is similar to discussing politics or religion. Everyone is an expert, feelings run deep, differences become personal affronts, and conversation, civilized or not, rarely changes minds. Rather than enduring never-ending phone calls and e-mail messages, consider organizing a family conference call or a gathering at a local restaurant or coffee shop.

Try to have an impartial person, such as a family friend, medical social worker, or eldercare manager, present to guide discussion. The presence of a third party, in addition to acting as a moderator, may reduce angry outbursts. Meeting in a public place like a coffee shop or a restaurant is another way to quiet difficult behaviors. But do remember, as your loved one's POA or guardian, you are the person ultimately responsible for making the end-of-life decisions.

TURNING ANOTHER CORNER

Dorothy never spoke directly to me about her end-of-life wishes. The little conversation we did have occurred many years ago and was in reference to other people. Sometimes she would say, "It is sad when people have to suffer." Other times she would say, "Where there is life, there is hope."

I do know that when doctors asked about a living will, she would laugh at the silliness of needing such a document. She always said she could wait until a change in her health made a living will necessary.

For similar reasons, arranging the medical power of attorney was another stumbling block. Many people tried to help her understand the importance of "just in case."

Fortunately, I managed to avoid guardianship and conservator proceedings when I found a lawyer who knew Dorothy and felt she was competent enough to know what she was signing (see chapter 6); however, Dorothy stated in her advance directive that she wanted her life to be "prolonged for as long as possible within the limits of generally accepted health care standards." Obviously, she did not sign a DNR.

It no longer surprises me that Dorothy chose life-prolonging measures over something more neutral like "letting my agent decide." Still, it worried me that a person who claimed to understand the consequences of life-prolonging measures fought against wearing postsurgical compression stockings. Did she really understand the reality of tube feeding, respirators, and cardiac defibrillation?

Not having a DNR was another source of deep concern. Because Dorothy had severe and debilitating osteoporosis, any resuscitation attempts would crush her ribs. To me, what Dorothy had defined for her end-of-life care was totally incompatible with any measure of quality of life or a death free from pain and suffering. Her decision left me feeling ethically compromised and emotionally spent.

JUST ONE SIGNATURE

It didn't take long for my inner turmoil to emerge as an ongoing dinnertime monologue. At first my husband listened. But it didn't take long before he directed his attention elsewhere. My friends didn't run, but I am sure they became tired of hearing about Dorothy and her (lack of) living will. My therapist didn't have a choice. She sat demurely in her chair and nodded in agreement to what I said.

Dorothy's doctor assured me things would work out in the end. He told me clinicians interpret the part about "generally accepted health care standards" to prevent the "grisly" situation I envisioned. Slowly, I calmed down.

A few days after Dorothy entered the assisted living facility, her new doctor and I spoke at length about his findings and her care. It was interesting to hear what he had to say. He described Dorothy as having "severe dementia and delusions of grandiosity." He also said that smart people who have dementia can be very difficult patients.

I mentioned my concerns about Dorothy's advance directive. He responded by saying that, as Dorothy's POA, it was my responsibility to make decisions that were in her best interest. Period. His approach made everything seem so simple!

The facility nurse expressed her concern about Dorothy's request for resuscitation. Apparently, Dorothy was the only resident in the facility who did not have a DNR. The nurse went on to say that she would be the one called in to do the resuscitation. She described how awful it is hear the noise of ribs cracking with each chest compression. A few moments later, and without any second thoughts, I signed Dorothy's DNR order.

DEMENTIA AT ITS TERMINUS

It's hard to think of dementia as a terminal illness. After all, the first symptoms seem to be nothing more than memory loss and difficult behavior. And unlike many other life-threatening diseases, people can live as long as ten to fifteen years after receiving a diagnosis of dementia. There is a good chance that heart disease, diabetes, or cancer will cause death long before the arrival of late-stage dementia.

Dementia is a progressive disease that destroys the brain bit by bit. Dementia first affects the parts of the brain that form memories and control behavior, cognition, and executive function (see chapter 2). With time, and as the disease destroys other brain functions, people lose the ability to swallow food, speak, and maintain balance. Eventually, your loved one will lose the ability to control their bowel and bladder and regulate body temperature. Death occurs when the brain can no longer regulate heart rate, breathing, and other fundamental body functions; however, most people—even if they are otherwise healthy—do not live that long. Something else happens that puts them into a downward spiral.

Eating and swallowing difficulties are often the "something else." An early sign of ensuing eating problems is the inability to coordinate using a fork and knife. Eventually, your family member will transition to finger foods and then to needing another person to hand- or spoon-feed them.

One day, Dorothy stopped using her dinner knife. Rather than using a knife and fork together, she used the side of her fork to cut food into smaller pieces. The noise of the fork scraping against the plate was painful. Watching her struggle to eat her dinner was painful. Resisting the temptation to take over, I asked if she would like some help.

Not unexpectedly, she declined and blamed tough chicken for her difficulties. Up until then, not driving and having to use the walker were her biggest insults and ones I could pass off as her doctor's orders. Somehow, the "doctor excuse" did not translate well in this situation.

The easy solutions were to serve foods that didn't require cutting or could be easily cut with a fork. One night, I cut everyone's food into bite-sized pieces before serving. Although far from a good solution, that strategy helped me and my husband understand that eating cut-up foods that we normally cut ourselves is both strange and remarkably unsatisfying.

Eating Difficulties

Eating difficulties become more serious when the person in your care can no longer synchronize chewing, moving food to the back of the mouth, and then swallowing. Pocketing, when food accumulates between the teeth and cheek, is a related difficulty.

It's hard to imagine that chewing and swallowing, something we do without thinking, could be the problem that makes us wonder, "What else could go wrong?" As it turns out, chewing and swallowing is a surprisingly complicated process. Nerve bundles coordinate communication between the brain and the more than fifty muscles it takes to chew and swallow food.

At this point, your family member's doctor might mention dysphagia, the medical term for difficulty in swallowing. The doctor may also recommend that your family member undergo one of several swallowing tests. The X-ray with contrast media requires that your family member drink a barium solution. The barium coats the esophagus, enhancing light and dark contrast, which makes it easier to see areas where food accumulates.

Some people say the barium solution tastes and feels like drinking ground-up chalk in water. It's not terrible, but it may be difficult to convince a person who has dementia to drink enough of it.

A variant of the barium swallow test involves having your family member swallow barium solutions of various thicknesses or a pill or solid food coated with barium. A speech pathologist will watch the muscles in your family member's throat, noting any problems with sputtering and coughing, as they swallow the liquid or barium-coated substance. A radiologist will evaluate the X-ray.

Unlike the still X-ray examinations most of us have experienced at one time or another, the barium swallow test is dynamic in that it shows moving parts.

A third swallowing assessment option is a visual examination. For this test, a doctor uses an endoscope, which is a thin, flexible, lighted instrument placed in the nose or down the throat. The view from the nose allows the clinician to see the esophagus and observe your loved one's ability to coordinate a swallow.

To learn more about swallowing and swallowing difficulties, use your internet browser and various combinations of the following keywords: "dysphagia," "barium," "swallowing test," "endoscope," "dynamic X-ray," and "video."

Many dysphagia treatments require the ability to follow and remember directions; therefore, exercises to help coordinate swallowing muscles or learning different ways to place food in the mouth may be too complicated for people who have dementia. Other options include hand-feeding small amounts of soft or liquefied foods.

For caregivers, solving feeding problems may be the first of what will become many end-of-life decisions. The immediate goals are to provide enough calories to prevent weight loss and malnutrition, as well as to prevent choking and aspiration. Respect and preserving dignity also figure into these decisions, as do the differences among quality of life, extending life, or saving a life. The combination of coordination problems and nerve dysfunction can cause people who have advanced dementia to inhale food, saliva, stomach acid, and expelled vomit into their lungs. Having food and other substances bypass the esophagus and enter the lungs through the trachea can cause lung inflammation, abscesses, and aspiration pneumonia.

Some doctors believe tube feeding will avoid these complications; however, research shows that using feeding tubes in patients with late-stage dementia neither prevents complications nor improves quality of life. Intravenous antibiotics to clear the infection are a usual treatment for aspiration pneumonia. If your family member lives in an assisted living facility, you may discover the facility does not have nursing staff qualified to start or monitor an intravenous (IV) line. Nursing homes, although they do have registered nurses who can manage an IV line, may claim they are too busy to provide the extra care your loved one needs. For these reasons, the doctor may suggest hospitalization.

Less Aggressive Care

It can feel a little strange to be the first person to mention less aggressive care. You wonder if it makes you seem uncaring or perhaps a little ghoulishly wishful. Some of your family may agree to less invasive management, or they may become angry with you. Other close family members might be very quiet and then appoint one of them to discuss the situation with you.

The topic of less aggressive care is a delicate matter. Family members who have not been a part of day-to-day care may not realize the depth of illness. They may not understand that dementia, more than memory loss and confusion, is terminal. Maybe the last time they saw their loved one she seemed like she was doing well—maybe a little repetitive—but basically okay.

Some family members are not ready to let go. They cannot believe their loved one is failing. They do not understand that dementia often takes a slow and somewhat unpredictable path.

Mentioning less aggressive care with the doctor in charge of your loved one's care may create another set of challenges. Some doctors are clearly uncomfortable talking about end-of-life care with their patients or their patients' families. Some clinicians, instead of speaking openly, will use code words or phrases like "Would you like us to divert food?" No, they are not asking permission to give your mother's lunch to the lady down the hall. "Tube feeding" is the phrase they are trying to avoid.

If you should speak to a physician or other clinician who talks in code, ask questions! Tell them you don't understand. Ask them to clarify who the "us" is who will divert food and if tube feedings reduce or create problems that impact length or quality of life.

Many clinicians prefer to take an advisory role. So, rather than telling you what to do, they will help you make well-informed decisions compatible with your personal beliefs. Again, it is important to ask questions and to discuss your thoughts with family members. Inquire about the pros and cons of each alternative the doctor presents and the likelihood of a particular treatment extending or improving quality of life.

Talking with other family members can be helpful. It feels good to get their support. Even disagreements, because they both test your conviction and introduce new ideas for consideration, can be useful. In the end, as your loved one's POA, it is important you feel comfortable with your decision.

END-OF-LIFE AND PALLIATIVE CARE

We often hear about people who undergo arduous treatments and interventions, such as surgery and harsh medications, in the belief that doing so will allow them to live longer. Often, rather than enjoying time with their family or attending to their "bucket list," many spend their remaining days in incapacitating postsurgical pain or in a drug-induced fog.

How many of us, if asked or given a choice, would say, "Let's go for the bucket list." Somehow we find it difficult to say the same when a family member or a close friend faces a similar situation.

In chapter 5, you read about the benefits of palliative care during the early stages of a life-threatening disease like dementia. Palliative care, or comfort care, takes on a different focus as your loved one transitions into the mid and late stages of the disease and can no longer speak on their own behalf. Now, all discussions are between you and your loved one's health care team.

Many comfort care decisions are difficult ones. When family disharmony interferes with the ability to take next steps, a palliative care team professional can guide meaningful and productive conversation among family members.

Dorothy had an informal palliative care team. The doctor she had seen for many years continued to provide care. Because he practiced at a large university hospital, a nurse case manager and a medical social worker were also available to her. Both were very helpful and often acted as intermediaries between Dorothy and me. Calling either of them with questions or concerns was considerably more efficient than trying to reach her doctor by phone. Fortunately, Dorothy's doctor was willing to correspond by e-mail and the clinic's Patient Portal system. The nurse case manager and the medical social worker became important elements in my support system. They listened, were empathetic, and made useful and practical suggestions.

At one point, Dorothy's doctor felt she might be better served in the geriatric clinic where they had a formal palliative care team. We gave it a try, and as I mentioned in chapter 6, it did not work. There were too many new people involved; Dorothy simply could not tolerate having strangers taking a too-kindly interest in her.

Dorothy's last straw was the well-meaning counselor who invited her to come and talk about anything that might be bothering her. Most people would welcome that kind of attention. But to Dorothy, that raised the paranoia flag. For many years, Dorothy assumed anyone who asked how she was doing meant other people were talking about her. Needless to say, her brief encounter with the counselor made the rest of the day very difficult for everyone.

PALLIATIVE CARE AND DIFFICULT DECISIONS

Feeding difficulties and aspiration pneumonia are often the first test of your ability to make end-of-life decisions for another person. Insufficient calories and nutrients make death a certainty. The alternatives to imposed starvation are spoon-feeding, hand-feeding, and tube feeding. Although tube feeding does deliver calories and nutrients, research shows that this practice may actually increase risk for aspiration pneumonia.

Spoon-feeding, although time consuming, addresses the patient's comfort. In comparison to starvation or tube feeding, hand-feeding contributes to a positive quality of life. If the person in your care can no longer sit, providing hydration with ice chips or a dampened cloth may be the most appropriate next step.

The swallow test mentioned earlier is another decision point. Choking makes it obvious that the person in your care is having difficulty chewing food and moving it to the back of the mouth. The swallow test is invasive and causes mild discomfort. It may be difficult to get a person who has dementia to follow directions and cooperate. Will undergoing a swallow test do more than confirm what you already know? Will it change your loved one's care?

Table 13.1.   Palliative or Nonpalliative Care for People in Late-Stage Dementia

Palliative Care	Nonpalliative Care
Hand-Feeding	Tube Feeding
Improves oral hygiene	May increase risk for aspiration
May lower risk for aspiration	Does not prevent malnutrition
Provides social contact and comfort	Does not improve comfort or quality of life
Respects the patient's dignity	Does not extend life
Improves quality of life	
Restricts cardiopulmonary resuscitation	Cardiopulmonary Resuscitation
Recognizes stages of active death	Futile effort
	Most die within twenty-four hours
	Causes injury
	Traumatic for family and other witnesses
Hospitalization	Hospitalization
Palliative care unit within a hospital	Often does not extend life
Provides on-site treatment	Causes confusion and psychosis
	Increases risk for infection
Antibiotics	Antibiotics
Reduces pain of infection	Less likely to be effective
Low relative harm	May or may not prolong life
Reduces fever and delirium	Antibiotic resistance
Respects family's need to "do something"	

Whether to use antibiotics is yet another difficult decision. Again, patient comfort and potential for regaining an acceptable quality of life are the palliative care guideposts. Aspirin or Tylenol (acetaminophen) may be sufficient to reduce fever. Conversely, if the patient is delirious and agitated, then antibiotics do become a comfort treatment (table 13.1).

Hospitalization also weighs in as part of the overall decision. Even though research shows that hospitalization does not extend life, many clinicians do not feel comfortable providing care in another setting. Many clinicians and families do not consider replacing hospitalization with private health care services. Home health care agencies can send a health care provider to your loved one's home who is qualified to administer antibiotics, give inoculations, and start and manage intravenous lines. And do remember, "home" also includes your loved one's assisted living facility.

Medicare does not pay for home nursing services. So unless your loved one has additional insurance that covers the added expense, affordability often becomes part of the equation.

Aspiration pneumonia, although common, is not every caregiver's test of their ability to make hard decisions for the person in their care. Worksheet 13.1 poses some general questions that can help define your decision-making processes.

TRANSITION TO HOSPICE

Not unexpectedly, end-stage congestive heart failure (CHF) caused rapid changes in Dorothy's health. Dorothy rarely got out of bed. She slept for most of the day and seldom spoke. When she did speak, it was to ask when she could go home. It seemed as if going home was the only thing on her mind.

Saying, "When you heart gets better" was a mistake. It made her angry.

When, a few seconds later, she repeated the question, I resorted to the old standby, "When your doctor says it is okay."

Dorothy fought the supplemental oxygen. She demanded that the caregivers remove it. Sometimes Dorothy removed the tubing herself. It only took a minute or two before she became short of breath and frantic. Dorothy couldn't associate one with the other.

To relieve distressing symptoms, Dorothy received medications to help her heart work more efficiently, to reduce the accumulation of fluid, and to relieve shortness of breath and feelings of fatigue and weakness. She also received medication to calm increasing restlessness.

For all practical purposes, Dorothy stopped eating. The combination of CHF with having some degree of difficulty chewing and swallowing food made eating too much work. The split second when one holds their breath to swallow was too much for her.

The facility caregivers began hand-feeding foods like gelatin, clear broth, and pudding. Not a balanced diet by any means. Just some calories to keep things going.

It seemed like I received phone calls on an hourly basis. Dorothy refused her medication. Did I want them to try again? Dorothy insisted on getting out of bed without help and fell. What did I want them to do?

I suggested bed rails. I was surprised to learn that restraints, which include bed rails, are not allowed in assisted living facilities. As the facility nurse put it, according to the state regulations they had to follow, "residents have the right to fall out of bed." After discussing other solutions to prevent Dorothy from hurting herself, we finally arrived at attaching a motion sensor to her bed. A buzzer would let caregivers know when Dorothy was becoming restless and perhaps attempting to get out of bed without assistance.

At first, these "what to do" questions surprised me and made me realize that I, as Dorothy's POA, was the person responsible for overseeing her care. In the end, these relatively simple questions helped prepare me for the really difficult ones.

With this turn of events, I visited more often and stayed longer. Most of the time, I was little more than a presence. During those quiet moments, I wondered if Dorothy and I would have one of those conversations. You know—the kind you read about in novels or see in movies—the kind where people say things to clarify a lifetime of painful misunderstandings. I figured dementia pretty much made that impossible.

A few days later, the doctor asked to speak with me. "Your mother has given up."

At first, I didn't realize he was using code. Then, I realized what he really meant was, "Your mother is dying."

I said, "It's time to call hospice."

HOSPICE

Hospice is a place, but mostly hospice is a philosophy of end-of-life care. Hospice is like the "Part B" of palliative care. People often receive hospice care in their own home. Hospice nurses and other support caregivers also provide care in assisted living facilities, nursing homes, and hospitals. Some people choose to go to a freestanding hospice center to receive their end-of-life care.

Most hospice caregivers work for an agency similar to the home care organizations you may have used earlier in your loved one's illness. Others work for hospitals that provide hospice care. Usually your loved one's doctor, or the facility where they are currently staying, will give you a list of recommended hospice agencies to contact. As always, friends are another good resource. Be sure to ask if the organization is certified by the Centers for Medicare and Medicaid Services (CMS). Only CMS-certified agencies can receive Medicare and Medicaid reimbursements.

Hospice caregivers include palliative care physicians, physician assistants, nurses, and nurse practitioners who have the training and the licensures required to provide specialized care. Other caregivers include medical social workers, home health aides, psychologists, physical therapists, chaplains, and bereavement specialists.

Because volunteers founded the hospice movement in the United States, there is an ongoing commitment to volunteerism. According to the National Hospice and Palliative Care Organization, in 2019, 420,000 trained volunteers contributed nineteen million hours of service to more than 1.5 million patients and their families. Volunteers spend time with patients and families, provide patient care and clinical services, help with fund-raising efforts, and serve on the hospice board of directors.

The focus of palliative and hospice care is to provide medical and emotional comfort for people who have life-threatening illnesses; however, unlike the palliative care described earlier and in chapter 6, hospice is for people who have less than six months to live. Hospice patients who outlive the six-month period can be recertified for additional sixty-day periods. It's not unheard of, but sometimes people do receive hospice services for one year or longer. It is also true that some people leave hospice when their prognosis improves or if they opt to receive curative treatments.

With home-centered hospice care, the next of kin (spouse) or the designated caregiver—with the guidance of hospice professionals—makes decisions if the terminally ill family member cannot speak for themselves. But family members and friends are welcome to feed, read, sing, or in other ways lend a comforting presence.

Hospice staff members make regularly scheduled visits to assess the patient and provide care that requires special training or skills (table 13.2).

Table 13.2.   Overview of Home-Based Hospice Services

Meet with family.
Develop a care plan.
Manage pain and symptoms.
Assist patient with the emotional, psychosocial, and spiritual aspects of confronting death.
Provide medicines, medical supplies, and equipment.
Give family caregiving instructions.
Provide special services (e.g., speech and physical therapy).
Provide short-term inpatient care when pain or symptoms are too difficult to treat at home.
Provide short-term respite care.
Provide bereavement care and counseling to family and friends.

In many ways, hospice care in assisted living facilities or freestanding hospice centers is similar to home-based care; however, the POA caregiver is still responsible for making decisions when the terminally ill family member cannot speak on their own behalf.

For the most part, the hospice services Dorothy received were those above and beyond what the assisted living facility could offer. Hospice nurses gave Dorothy medication to help her breathe and to prevent anxiety and restlessness. They also provided oxygen, a more comfortable bed, disposable gloves, mattress protectors, and other sundries.

A hospice caregiver bathed her, gave massages, and put lotion on her dry skin. The assisted living caregivers didn't disappear and often stopped by to keep her company.

Dorothy did not know that she was receiving special care; however, she must have realized something was different when she told me about all those nice people. Hearing those few words helped me feel better about moving her to the assisted living facility.

Dorothy was more than a loner. She shunned contact and the kinds of things caring people do for one another. It made me happy to hear that she accepted those small tokens of uncomplicated human kindness.

A friend told me about her experience when her mother went to a dedicated hospice center. She praised the emotional support she and her mother received and reminisced over the little things that made such a wonderful difference: hospice cooks who made favorite foods for patients who could do little more than enjoy the aroma, homemade comfort foods for family members, quiet gardens for escape and respite, and the volunteers who were always there to lend a helping hand. My friend called hospice a very life-affirming experience.

Hospice Criteria

Before your loved one can transition into hospice care, they must meet statistically determined criteria for living roughly six months or less. Another requirement is a signed statement affirming the use of palliative care and not curative treatment. Medicare calls these eligibility standards the Conditions of Participation.

The Palliative Performance Scale (PPS) is one of several assessment tools doctors use to determine eligibility for hospice care (see table 13.3). The PPS scale evaluates five characteristics: the ability to walk, work, perform activities of daily living, eat, and converse with others. The lower the PPS score, the more likely death will occur within six months.

As an aside, you might find it interesting to know that the last skills acquired in childhood—the ability to perform sequential and complex tasks—are some of the first noticeable losses linked to dementia, whereas the ability to smile, something babies learn at about six weeks of age, remains almost to the end. Barry Reisberg, MD, coined the word *retrogenesis* to describe the sequentially reversed developmental steps dementia causes.

Hospice and Dementia

It's never easy to tell how long a person with a terminal disease may live. Some diseases, such as cancer and congestive heart failure, take a fairly predictable downhill path. Other diseases, such as dementia, do not. Because it is hard to tell how long a person with dementia will live, relatively few people who enter hospice have dementia as their primary diagnosis. According to the 2019 National Hospice and Palliative Care Organization report, of the people who choose hospice care, 31 percent have cancer, 18 percent have heart disease, and 15 percent have dementia as their primary diagnosis.

Table 13.3. Palliative Performance Scale (PPS)

Percent	Ambulation	Activity	Self-Care	Food Intake	Consciousness
100	Full	Normal	Full	Normal	Full
90	Full	Normal, some evidence of disease	Full	Normal	Full
80	Full	Normal activity with effort, evidence of disease	Full	Normal or reduced	Full
70	Reduced	Unable to do normal work, evidence of disease	Full	Normal or reduced	Full
60	Reduced	Unable to do hobby or housework, significant disease	Occasional assistance	Normal or reduced	Full or confusion
50	Mostly sit/lie in bed	Unable to do any work, extensive disease	Considerable assistance	Normal or reduced	Full or confusion
40	Mostly in bed	Unable to do any work, extensive disease	Mainly assistance	Normal or reduced	Full or drowsy +/– confusion
30	Bed bound	Unable to do any work, extensive disease	Total care	Reduced	Full or drowsy +/– confusion
20	Bed bound	Unable to do any work, extensive disease	Total care	Minimal sips	Full or drowsy +/– confusion
10	Bed bound	Unable to do any work, extensive disease	Total care	Mouth care only	Drowsy or coma
0	Death				

Note: Adapted from L. Scott Wilner and Robert Arnold, "The Palliative Performance Scale (PPS)," Palliative Care Network of Wisconsin, accessed June 6, 2020, https://www .mypcnow.org/fast-fact/the-palliative-performance-scale-pps/.

Other diseases like HIV/AIDS and lung, kidney, and liver diseases constitute the remainder of admissions.

The six-month rule is certainly one reason that makes it unlikely that people who have dementia as their only diagnosis will receive hospice care. Another reason is that family members and some physicians alike wrongly assume hospice is only for people who have cancer. The same National Hospice and Palliative Care Organization report mentioned earlier shows that people who have diseases other than cancer constitute nearly 67 percent of the people in hospice care.

Another reason for low representation in hospice is that dementia is not always recognized as a fatal disease. Death is often attributed to secondary causes (such as pneumonia or malnutrition) or a coexisting condition (such as cancer or cardiopulmonary disease). Research shows that people in late-stage dementia, similar to people who have terminal cancer, experience distressing symptoms like pain, shortness of breath, pressure ulcers, aspiration, and agitation.

Cost of Hospice Care

As one assisted living facility director put it, "Hospice is your last gift from the government." Medicare and Medicaid are the payers for nearly 90 percent of people receiving hospice care. Those not covered by Medicare or Medicaid receive coverage from managed care plans, private insurance, or, in a few instances, charity. The bottom line is that nearly everyone can receive hospice care regardless of their ability to pay.

According to the National Hospice and Palliative Care Organization, more than 90 percent of hospice agencies are certified by the CMS to provide services under the Medicare hospice benefit. Noncertified agencies are those currently seeking certification and those that are donation-based and all-volunteer programs.

Medicare and Medicaid pay for comfort care and other services directly related to the illness that made your family member eligible to receive hospice care. Hospice expenses unrelated to the primary diagnosis are usually covered by your family member's private insurance carrier. If your family member does not have additional insurance, then other payment sources, such as donation funds marked for such purposes, may be available.

LONG-LASTING WORDS

I know he was just trying to be kind. But those words "Your mother has given up," took on a different meaning. Maybe Dorothy gave up because the daughter she trusted couldn't find a way to get her out of there. Maybe, if I hadn't taken Dorothy from her home in the first place, she would have had many more months of enjoying the wild birds that came to her window and listening to the National Public Radio station. Maybe Dorothy would have had the good fortune to die in her own bed. The emotional side of me still hangs on to those thoughts and makes me feel like I failed her.

My intellectual side tells me otherwise. Her caregivers and I were getting worn out from trying to stay ahead of progressively bizarre and difficult behavior. Falls and nocturnal wandering meant that thirteen hours a day of home care was neither sufficient nor safe.

In retrospect, it is obvious that end-stage congestive heart failure no longer was a silent partner. I cannot imagine the difficulty of getting her to the doctor when breathing problems and edema took over. More than likely Dorothy would have ended up in the hospital, a place where the goal is to cure people. Undoubtedly, she would have had to endure many last-ditch and futile efforts to stabilize her condition.

I wonder if the transition to hospice care, either at home or at the hospital, would have occurred as seamlessly as it did in the assisted living facility. Having an on-staff physician made the difference. The assisted living facility doctor evaluated Dorothy daily—and sometimes more frequently than that. Unlike many clinicians, he was comfortable with end-of-life care.

The assisted living facility wasn't Dorothy's true home, but a favorite chair and being surrounded by a collection of family mementos hopefully made it comfortable enough for her.

Without question, I passed many invisible lines miles and miles ago. Moving her to an assisted living facility, even though it was difficult, was the right thing to do.

FREQUENTLY ASKED QUESTIONS

1. My mother is in early-stage dementia. She likes the idea of palliative care but is afraid it will prevent her from having the latest treatments. I am trying to convince her only good things can happen when doctors focus on the patient's comfort and well-being. Is there anything else I can say to her?

First of all, until we find a way to cure dementia, all dementia care is palliative care. But what you can tell your mother is that palliative care patients frequently do receive treatment for their condition. You can also tell her that she is not obligated to stay in a palliative care program.

2. My father's health is failing. He is in mid-stage dementia and end-stage kidney disease. Is he eligible for hospice?

This is a bit of a tricky question. For your father to be eligible for hospice, his doctor must provide evidence that your father is not likely to live for another six months. Mid-stage dementia does not qualify as it is not possible to predict the likelihood of death occurring within six months.

End-stage kidney failure is another matter. The Medicare Conditions of Participation include no dialysis treatment, as well as blood and urine tests that demonstrate significantly impaired kidney function.

3. My father has early-stage dementia and end-stage emphysema. My sister, who is my father's POA, refuses to consider hospice. She says hospice means we are giving up. She calls hospice a "death watch" operation. It saddens me to see how much my father suffers. In the past, he told me that he is ready to die but that he is afraid of pain and struggling to breathe.

You and your sister have opposing deep-seated convictions and beliefs. Perhaps your father's siblings can provide helpful input; however, as POA, your sister is the person responsible for making health care decisions for your father.

If competent, your father can retract his POA and reassign it to you or another person. Your sister, claiming lack of competency and cohesion, may fight his decision and take you to court. You, of course, can begin guardianship and conservator proceedings. As you can see, for many reasons it might be better to leave things as they are.

Do take advantage of this difficult time to speak with your immediate family. Tell them how you feel about your father's situation and what you would want for yourself. If you haven't already, write your advance directive and assign POA responsibilities. Our behavior during these trying times has a tremendous influence on the next generation. Give them the opportunity to learn from your actions.

WORKSHEET 13.1:
Difficult Questions

Sometimes answers to smaller questions can help reveal a logical answer to a big question.

1. Is this the first time the person in your care has required emergency care or hospitalization (for any reason) in the last six months?
2. Is this the first time the person in your care has required emergency care or hospitalization for a particular condition or illness?
3. How many times has your loved one required emergency care or hospitalization for this particular condition or illness?
4. Did stabilization or treatment improve comfort or quality of life?
5. Has the doctor suggested easier ways to provide comfort and improve quality of life?
6. Are you comfortable speaking to the doctor about comfort care?
7. Do you feel you have a good understanding of the complications and prognosis associated with having dementia?
8. Are you receiving pressure from other family members to provide a different kind of care for your loved one?
9. List three or four questions you would like to ask the doctor.
10. What advice would you give to another person in your same situation?
11. What decisions would you make for yourself if you were in the same situation as the person in your care?

14

PASSING

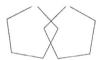

Woman, age seventy-three, pentagon.

I had always believed that when people said "passed" it meant they were too afraid to say "died." I now know they were describing something real. Unlike people who die suddenly as a result of an accident or a massive heart attack, Dorothy stopped eating, became distant, wandered in and out of consciousness, and finally, when breathing became nothing more than an inefficient reflex, she slipped away.

I feel fortunate to have been there for her passing. I don't know if she felt my presence—it was perhaps too strange a concept for her. My focus was intense. I listened to her labored breathing. I counted the moments of silence until I heard another inhalation. I heard crackles as liquid seeped into her lungs. I counted forty-one, forty-two, forty-three seconds until I heard another heave. I counted fifty-eight, fifty-nine seconds, one minute, and then no more.

We often talk about quality of life and rarely the quality of dying. We hope it is painless and without fear. We believe that something grand and wondrous may happen in those last moments—peace, serenity, or even visions of a heavenly warm glow. I don't know if any of that is real. Maybe it is just something bystanders create to justify their presence, calm their own fears, and reduce an inborn abhorrence of the situation.

A good death—what does that mean? Family nearby? Touching, caressing, calming words, music, or singing? Medication to reduce pain and anxiety and to ease breathing? Doctors say, rather than terminating life more quickly, medication may extend life and provide a bit of time for last words and reconciliation.

Medication to make breathing less difficult did give Dorothy a small gift. I have to admit that her rebound was not entirely welcomed. I had prepared myself for the end, and now it seemed as though there might be more. A nurse said this could go on for weeks, and yes, it was hard on the family. My mother had a blood pressure so low it was not measurable, and yet she insisted on getting out of bed to use the toilet. She asked for water, had some soup, and slipped back into that place between wakefulness and sleep.

Then, after many days of comparative silence, she spoke. Rather than gestures, grunts, and "yes" and "no" responses, my mother had things to say. Over and over again she said she loved my vegetable garden. She stated she wanted to go home and wondered when the doctor would allow her to drive. Death came the next day at 4:48 p.m.

At first, I was grateful that her last words didn't include her usual tirade about my hair or clothing. But the business about the vegetable garden stuck; it hung in the air. Why did she say that, and was there a larger significance to her words?

I know she appreciated the fresh produce I frequently brought to her home. Later, I recalled that her mother, my grandmother, fed a family of seven children from a kitchen garden. And I remembered how much my children enjoyed hearing Dorothy's stories about making homemade root beer and sauerkraut and the antics of their great-grandmother's chickens. And then I knew. This was Dorothy's way of connecting the generations. It was her way of saying that by some measure we had shared a good life together.

DYING OF DEMENTIA

Dying of dementia is not the same as dying of cancer or pneumonia. With dementia, the dying process begins many years before the physical signs of impending death. From the perspective of family members, the dying begins when a loved one no longer remembers the history they once shared with you.

As the disease progresses, one begins to see a separation between the personality you once knew and the body that contains your loved one. The memories that form bonds between family members and friends are the first to go. Then, when executive functions fail, the special abilities—gardening, cooking, making art, composing music, woodworking, and sewing—depart. As late-stage dementia approaches, we mourn the loss of our loved one's infectiously warm smile, mischievous expression, or wonderful laugh. It's a little less than terrifying, but those losses help us appreciate that people are more than an appearance.

Sometimes it almost seems that dementia is catching like a cold or strep throat. Your family member's seemingly distorted memories can make you feel confused and perhaps ungrounded.

One friend said that her father's dementia made it difficult for her to remember the words for common objects. Her doctor did an MR scan just to make sure her word loss problem wasn't anything more than stress.

Long before the death of a loved one, families may feel a profound sense of loss. People grieve for the person they once knew, the loss of future plans and dreams, and the companionship and relationship they once shared. They grieve over the loss of personal freedom and perhaps the finances or lifestyle they once took for granted.

Caring for a person who has dementia is an emotionally difficult job. Feelings run rampant and swing from despair and denial to anger and resentment. Sometimes the family caregiver wishes for their loved one's death. Anyone who has been a caregiver for a person who has dementia will admit to experiencing some or all of these emotions.

When death (finally) arrives many years later, the family caregiver may feel unburdened and relieved. Other people may be surprised at the apparent lack of sadness. They wonder if there is something wrong and ask too many personal questions.

The family caregiver may have a difficult time connecting their sense of loss to grief and grieving. Some family caregivers do respond to well-wisher inquires by saying, "No, I don't feel particularly sad." Then, to counteract surprised looks, they follow up by explaining they started grieving years ago.

Relief often gives way to guilt and self-doubt. It's important to find ways to help yourself understand that you did the best you could. Talking with understanding friends and family can be helpful. Seeking counsel from clergy, a medical social worker, or a psychologist can make a wonderfully positive difference.

STAGES OF DYING

Just like birth, growth, and development, dying is a process described by a continuum of smaller, somewhat orderly, steps. Withdrawal from social contact is often the first clue that indicates a person has begun to die. This step, which occurs one to three months prior to death, is probably easier to recognize in retrospect.

Some say withdrawal is a mental processing stage when the person who has a terminal disease begins to separate from the world around them. Some use phrases like "withdrawal from outside influences" and "go inside to evaluate self" to describe what happens during this phase.

A person who is beginning to turn inward may speak less frequently, lose interest in pleasurable activities, and stop reading newspapers, watching television, or accepting visits from neighbors and friends. Spending all day in bed and more time asleep than awake becomes the new normal. In a way, their inward isolation helps prepare everyone for what happens next.

It's hard to say if the withdrawal step translates well to people who are in the later stages of dementia. Do people who cannot recognize themselves in the mirror or who believe they are living in their childhood home have the capacity for this kind of deeply self-reflective and meditative thought? It's hard to know and even harder to definitively prove or disprove. Maybe knowing one way or the other really isn't important.

A quick review of Dorothy's caregiver's notes shows that, shortly before her move to the assisted living facility, Dorothy was sleeping for the greater part of the day. When awake, she sometimes spoke about vivid dreams and visiting with people who were long dead. Other times she would wake up fearful, angry, and unable to separate from deep sleep and dreams.

A week or two before death, people enter a phase that palliative care practitioners call "active dying." During this time, body functions begin to shut down. The signs of approaching death are specific to the dying process and are distinct from the effects of a particular illness the person may have. Most people experience some or all of the eleven signs of impending death.

As energy needs decline and the ability to digest food wanes, your loved one may resist or refuse to eat. There may be times when they will eat small amounts of bland foods, such as clear broth or mashed potatoes. It's important to follow their cues and not try to force food. Tube feeding is both unwarranted and inappropriate at this time.

Do offer ice chips, a frozen juice bar, or sips of water. You can use a moistened towel around the mouth and apply lip balm to the lips to keep their mouth and lips moist and comfortable. Near the very end of life, and for reasons not related to having dementia, your loved one may lose the ability to swallow.

Soon, as metabolism slows further and the decline in food and water consumption contributes to dehydration, your loved one will enter a deep sleep for the majority of the day and night. Do not try to waken them. But do assume they can hear what you say. Many clinicians believe people do hear when unconscious or in a coma. Although your loved one can no longer respond to your words, speaking in a soft, comforting tone creates a soothing setting and lets them know they are not alone.

Soft music, comfortable lighting, gentle massage, and perhaps a little incense or the aroma of a favorite food are all ways to create a comforting ambience for everyone. Tactile stimuli are especially good if your loved one is hard of hearing. As you can see, communication is now entirely sensory—soft sounds and lighting, gentle touch, and pleasant aromas.

I didn't know how I would respond when Dorothy entered active dying. Our relationship was never one that included hugs or comforting words. I had heard that some daughters get into bed with their dying mother. Now, many years later, I wish I could have done better.

Quiet murmurs and gentle massage were my intuitive and heartfelt response. Dorothy's favorite National Public Radio station played in the background. No incense. Neither of us cared for that sort of thing.

Attention to comfort becomes even more important as energy levels decline further and your loved one can no longer move in bed, raise their head from the pillow, or sip from a straw. With the help of the hospice caregiver, reposition your loved one several times a day to prevent bedsores and other breaks in the skin. It is also important that the hospice nurse keeps your loved one clean and regularly changes their clothing and undergarments.

Your loved one will become confused and disoriented as organs, including the brain, begin to fail. Some of these mental changes are caused by kidney and liver failure and the accumulation of toxic metabolic by-products. Urine will be scant and brown or tea colored.

Your love one may not be aware of their location or if there are others in the room. Your loved one may mutter, cry out, grimace, become restless, or pick at the sheets. Your loved one may feel anxious, struggle to breathe, or appear uncomfortable or in pain. The hospice nurse or doctor can give medication to manage these symptoms.

You will also notice changes in your loved one's breathing pattern. Rather than a steady rhythm of inhalations and exhalations, you may hear a deep and loud inhalation followed by a period lasting as long as a minute when breathing ceases. Another change is hearing loud crackling or gurgling noises. These noises, sometimes called a "death rattle," are caused by secretions that accumulate at the back of the throat and in the lungs.

Although you and the other people in the room may find these noises disturbing, your loved one is unaware of the changes in their breathing. Again, comfort care is the best approach. Use a pillow to elevate the head and move your loved one onto their side to let secretions drain from the mouth. You can also ask the hospice nurse for medication to reduce excessive secretions and to ease breathing.

At times, your loved one may mutter unintelligibly, may not respond, or may simply turn away when you speak to them.

These behaviors are a natural part of dying. Your loved one is not purposefully ignoring you; however, do continue your gentle touch and quiet and loving words.

Interspersed with deep social withdrawal, there may be brief moments of lucidity and attentive behavior before finally receding into that other world for the last time.

I don't know how well this aspect of dying translates for people in the later stages of dementia; however, Dorothy did experience one of those energy bursts, and I am very grateful to have been present for those few moments. It made a big difference. Her words helped undo some of the pain of our past history.

Death usually occurs within a day of the energy burst. Ongoing organ failure and the continued buildup of toxic waste products will cause your loved one to drift off into a peaceful coma. Other than maintaining your loving presence, there is nothing else you need to do. These changes are part of the natural dying process.

A few hours before death, blood circulation begins to pull back from the extremities in efforts to maintain the vital organs. When this happens, you may notice your loved one's fingers and toes feel cool, the nail beds may look pale or bluish, and the soles of the feet take on a mottled appearance.

The day after Dorothy's burst of energy, her breathing became more labored, and the time between breaths became longer. Then came a final exhalation and nothing more. I turned to my husband who, for the past few days, had sat quietly in the background. We embraced, and I said, "It's over."

PRACTICALITIES

Planning ahead for this last day will make things easier for you and your family (worksheet 14.1). A designated "home" manager should have sufficient information to free you and your family from unnecessary distraction.

Even when it seems certain that death will occur soon, it is difficult to predict if death will happen within a few hours or a few days. As much as you may want to stay with your loved one, it's neither possible nor good for you to be at the bedside twenty-four hours a day. It is important that you eat and sleep so you have the energy to get through the death, the funeral, bereavement, and the paperwork that follows. Remember to be kind to yourself.

If you feel your loved one should always have someone with them, tell your designated manager to schedule other people to take your place.

Although friends and family will want to know what is happening, you and other immediate family members should limit the amount of time spent making phone calls or sending e-mails or text messages. Your "Planning in Advance" worksheet (worksheet 14.2) should contain the information your designated manager needs to set up a communication tree.

The days I spent by Dorothy's side were important ones. The quietness provided space for self-reflection and reconciliation. I felt it was a privilege to share this most intimate time with my mother.

While sitting with Dorothy, I realized that, with her death, my husband and I had lost our status as "the kids." Yes, we were parents, but up until now there were people who still considered us their children. That realization did give me a moment's pause. The expression "passing the torch" came to mind.

The relative quiet gave me the time to consider the real-world changes. With her death, my role as power of attorney would cease. So one evening, in addition to my attentive presence, I paid her bills. While it might make me seem insensitive, I knew it could take up to six weeks before I had the legal right, this time as the personal representative of the estate, to sign checks. I also made the time to go to the bank and move important documents, such as the deed to her house, from her bank vault box to mine. Again, it was important to have access to those documents during that limbo time when I was neither her power of attorney nor the personal representative of the estate.

A GOOD DEATH

Karen Steinhauser, PhD, and colleagues at the Duke University School of Medicine and the Duke University Center for Aging used focus groups and in-depth interviews to identify six distinct attributes of a good death. Study participants included physicians, nurses, social workers, chaplains, hospice volunteers, patients, and recently bereaved family members.

Not surprisingly, freedom from pain and distressful symptoms was a theme that quickly emerged. Not unexpectedly, their study revealed an important aspect to pain and symptom control. Many patients volunteered a deep fear of waking up in the middle of the night in pain and gasping for air. In other words, patients wanted caregivers to anticipate and prevent distressing events.

Study participants felt that fear of pain and inadequate symptom management could be reduced by improved communication among the physician, the patient, and the patient's family. What the authors call "clear decision making," then, is another attribute of a good death.

Terminally ill patients said they want more preparation for what might happen next. They also wanted to plan ahead and do such things as write their obituary and invite friends and family to their funeral. Family members stated they wanted to learn more about the physical and psychosocial changes that occur as death approaches. All agreed that talking about death did not take away hope.

Completion—the importance of spirituality, life review, conflict resolution, and time to say good-bye to friends and family—was another theme revealed by Steinhauser's study. The authors state that completion is an important, and often overlooked, final quality-of-life factor.

"Final contributions to others" and "affirmation of the whole person" were two unexpected outcomes of the Steinhauser study. Terminally ill people not only need care but also want to reciprocate with gifts or by passing important life lessons on to others. All study participants mentioned "affirmation of the whole person," or the importance of upholding the patient as a unique person not defined by disease or relegated to nothing more than "a case."

The Steinhauser study shows that a good death provides physical and emotional comfort to the patient and their family. A good death incorporates many people and is as much for the benefit of the person with the terminal disease as it is for the people left behind.

IMPORTANT DETAILS

We joke about death and taxes as the two things we can always count on. As it turns out, there is more truth to that than one might expect. In addition to always counting on the intrusiveness of death (and taxes), there is the paperwork that accompanies this final life cycle event.

A person just doesn't die; there must be medical professionals who either expect the impending death to occur or who are present to witness the event. Afterward, there must be an official written pronouncement stating the person is no longer living.

Unattended Deaths

In some states, an unattended death is one where the deceased has not been under a doctor's care for the past thirty days. In other states, an unattended death is one where a health professional does not witness the death. Unattended deaths that involve elderly people are more likely to occur at home or in an assisted living facility.

The consequences of an unattended death vary. Usually the Office of the Medical Investigator (OMI), or in some communities the Coroner's Office, gets involved. Their job is to make sure trauma or negligence are not contributing factors. As part of their investigation, the OMI field officer may take fluid samples from various parts of the body. Testing blood and fluid removed from the eye and the knee joint for various substances can help determine time of death.

If everything indicates natural causes for death, the field investigator will release the body to the funeral home. If the field officer feels circumstances warrant a more detailed evaluation, the officer will take the body to the Office of the Medical Investigator.

Pronouncement and Time of Death

A person is not officially deceased until a clinician or other health care professional signs a death certificate. Before signing the form, a health professional—usually a doctor, hospice nurse, or paramedic—makes sure there is no detectable pulse, signs of respiration, or response to verbal or tactile stimuli. The time of death can be either the time breathing stopped or the time when the doctor or other health care professional makes the pronouncement.

Autopsy: A Personal Decision

You want to believe your loved one is finally at peace. An autopsy can seem out of place with the philosophy of palliative care and hospice.

Cultural and religious beliefs and practices are often given as reasons why families do not consent to having their family member undergo a clinical autopsy. Jews and Muslims object outright, citing that a body must be returned to the earth as it entered—clean, pure, and intact; however, Jewish and Muslim law does accept the procedure when autopsy is required by local authorities or if the knowledge gained will benefit others.

Research shows that postmortem CT and MR scans (see chapter 4) often reveal more information than a traditional autopsy. In addition, these minimally invasive procedures leave the body intact and provide an electronic record available to clinical researchers.

In most cases, an autopsy is a personal choice. Families may request one to clarify unanswered questions, to learn about conditions that may affect other family members, or to rule out suspected medical mismanagement. Participation in research studies may require that the patient agree to have an autopsy. Local authorities may require an autopsy if there is reason to believe that trauma or neglect contributed to the death.

What Is an Autopsy?

Autopsies are performed either for forensic (legal) or medical reasons. The purpose of a forensic autopsy is to determine if criminal activity, such as trauma, neglect, or poisoning, was the cause of death. A clinical autopsy determines the medical causes of death and, in the process, may reveal misdiagnoses or missed contributing factors. Because of the expense, clinical autopsies are not a routine procedure and most often occur when the cause of death is unknown or uncertain, if the patient died of a rare disease, or if the patient was part of a research study.

An unattended death may warrant an autopsy if there are reasons to suspect trauma or neglect. In most cases involving dementia, an external autopsy, when the body is photographed, examined for wounds, washed, weighed, and measured, is sufficient.

An internal autopsy is a surgical procedure. The pathologist and other medical professionals weigh the internal organs and inspect their appearance. They take tissue samples and test them using various microscopic and biochemical assessment methods. After inspection and sampling, the pathologist stitches together the incisions and makes the body presentable for viewing. The autopsy usually takes less than two hours to complete; however, it may take several weeks before the laboratory results are available.

A brain autopsy is an option when the doctor or the patient's family wants to confirm Alzheimer's disease or dementia with Lewy bodies. A brain autopsy does not disfigure the face, and the family can proceed with any plans they may have for an open casket viewing. Looking at brain tissue under the microscope is the only way to see the structures associated with having either of these two kinds of dementia (see chapter 3).

Brain Donation and Clinical Trial Programs

Donating a brain for a research study is different than having a clinical brain autopsy to confirm a diagnosis. Each clinical research program has certain criteria for enrollment, such as participation in a drug study or having an uncommon dementia (e.g., dementia with Lewy bodies or AIDS dementia complex).

Brain harvesting can take place in the hospital or in the funeral home. The designated study center receives half of the tissue, and the other half is preserved and stored in a brain bank for future research. Usually, the family incurs little or none of the cost of the brain-harvesting procedure.

Researchers from around the world can use brain bank tissue in their investigations. Studies require only small amounts of tissue, so each donated brain benefits a large number of research programs. The combination of your generosity and worldwide scientific research efforts will advance knowledge regarding the risk factors associated with the disease, as well as the medications used to manage dementia signs and symptoms.

The majority of brain donation programs require that the patient enroll months or years in advance of making the donation. That way there is ample time to do a complete diagnostic assessment of the patient as well complete the legal paperwork necessary for participation.

The Helpful Resources section at the end of the book contains links to several brain donation and clinical study websites, including the ClinicalTrials. gov website, as well as the Brain Donation Project and National Institute of Neurological Disorders and Stroke websites (see Helpful Resources).

Death Certificates

Like a birth certificate or a marriage license, a death certificate is a permanent life cycle record. The information contained in the death certificate includes demographic data, such as your loved one's place of birth, race, occupation, and the names of their parents, as well as the time and place of death. The funeral home uses the information that you provided earlier to complete this part of the death certificate. Plan ahead and compile your family member's demographics to reduce stress and lighten your workload (worksheet 14.3).

Your loved one's doctor, or the Office of the Medical Investigator (OMI), will list the diseases, injuries, or other complications that directly caused or contributed to your loved one's death on the second portion of the death certificate. Your loved one's doctor or an OMI pathologist will sign the death certificate.

Usually it takes seven to ten working days before you receive copies of the death certificate issued by your state Office of Vital Records. The funeral home takes care of delivering the completed death certificate to you. In situations where an autopsy, toxicology studies, or other investigations are necessary, it may take several months before the OMI can issue a certified or legal death certificate.

The death certificate serves many purposes. It is the legal proof that Social Security, Medicare, banks, credit cards, pension funds, and life insurance plans require before they can take appropriate next steps. You need a death certificate to begin the legal process of settling your loved one's estate.

Most organizations require an original copy. Others are willing to accept a paper reproduction or an electronic version that you can send attached to an e-mail. Many funeral directors suggest that you request at least ten death certificate originals. If needed, you can always request more, either by contacting the funeral home or getting them directly from your state Office of Vital Records.

Death certificates are a reference for medical researchers, historians, and people interested in family genealogy. Medical researchers use death certificate information to link such things as location, age, or occupation with cause of death. Historians use these records to tie events to the condition of the people living at that time. Genealogy enthusiasts use death certificate records to learn about their family history. And finally, government entities use death certificates to make sure the names on petitions, voter registration applications, or ballots are of people eligible to vote.

DEATH AT HOME

While dying at home is often a preference, few people get their wish, and fewer family members know what to do when death does occur at home. What happens next largely depends on local state laws and the particular circumstances.

Calling 911 or the local police department is a good starting point. In most cases, the 911 operator will inform the Office of the Medical Investigator or the Coroner's Office. Be prepared to give the operator the street address and a phone number where they can reach you. Often a law enforcement officer and an OMI field investigator or a paramedic will come to the house. The field investigator will have questions regarding your loved one's medical history and will want to know the name and phone number of their primary care doctor. This is another situation where having completed worksheet 14.2 will make things easier for you.

If there is no reason to suspect trauma or neglect, the field investigator will call your loved one's doctor, and if they agree to sign a time-of-death certificate, the OMI will either release the body to the funeral home, or if you don't have a designated funeral home, take the body to the morgue. Once you have made funeral home arrangements, the OMI will release the body to the funeral director.

DEATH AND HOSPICE

Home hospice care can prevent the drama an unattended death often creates. When death is imminent, a hospice nurse will be present to provide the comfort care your loved one may need. The hospice nurse will record the time of death and sign the pronouncement document. The nurse will inform your loved one's doctor of the death and call the funeral home.

If the hospice nurse did not witness the death, simply call the hospice agency. The agency will send a nurse to pronounce your loved one and then inform the funeral home.

In either case, hospice will help you through the next days and arrange for any emotional support services you and your family may need.

HOURS AWAY

Dorothy died in the assisted living facility. Hospice caregivers, although respectful of our privacy, were there to provide any needed comfort care. They massaged body lotion into her skin. They moistened her mouth with a damp cloth and used lip balm to prevent sores. They moved her to prevent painful bedsores. And after asking us to leave the room for a few minutes, the hospice nurse gave Dorothy a sponge bath and changed her clothes and bed pads. It was good to see the ongoing attentiveness to patient comfort, respect, and dignity.

The assisted living facility caregivers frequently dropped by to spend a few minutes with Dorothy. Some asked if they could bring us anything to eat or drink. All offered to keep an eye on her so we could leave for a few hours or go home to sleep.

The day when it seemed quite certain that death was just hours away, the hospice nurse checked in more often. She told us to report behaviors like grimacing or restlessness, which can indicate pain or other kinds of discomfort. The nurse always responded quickly and adjusted Dorothy's oxygen flow and medication to restore comfort. After all these years of agitation and anxiety, it was good to see Dorothy relaxed and at peace.

Later that afternoon, the hospice nurse said, "I think it is time to turn off the oxygen." I knew it was the right thing to do. For the next hour or so, the sound of Dorothy's breathing replaced the noise of the oxygen tank. She didn't struggle.

My husband and I sat with Dorothy for a short while before telling the hospice nurse of her death. The hospice nurse checked for vital signs and signed the pronouncement document.

We talked for a bit and thanked everyone for their hard work and thoughtful care. Just as we were about to leave, one of the assisted living facility caregivers came up to us and, in halting English, asked if she could kiss Miss Dorothy good-bye.

SOMETHING UNEXPECTED

My husband and I went home and made a few phone calls to family and friends. I called our rabbi and discussed the day and time for Dorothy's funeral—a simple affair involving a graveside service followed by an open house at our home for family, friends, and neighbors.

Both hospice and the assisted living facility knew to contact the funeral home. The only remaining detail I had to attend to was finding pall bearers. I was surprised at how many people volunteered. Women, in particular, were honored to participate in a tradition reserved for men.

Long ago, I had decided that rather than cremation or embalming, I wanted Dorothy to have a "Tahara," or the traditional purification ritual used to prepare a Jew for burial. Trained community volunteers, all members of Chevra Kadisha, or the sacred society, gather at the funeral home and perform a physical cleaning to return the body, as close as possible, to its natural state followed by a ritual cleansing that includes washing the body with a measured amount of clean water. They dress the body in white cotton or linen burial garments and place the deceased in a wooden coffin. Natural processes return the deceased, the burial garments, and the coffin back to the earth. To respect modesty, women volunteers prepare deceased women, and men volunteers do the same for deceased men.

For many years, I have been one of these volunteers. It is a beautiful tradition. I wanted Dorothy to experience the loving kindness that she never permitted for herself. I also wanted to be one of the five women at her side.

Some people were quite horrified at the idea. Others were concerned the experience would be harmful. I spoke with the rabbi who oversees the Chevra Kadisha volunteer program. At first, she was a little resistant. Then, she mentioned that it was once traditional for family members to prepare the body of the deceased at home—often on the kitchen table. Then she said, "I think you can do it. And if you get into trouble, you know where the door is."

I asked if she would be one of the five and then named three other women who I hoped would join me. One is a very close friend; the other two were women who, I felt, would lend a peaceful ambience to the service.

I have to say, for me, it was a very right thing to do. No, it wasn't closure or any of those other buzzwords. It was just "right." An unexpected bonus was that the Tahara gave Dorothy a chance to make a "final contribution to others."

At the end of a Tahara, we always gather around the plain pine casket and say a few words to the woman we have just washed and dressed. Usually, we don't know the person, so each of says a few words of thanks for the honor of performing her Tahara and wish her well on her journey. This time it was a little different. Everyone knew me, and two of the others knew Dorothy.

It was one of the women who did not know Dorothy who said the magical words. She said that because of the Holocaust, she never had the chance to know the women of her mother's generation. Saying good-bye to Dorothy gave her the chance to say good-bye to them as well.

GOOD GRIEF

The grief associated with dementia care is an ongoing process that for many begins long before death. In the beginning, you may swing between despair and anger. You may deny there is anything wrong and do your best to suppress your feelings.

Later, as the disease progresses, you may feel overwhelmed by sadness or resentful of the changes this disease has imposed on your life. Oddly enough, when it becomes necessary to put the person in your care into an assisted living facility or a nursing home, the relief you first felt may be replaced by another round of grief mixed with a good dose of guilt.

The days and months following the death can be an awkward time. Some people do feel sad and grieve again. Others will acknowledge they aren't sad. The person who was your parent, partner, spouse, sibling, or best friend died a long time ago. The apparent lack of sadness is often difficult for others to understand.

NOT SO GOOD GRIEF

Grief is a natural emotion we feel in response to a major loss like the death of a loved family member. Although everyone feels grief in their own way, there are definable stages—beginning with recognizing the loss and ending with acceptance. The in-between part varies with the person and the circumstances. Anger, despair, bargaining, sadness, guilt, and resentment are just a few of the emotions people in mourning may feel at one time or another.

Most people believe that grief is something that only happens after a death; however, for people caring for a person who has dementia, grief and grieving tracks with degeneration. By the time their loved one dies, there is nothing left.

There are situations when the feelings of loss become debilitating and do not resolve with time. Called "complex grief," this response to a death has symptoms that overlap with depression and post-traumatic stress disorder

(PTSD). People whose grief follows a more difficult path may have ongoing thoughts and images of the deceased and overwhelming yearnings for his or her presence. Denial of the death, believing the dead person is alive, and feelings of desperate loneliness, helplessness, anger, and bitterness, as well as wishing for their own death, are other symptoms associated with complex grief.

A study by Richard Schultz (professor of psychiatry and director of the University Center for Social and Urban Research at the University of Pittsburgh) and colleagues reveals the risk factors associated with complex grief among dementia caregivers. In their study, they found that as many as 30 percent of family caregivers were at risk of experiencing clinical depression for as long as one year after the death of the person in their care. Of these, 20 percent experienced complex grief.

Some of the predicative risk factors for post-death depression and complex grief include anxiety and depression before the death, caring for a spouse, a long and loving relationship, and loss of benefits (money or status) derived from caregiving. Other risk factors include high levels of burden, feeling exhausted, lack of support, and having additional home and work responsibilities. It comes as no surprise that caregivers who use hospice care services are less likely to experience complex grief.

Treatment for complex grief is not yet well defined. Currently, treatment includes psychotherapy to help people adjust to their new circumstance. Some clinicians use medication to relieve symptoms of depression and anxiety. Others are of the opinion that grief, even if complex, is not an illness and, therefore, medication is not warranted. These clinicians stress the value of talk-therapy to encourage self-reflection and discussion about the relationship they once had with their loved one.

When Dorothy died, my overwhelming emotion was relief. I was so thankful the turmoil of the past few years was over. Compared to what I had experienced, the paperwork and the physical labor of settling her estate was easy and also very distracting.

Now, more than ten years later, I feel an unexpected sadness. I remember and appreciate the person I, and so many other people, lost before dementia became her dominant feature. I tell my children and grandchildren about their very intelligent and interesting grandmother.

FUNERALS

Many people do not preplan their funeral. When this happens, the responsibility falls to the family. Most family members find that making the decision to plan their parent's or other loved one's funeral is difficult. In addition to overcoming the emotional hurdle of accepting the reality of an impending death, funeral homes are not familiar places. For most, planning a funeral with the help of a funeral director is a first-time experience.

It's almost funny, but funeral directors are very much like the ones you see in movies and television shows. They wear dark suits, speak softly, and avoid harsh-sounding words. Sitting in their office, you will notice a box of pastel-colored tissues, drinking water, and a dish of hard candies within reach. The reason for the box of tissues is obvious. The drinking water and candy are there to calm emotions. It's impossible to cry when there is something in your mouth.

Funeral directors are very good at explaining the services they offer. You may be surprised to learn that, in addition to body preparation and the burial, the mortuary offers what one funeral director described as "all-encompassing attention to detail and comfort." Services range from giving the eulogy and writing the obituary to arranging flowers and coordinating transportation for the bodies of those who will be buried in another state or country. Many funeral homes provide a limited number of complimentary grief counseling sessions.

When you feel ready to plan the funeral, call a local mortuary. By way of a brief introduction, give your thoughts about the kind of funeral under consideration, as well as the inclusion of specific cultural or religious traditions. Some people find it helpful to have a friend or family member accompany them.

Cost is a realistic concern. Be upfront and discuss your cost requirements with the funeral director. Most funeral directors understand the apprehension people have in talking about funeral expenses. Most will respect your requirements and will not "upsell" their services. Many funeral homes offer a discount to veterans.

When choosing the various funeral service and casket options, try to keep in mind that funeral rituals comfort the living. Purchasing the most expensive casket will not necessarily help you or the other people important to your loved one feel better.

The funeral director will want to know a little about your family. They will want to know if you are considering a casketed burial, cremation, or an environmentally friendly green burial, and they will want to be aware of any specific religious or cultural needs. If you are unsure of what you and your family may want, the funeral director will explain and describe the various options. Do not be afraid to ask questions!

Come prepared with the information the funeral director needs to fill out forms and to write the obituary (worksheet 14.4). In addition to your loved one's date and place of birth and Social Security number, the funeral director will need family and personal information to include in the obituary. An obituary is an option and not a requirement. Be sure to proofread the obituary before the funeral home submits it to the newspaper.

PREPLANNED FUNERALS

It's always better if you can preplan your loved one's funeral. It's even better if your loved one did it for or with you. Although it is a difficult task to face, doing so reduces stress. Having this one very big undertaking out of the way means you don't have to think about it anymore. And months, or even years, later, a single phone call takes care of everything.

When you are ready, ask your friends to recommend mortuaries they may have used. An internet search using such keywords as "mortuary" and "funeral home," as well as the town and state where you need services, will give you enough information to take next steps.

Some mortuaries cater to specific religious or cultural groups. Others accommodate a spectrum of specific religious and cultural needs. "Green" or environmentally conscious burial is another kind of funeral many mortuaries provide. Some mortuaries only do cremations.

There are two ways to preplan a funeral. One is to have the funeral director develop an emergency record guide, or ERG. The ERG includes your family member's vital information, such as the date and place of birth, Social Security number, and the names of their parents (worksheets 14.3 and 14.4). The ERG also lists your wishes for your family member's funeral. The ERG does include a cost estimate but does not guarantee that same price months or years later.

The other way to preplan a funeral is to work with an insurance company who, in partnership with the mortuary, helps you make funeral arrangements. There are advantages to this approach. First of all, the insurance policy guarantees the price of the services the funeral home provides. The policy does not guarantee costs associated with such things as the newspaper obituary, certified death certificates, or new sales tax rates; however, the funeral director will build a small cushion into the insurance plan in anticipation of these increases.

In addition to being preplanned, the insured funeral is prepaid. Again, the advantages of doing so are many, and they include a hedge against inflation and the circumvention of probate, periods when funds are not accessible, and the need to make a "gift to the estate" to pay for your family member's funeral. Ask if you can transfer the insurance policy to another mortuary. If you do decide to take the preplanned and prepaid route, the funeral director will put you in contact with an insurance agent who will meet with you a few days later.

Do note that the American Association of Retired Persons (AARP) has words of caution regarding the purchase of the prepaid packaged plans many funeral homes sell. According to the article, not all packaged plans transfer to another state. Another concern is the inability to get a refund should you change your mind about the kind of funeral or decide to use a different mortuary.

BURIAL OPTIONS

Most people have a sense of how they might like their own remains treated; however, making a similar decision for another person is difficult. Your family member may or may not have told you about their burial wishes. Sometimes, requests are impractical or clash with your own views. Sometimes, you don't have any idea what your family member may have wanted.

Burial wishes are closely tied to cultural, religious, and personal views about the afterlife. Some people have strong feelings about what does or does not happen after death. While embalming and casketing may seem right to some people, others may find the practice abhorrent.

It is the funeral director's job to help families overcome disharmony when opposing opinions make it difficult for the family to make a decision. As one funeral director stated, "Funerals are part of the healing process and shouldn't cause harm." So even when the majority of family members have one opinion, it's important that the family tries to make decisions that are acceptable to everyone.

The funeral director will offer many options. Cremation and embalming are the usual body preparation choices; however, some traditions require that the body remains in its natural state. If cremation is your family's wish, the funeral director will want to know if you want to put the ashes into an urn or biodegradable box. He will ask if your family wants to disperse the cremains, deposit them in a cemetery, or bring them home. If dispersal at a home garden or favorite location is the request, the funeral director will inform you about any permits you may need.

Many people, rather than dispersing the cremains, take the ashes home. If this is your choice, be sure to consider how you will keep your loved one's ashes safe. Some people put the urn in a place of honor. Others, unsure about what they want to do next, don't get any further than the cardboard box the funeral home presented to them.

Placing a label on the small and nondescript cardboard box will reduce the possibility that a person will unknowingly put the cremains in the trash. A house break-in is another worry. Put an identification marker on the urn to increase the possibility of having it returned to you.

Many cemeteries and memorial parks now offer mini-plots and wall vaults designed specifically for cremains. This option both removes the possibility of misplaced or stolen ashes and creates a physical memorial that everyone can visit.

Embalming with or without an open casket involves another set of related choices. An open casket presumes embalming to make the body presentable for public viewing. Embalming also reduces odors and prevents the transmission of infectious diseases. The effects of embalming last only a short time and do not permanently protect the body from decay.

A closed casket, where mourners do not view the body, often reflects religious or cultural preferences. A closed casket is sometimes the only choice when trauma or disease makes cosmetic restoration impossible and viewing the body disturbing.

Embalming is not a requirement; therefore, you can ask to have your family member casketed without having to undergo the embalming step.

Casket choices range from simple pine boxes and wicker baskets to caskets made from highly polished mahogany, other exotic woods, and metals like bronze or stainless steel. The funeral director will take you into the showroom so, just like buying a car, you can choose a model and the various options.

An ethical funeral director will help you chose a casket within your price range. A sensitive funeral director will make you feel good about the choice you made.

Natural or green burials are another choice for families interested in reducing the environmental impact of burying their loved one. Environmentally friendly embalming fluids, if used at all, do not contain formaldehyde, and the casket and any cloth body coverings are all made from renewable, recycled, and biodegradable materials. The idea is to allow natural decomposition processes to return the body to the earth. Compared to the highly manicured memorial parks, green burial cemeteries, with an abundance of wild flowers and native grasses, look more like a nature preserve.

CEMETERY PLOTS

Where to bury your family member is often another difficult decision. The easiest scenario is one where your loved one purchased a plot in or near the community where they died. In that case, you simply tell the funeral director the name and location of the cemetery and, if possible, the plot location number. If you are lucky, you will know where to find the cemetery contract that contains all of those details. If not, the cemetery manager can go through records and find the plot your loved one purchased many years ago.

Another scenario is one where, in addition to planning and paying for your loved one's funeral, you also need to purchase a cemetery plot. The mortuary director can guide you through that step.

Some funeral homes either own or have an affiliation with a local cemetery. Other options include churches, mosques, synagogues, and burial societies. Many religious groups do sell plots to nonmembers for a slightly higher fee. Usually, the church or synagogue requires your loved one be of their faith. Burial societies are another kind of membership or kinship group, such as union members and people who have a country of origin in common.

If your loved one was a veteran, or was married to a veteran, they may be eligible for interment in a U.S. Department of Veterans Affairs national cemetery.

Another common situation is one where your loved one purchased a burial plot in the community where they once lived. Perhaps other family members are buried there; however, for any number of reasons, you may decide to bury your loved one closer to where you live. It is possible to sell the distant plot to help pay for the local one. You can post the sale on the cemetery website, in the classified section of a local newspaper, or in a church or synagogue newsletter.

A plot exchange program is another solution. Many cemeteries, understanding that people move and circumstances change, will help clients exchange a plot for one located in a more convenient location. Use the keywords "cemetery plot exchange" to find internet exchange services. You can also call the cemetery and ask about their plot exchange plan. They will be happy to provide you with their exchange program details.

Most cemeteries require a distance of seventy-five miles between the two plots. The rate of exchange is usually based on applying a percentage of the price paid for the original plot to the new purchase. If your family member bought their plot many years ago, the exchange rate may not do much to offset the price of the new one. In that case, consider donating the plot to a nonprofit organization.

TRAVEL TO A FINAL RESTING PLACE

When people die in a community far away from the place where they want to be buried, distance doesn't have to be a stumbling block. The local funeral home will prepare the body and coordinate the permits and transportation services needed to deliver the body to the receiving mortuary.

Here too, embalming is not a requirement. The funeral home will surround the body in frozen cold-packs when family preferences or religious prohibitions prevent the use of embalming fluids. The funeral home uses special containers to ship bodies. Air cargo is the usual means of transportation.

BE AWARE OF YOUR FEELINGS

A few days after Dorothy's death, a friend asked how I was doing. "Fine," I said, and then proceeded to tell her about the things I was doing or planning to do. "Be aware of your feelings," she said. I took her statement as a not-too-subtle warning to take care of myself and to slow down.

FREQUENTLY ASKED QUESTIONS

1. My mother's doctor suggested that when my mother dies that she undergo a brain autopsy to confirm dementia with Lewy bodies. In some ways I want to have a real answer, too. But what if the autopsy report is normal? I know this is an irrational thought, but it scares me, nonetheless.

Unless your mother was part of a clinical study where a brain biopsy was a condition for participation, this procedure is optional.

Although the signs and symptoms of dementia with Lewy bodies are quite distinct, looking at brain tissue under a microscope is the only way to confirm the diagnosis. Your mother's test results may contribute to a better understanding of the disease, or they may someday help family members get the care they need.

I can, however, understand your fear of a negative result. Dementia of any kind is difficult to understand and accept. Even after years of caregiving, we may still harbor thoughts that our parent had a curable illness, such as a chronic bladder infection. Perhaps getting the support and input from other family members will make it easier to evaluate how to respond to the doctor's suggestion.

2. My father-in-law, who is in the earlier stages of dementia, is dying from cancer. When I visit, he wants to talk about his death and how he would like to be buried. When his daughters heard about these conversations, they were furious. They said talking about death and dying took away all hope. I don't feel like I did anything wrong.

People in the early stages of dementia are quite capable of knowing what they want for themselves. Your father-in-law understands that you are a person who is willing to take the time to listen and takes what he has to say to heart. Talking about end-of-life wishes is something terminally ill people desire. Rather than taking away hope, talking about these matters allows terminally ill people to live the rest of their life in peace. What you did for your father-in-law was a kindness.

3. I am in the process of preplanning my mother's funeral. I was surprised to discover that my sister and I have very different views about cremation. What can I do so that one of us isn't left feeling unhappy or angry?

People tend to have strong feelings one way or the other about cremation. Some people feel cremation is an environmentally responsible choice. Others like the idea of returning their ashes to nature. On the other hand, some people feel cremation is not an environmentally responsible alternative and is distasteful because it accelerates a natural process.

Families often have differing opinions about their loved one's body preparation and funeral. If at all possible, both you and your sister should meet with the funeral director. If your sister's physical presence is not possible, a conference call will be sufficient. Funeral directors are experts at helping families make comfortable decisions.

If a family is considering cremation *only* because of financial limitations, then it is well worth inquiring about less expensive ways to give your loved one another kind of funeral. Many funeral homes give discounts to veterans. There are "discount" and "flat-fee" funeral homes that provide less expensive funeral services. Many churches, synagogues, and community service organizations have funds set aside for families who may need a little financial assistance at this time.

4. Shortly after my mother died, my father became friends with a woman who lives in the neighborhood. It didn't take long before they became a couple. Now, twenty years later, he is in mid-stage dementia and end-stage kidney disease. His girlfriend, although good for him, never got along with the rest of the family. My sisters and I are wondering if she should be mentioned in the eulogy and be invited to sit with the family during the service.

Undoubtedly, many people attending the funeral will know about the relationship these two people enjoyed together. While she may not be part of the family, she and your father did have a twenty-year relationship. Think carefully what ignoring her says about you and your family if you do not acknowledge their relationship. To repeat what a funeral director told me, "Funerals are part of the healing process and shouldn't cause harm."

5. My brother, who is gay, is in the advanced stages of early-onset dementia. My husband and I are very close to him and his husband; however, my parents have made it very clear they do not approve of what they call "your brother's sinful lifestyle" and want nothing to do with him. Telling them my brother, their son, will die soon, did not soften their stance. Is there anything I can do to bring our family together during this difficult time?

Try contacting a local branch of the Parents, Family and Friends of Lesbians and Gays (PFLAG). There is always the possibility that having your parents meet with other parents of gay adult children may be helpful; however, the parental rejection you describe frequently happens, and while it is understandable that you want to reconcile family differences, it may not be possible. Whatever the outcome, do continue to give your brother and his husband the support they both need. Doing so will enrich your life, too.

6. My mother's brother, my uncle, is a family outsider. He doesn't get along with any of us and is a violent and abusive person. We are worried that his presence at my mother's funeral will be disruptive and maybe even dangerous. What can we do?

Funeral directors say many families are worried about a particular family member or guest who they feel may become disruptive or violent. In circumstances like the one you describe, funeral directors suggest either hiring security guards to lend a presence or having a funeral home employee stand or sit near the person who is the cause for concern. In most cases, using either or both of these strategies prevents any altercations.

7. A few months after my father died, my brother and I found a contract for a prepaid funeral he purchased thirty years ago. Is there a way to get a refund?

Modern life insurance and burial policies generally don't have expiration dates. Some older policies may have "redemption clauses" requiring a claim within a certain period; however, these restrictions are rarely binding. You may get help from the state association of funeral directors and from the policy underwriter.

WORKSHEET 14.1:
Quiet Time

The estate sale can wait. Once you complete the preliminary steps to close your loved one's estate, it's time to relax and clear your brain. No lists, no reflective writing assignments, and no family meetings.

Some people find meditation, yoga, or other kinds of slow motions calming. Others prefer swimming or working out in the gym. Music, art, cooking, and gardening are other options; do what feels good and places you in a mindful place.

WORKSHEET 14.2:
Planning in Advance

My phone numbers(s) and e-mail:

Name, phone number(s), and e-mail of your designated "home" manager:

Name, location, phone, or e-mail for the care facility:

Location of extra house and car key/fob:

Work

Inform appropriate individuals of your dates of absence and make arrangements with human resources for illness and bereavement leave.

Home

Make a list of things that must be done—when and by whom.

Make a list of important names and phone numbers that include the following:

_____ close family members

_____ close friends

_____ neighbors

_____ taxi service

_____ your doctors

_____ take-out and delivery restaurants

_____ church or synagogue contacts

Legal Information for Family Use Only

Location of will:

Attorney name, address, and contact information:

Location of safety deposit box:

Location of safety deposit box key:

Name, address, and contact information of the personal representative of the estate (executor/executrix):

Prepaid funeral policy? _____ yes _____ no

Policy number: _____

Other pertinent information:

WORKSHEET 14.3:
Information for the Funeral Director

The funeral director will need information to complete the death certificate. In the case of an unattended death, the Office of the Medical Investigator will have questions for you as well. The funeral director can write the obituary for publication in the local newspaper. Be sure to proofread the obituary before the funeral director sends it to the newspaper. Of course, you can write the obituary yourself!

Death Certificate Information

Decedent's legal name: _____

If female, maiden name: _____

Date of death: _____   Time of death: _____

Sex: _____   Social Security number: _____

Marital status: _____   Name of surviving spouse: _____

Name of surviving spouse (if wife) maiden name:

_____

Date of birth: _____   Birthplace: _____

Served in U.S. Armed Forces? _____ yes _____ no

Decedent's race: _____   Tribe: _____

Decedent's residence county: _____   State: _____

Mother's full maiden name: _____

Father's full name: _____

Method of disposition (burial): _____

Disposition location: _____

Funeral service facility: _____

County of death: _____

Place of death: _____   Type of place: _____

(continued)

WORKSHEET 14.3:
Continued

Additional Information for the Office of the Medical Investigator (OMI)

The decedent's doctor:

Name: _____

Address: _____

Phone number: _____

Brief description of the decedent's medical history:

_____

_____

_____

Information to Include in the Obituary

Age at time of death and occupation:

Interests, hobbies, and accomplishments:

Name of spouse, parents, and other relatives:

List those who are predeceased:

Names of children and their spouses or partners and other special people:

Names of grandchildren, great-grandchildren, and other next-generation family:

Words to describe the deceased:

What you would like others to know about him/her:

WORKSHEET 14.4:
Information for the Obituary

Preplanning your loved one's funeral can make it a little easier if you collect the information you will need before meeting with the funeral director. The funeral director will use some of the information you provide during the preplanning meeting to write the obituary and complete the death certificate.

General Information

Full name and Social Security number:

Name of community, former community, and length of time living there:

Physician name, address, and contact information:

Date of birth and death:

Country, state, and city of birth:

Education and occupation:

Ethnic origin and race: _____

Mother's birth name: _____

Father's birth name: _____

How would the person want to be remembered?

Contact Information for Immediate Family

Name	Relationship	City and state	Phone number

(*continued*)

Emergency Contacts

Name	Phone number(s)

Funeral Service Instructions

Location of service: chapel, church, gravesite, other

Cemetery address:

Type of burial:

Clergy's name and contact information:

Music: _____ yes _____ no

Vocalist: _____ yes _____ no

Musician name(s) and contact information:

Vocalist name(s) and contact information:

Favorite religious passages or other readings:

Flowers: _____ yes _____ no

Clothing:

Jewelry:

Name and contact information of person to make decisions about clothing
and jewelry:

Participating organizations (fraternal, military):

Name, city, and phone number of pall bearers:

Portrait:

Special instructions:

15

PICKING UP THE PIECES AND PEELING BACK THE LAYERS

Man, age eighty-two, clock, 9:10 a.m.

Dorothy died on New Year's Eve. I am sure she was more than disappointed she didn't make it to 2011—the year of her one hundredth birthday. Maybe I could have told her it was 2011 in Europe, and that yes, she did make it to her one hundredth year in another time zone. Dorothy never did have a sense of humor, and I am sure she wouldn't have found what I said even a little bit funny.

Her death heralded more than just the changes associated with the upcoming New Year. My sibling and I were now members of the older—no, the oldest—generation.

And Dorothy's death had transformed me from caregiver and power of attorney (POA) to that of a funeral planner, personal representative of the estate, and self-appointed "domestic archeologist."

With the exception of a few details, the funeral pretty much took care of itself. My husband and I told the rabbi a little more about Dorothy. Yes, she was a difficult person, but she also encouraged her children to follow their interests. She had high standards and appreciated creativity and perseverance. The service was short, and one of the adult grandchildren, unable to attend, wrote and sent a poem for us to read. It was an honest poem that described her grandmother as a person who meant well and, if you looked a little deeper, was a loving person. Everyone received a copy of Dorothy's recipe for blueberry muffins. Unlike the sweet cake-like ones we eat today, hers—a recipe showing the frugality of the World War II years—are not at all sweet (see worksheet 15.1).

Her death terminated my role as her POA. A trip to the lawyer, a couple of signatures, filing a bunch of papers with probate court—followed by an unspecified waiting period—and voila, I was the personal representative of the estate. So, rather than speaking on Dorothy's behalf, my responsibilities now involved such things as ending her relationship with Social Security, working with the bank to establish a special estate account, and eventually, distributing estate funds and property according to the stipulations of her will. I have to admit, giving special presents to various friends and family members was an enjoyable task; however, to make that possible, I had to clean her house.

Similar to an archeologist, I found many curious things that made me wonder "why?" A pair of mismatched mittens last worn when I was nine or ten years old. A box containing increasingly complicated dental bridges and partial dentures. Drawers stuffed with mostly never-worn underwear. And then there were the things I couldn't find.

Where is the vintage face powder music box? I am five years old and seated at my mother's vanity. I smell the lingering aroma of my mother's face powder and hear "You Are My Sunshine" in the background.

Maybe Dorothy threw it out in an attempt to reduce household clutter. Maybe she put it in a very special place for me. Wondering about the whereabouts of the music box still brings tears to my eyes. It's interesting how an object can become so precious.

AFTERWARD

It's no secret that I like to cook. I find baking and cooking, especially for others, pleasurable and relaxing.

After the funeral, friends and family gathered at our home. I served "round foods" to symbolize the cycle of life. Bagels, of course, but also eggs, round cheeses, a spicy black bean soup, fruit, and a selection of homemade yeast breads, cakes, and cookies. Friends and neighbors brought many wonderful things to add to our meal of condolence.

It was good to spend the afternoon and early evening schmoozing with friends and family. Our gathering was a little like a real-time social networking event. Everyone knew our family, some knew each other, and many made new friends.

Dorothy was one of many topics of conversation. The neighbors knew her in one way and family in another. A friend, someone I have known since fifth grade, had a unique perspective based on our half century of friendship. All were pleasantly surprised to see photos of Dorothy as a young woman whose face didn't reflect the troubles and difficulties she would encounter later in life.

Circles of friends often have a way of expanding and encompassing the unexpected. The obituary published in our local newspaper resulted in a letter from an elderly woman. A few weeks later over lunch, she told us about the summer when, seventy years ago and 2,300 miles away, she sat on the beach with a handsome young couple and my then three-year-old sister.

WHAT'S NEXT?

The funeral is over, and your friends and out-of-town relatives have dispersed. You are left with a too-full refrigerator and wondering what happens next. And, as is often the case, the person who once was the POA is now the personal representative of the estate.

The personal representative (PR) of the estate—sometimes called the executor (male) or the executrix (female)—is responsible for distributing property and other assets according to the stipulations of the will. Usually, the personal representative seeks the guidance of an estate lawyer. If your loved one did not write a will or if the will did not name an administrator, the district court will appoint someone to settle the estate.

Whew! This is a lot to learn! Personal representative, estate, assets, wills, administrators, district court, estate lawyers, and banks—and I have yet to mention trusts, living trusts, probate, and probate court.

Because so much of settling an estate is dependent on state laws and the particulars of the estate or the will, I can do little more than get you started on the next leg of your unintended journey.

GETTING STARTED

It's a considerable understatement to describe the PR job simply as one that makes a person responsible for the distribution of property and other assets according to the stipulations of the will (see table 15.1). Even for an uncomplicated estate, it can take more than a year before you are finally able to distribute property and assets to heirs.

Table 15.1. Personal Representative Responsibilities

Follow the decedent's written instructions for body preparation, funeral
    arrangements, and funeral.
Arrange for the immediate needs of survivors.
Locate the will and other important information and papers.
Make application to probate the will within five days of the death.
If necessary, elect an attorney to handle the estate.
Give written notice to heirs of your appointment as personal representative.
Take care of estate property.
Notify Social Security and the decedent's life insurance companies.
Pay expenses for last illness, funeral, and any debts.
Have real and personal property appraised.
Prepare an inventory of the decedent's property.
Publish a notice in the local newspaper to creditors for debts about which
    the personal representative maybe unaware.
Prepare and file federal estate tax returns, if applicable.
Prepare and file state and federal income taxes for the last year of life.
Arrange for the family's immediate living expenses.
Make charitable donations as stipulated by the will.
Close bank accounts and open an estate account.
Distribute assets as required by laws of succession (no will) or by the
    decedent's will.

Estate Lawyers

The process of settling the estate will have fewer hitches and frustrations
if you work with an estate lawyer. Yes, hiring a lawyer is expensive. Fees vary
by location and are generally higher in urban areas.

Lawyers often charge a percentage of the estate value; however, if the
estate is small and uncomplicated, the lawyer may opt to charge an hourly fee.
If the lawyer doesn't mention options, ask!

If affordability is a concern, you can often find clinics or not-for-profit
legal organizations that specialize in elder law. Contact a local law school and
ask to speak with someone from their community or elder law clinic.

You can save a little money by doing some of the legwork yourself;
however, what you save in lawyer fees may not be worth the added expenses
of gas and parking, the frustration of finding the right building and office, and
the time wasted waiting in line.

The lawyer who, several years earlier, helped me with various issues
concerning oversight of Dorothy's care also practiced estate law; therefore,
it made sense to continue working with the person who already understood
our situation.

Some First Steps

Again, keep in mind what I describe may differ from what you need to do. Estate law varies from state to state, and wills often contain unique combinations of stipulations.

The first thing my lawyer did was file papers with probate court to establish the will as a legal document and me as the PR with the "power" to dispose of the assets. The next step was to apply for (another) Employee Identification Number (EIN).

Why? As the personal representative, your role is essentially that of an employee whose job is to administer the closing of the estate. In some states, the PR can draw a salary; however, the money you earn is taxable.

This EIN was my ticket to establish an estate bank account that allowed me to deposit estate income, pay estate bills, and eventually distribute estate funds.

Remember to scan the probate and EIN documents. Having an electronic file makes them easily accessible and can make things more efficient when banks or other entities want to see a copy before proceeding on to a next step. The bank or other institutions may request a hard copy as well.

Setting up the estate account was a lengthy and tedious process. The bank required that I provide a certified death certificate and copies of the probate court and EIN documents. Then, the bank representative and I spent several hours going through Dorothy's bank holdings. He combined the accounts that were solely in her name into a special estate account.

The combination of establishing the will as a legal document, me as the PR, and opening an estate bank account gave me the ability to begin the process of settling the estate. I now had an account where I could deposit refund checks from Dorothy's car insurance and newspaper subscription, as well as the money collected from selling her car and the proceeds from an estate sale. The checking account gave me a way to pay for certain estate-related expenses. I signed checks with my name followed by the phrase "PR for the estate."

KEEPING RECORDS

Record keeping is extremely important throughout the process of settling the estate. It's very easy to forget who you spoke with, what they said, and when they said it. Sometimes people at the other end don't do as they promised. Sometimes important documents disappear.

In addition to keeping track of correspondence, it is also important to record all expenses, income, financial transactions, and transferals of property, as

Table 15.2.   Sample Record Keeping Pages

Correspondence with Social Security, Medicare, and Other Organizations and Businesses		
Date of Correspondence	Summary of Discussion	Name/Contact Information

Payments and Receipts		
Date of Payment (–) or Receipt(+)	Description and Check Number/Cash	Dollar Amount

Gifts to the Estate		
Date of Gift to the Estate	Description and Check Number/Cash	Dollar Amount

well as listing all bank accounts and other estate assets (see table 15.2). Keep all the paperwork that accompanies any of these transactions. Scanning and filing is probably the easiest way to organize transaction receipts. Be sure to keep a hard copy in a safe and easy to remember location. Underline or use a marking pen to identify estate-related expenses on your monthly credit card bill.

Some expenses are called "gifts to the estate." Rather than a present, a gift to the estate is a loan that gets repaid before heirs receive their inheritance. People make gifts to the estate when estate funds are not yet available, or if it just happens to be more convenient to pay for services or products with personal funds.

The lawyer will tell you to make an inventory of the estate. In addition to such things as houses, land, and bank accounts, you should list particularly valuable or noteworthy items like art, musical instruments, and jewelry. It is also permissible to make categorical itemizations like "$7,000 for household furniture" (see table 15.3).

THE ESTATE

The estate is everything your family member owns, which includes real property—houses and land—and personal property, such as the contents of houses,

Table 15.3. Sample Inventory Page

Type of Item	Value	Total Value	Sell? Donate? Gift?
House			
Clothing			
Furnishings			
Car(s)			
Art			
Collectibles			
Stocks and bonds			

stocks, bonds, bank accounts, checking accounts, certificates of deposit, and life insurance policies.

Your family member's debts are also part of the estate. The estate pays for debts like car payments, mortgages, and unpaid bills. If your family member received Medicaid, the estate reimburses the state Medicaid Estate Recovery Program for a portion of the public money used to pay for care.

Some family members find it advantageous to put certain parts of their estate into trusts. Trusts can be pretty complicated. As an example, your father—the "trust maker"—enters into an agreement with a trustee, a bank, or a trust company to manage property or funds while he is still alive. The beneficiary, you or another person, receives the contents of the trust at a later time—often when the trust maker dies. Trusts, depending on how they are set up, may or may not be part of the estate. Your estate lawyer can tell you if the trust is part of the estate.

TRANSFER ON DEATH (TOD)

Your family member may have prearranged to have certain assets, such as the house or certain bank accounts, marked with the designation Transfer on Death (TOD) along with another person's name. The TOD stipulation removes those items from the estate and, at the time of death, the designated person is now the owner.

The person listed on TOD bank accounts, stock certificates, or other types of monetary assets takes ownership by presenting the financial institution with a certified death certificate and a photo identification card. The bank representative or stockbroker completes the paperwork to complete the transfer.

In many states, transferring ownership of real property, such as houses or land, involves a TODD or Transfer on Death Deed. You or your lawyer can file the TODD with the appropriate city or county real estate records office. You may have to wait as much as a few weeks before your name appears on the deed. Do not assume things will take care of themselves. It may take a couple of phone calls, and maybe an additional trip to the records office, to get the right name on the deed. The person whose name appears on the TOD or TODD is responsible for this task (see Helpful Resources).

NOTIFICATIONS

As soon as possible after the death, notify Social Security and any other state, federal, and private organizations that provided income, helped pay for care, or provided services. Often a verbal notification will get things started, but most will require a certified death certificate to close the file or send reimbursement for unused services. In addition to the death certificate, include a cover letter that contains your family member's date of death, Social Security and Medicare numbers, and any other relevant identification numbers.

Yes, most of that information is available on the death certificate, but like wearing a belt and suspenders, it never hurts to make sure things will happen as intended.

Make electronic and paper copies of all correspondences and save them as a hard (paper) copy and as a file on your hard drive. Sometimes it takes a while for the right person to receive and respond to your letter.

Be sure to get the name and contact information for the person you spoke to on the phone. Ask how long it will take to close the account once they have received the information they need. Give them an extra week, and if you don't receive what they promised, follow up with a phone call.

SOCIAL SECURITY

Even under less stressful conditions, navigating through the Social Security system is a challenge. In this section, you will find an overview of the steps one must take to report a death, stop Social Security payments, and determine eligibility for the surviving spouse and other family members.

In all likelihood, you will find the information contained in the following paragraphs a bit overwhelming. Please, it's just an overview! You will find all the information you need in the Helpful Resources section located at the end of this book.

Your first step is to report the death to your local Social Security office. Be prepared to give the person who answers the phone the decedent's Social

Security number. In addition, the representative will want to know your Social Security number, your date of birth, the city and state where you live, and your mother's maiden name. They ask for this additional information to protect identity and to safeguard the account.

Many people have their Social Security payment electronically deposited into their bank account. So, in addition to reporting the death to Social Security, you must also notify your family member's bank, credit union, or any other financial institution. The U.S. Treasury will automatically debit the account.

There are a couple of quirky things about Social Security payments: 1) your family member must be alive for the entire month, and 2) payment is one month in arrears for people who receive payment based on their or their spouse's work record. So if death occurred on August 31 at 11:59 p.m., then you would have to return the check deposited on September 1; however, if the death occurred at 12:01 a.m. on September 1 and they were therefore alive for the entire month of August, you do not have to return the payment.

Keep track of all Social Security communications and transactions. You don't want to mistakenly believe there is more money in the account than is actually available. Be sure to notify the Social Security office a second time if the bank receives another deposit the following month.

Things get fairly complicated when there is a surviving spouse. What happens next depends on how the surviving spouse is "recorded" on the decedent's Social Security. If you are a surviving spouse, make an appointment to speak with a local Social Security representative.

You cannot apply for survivor benefits online.

Many people are unaware of the $255 Lump Sum Death Benefit that an eligible surviving spouse or, if there is no spouse, eligible surviving dependent children may receive. Although there are many "if" and "must be" clauses, the main eligibility criteria are 1) spouses living together at the time of death, and, in the absence of a spouse, 2) children are eighteen years of age or younger and unmarried. Each child, or their representative, files for their Lump Sum benefit.

MEDICARE

The Social Security Administration (SSA) administers Medicare; however, unlike reporting cessation of Social Security benefits, you cannot report a death online. In most cases, the funeral home will report the person's death to the SSA; therefore, it is important the funeral home has your loved one's Social Security and Medicare numbers. A family member or person responsible for the care of the beneficiary may report the death as well. Social Security will remove your family member from Medicare upon receiving verification of their death.

LIFE INSURANCE AND ANNUITY BENEFITS

The beneficiary, rather than the personal representative, is the person responsible for filing a claim for their life insurance and annuity benefits. To claim benefits, the beneficiary should contact the company's local office and inform them of the death. Typically, companies ask the beneficiary to complete a claim form and submit it to the company along with a certified copy of the death certificate. If there is more than one adult beneficiary, each person should submit a claim.

VETERAN'S BENEFITS

Similar to life insurance and annuity benefits, the beneficiary is the person responsible for applying for veteran's survivors' pension benefits. Basic eligibility requires that the beneficiary is an unremarried spouse or an unmarried child of a deceased veteran (see table 15.4).

Although there are no age requirements for an unremarried spouse, there are income eligibility requirements. The U.S. Department of Veterans Affairs suggests that unremarried spouses file an application even if unsure of their eligibility. Use your internet browser and the phrase "VA Survivors' Pension Benefit form" to get the application.

There are age requirements for unmarried children. To be eligible for veteran's survivors' benefits, unmarried children must meet one of the following requirements: younger than eighteen years of age or a full-time student under the age of twenty-three. Disabled unmarried children must have been disabled before their eighteenth birthday and incapable of self-support.

Table 15.4. Eligible Active Service Branches

Air Force
Army
Coast Guard
Commissioned officer in the Environmental Science Services Administration
Commissioned officer in the National Oceanic and Atmospheric Administration (NASA)
Commissioned officer in the Public Health Service
Marine Corps
Merchant Marine
National Guard
Navy

Table 15.5.   Dates of Wartime Service

War	Dates
World War II	December 7, 1941–December 31, 1946
Korean War	June 27, 1950–January 31, 1955
Vietnam War	August 5, 1964–May 7, 1975
Vietnam War for veterans who served "in country" before August 5, 1964	February 28, 1961–May 7, 1975
Gulf War	August 2, 1990–a date yet to be determined

A wartime veteran is not necessarily someone who saw active combat. According to the Department of Veterans Affairs, the deceased veteran must have served at least ninety days of active military duty of which at least one day was during a wartime period. For those entering active duty after September 7, 1980, he or she must have served at least twenty-four months, or the full period of their call to active duty, of which at least one day was during a wartime period (see table 15.5). This includes people who served in World War II, the Korean War, the Vietnam War, and the Gulf War through a future date to be set by law or a presidential proclamation.

UNPAID BILLS

Earlier you read that debt is part of the estate. Debt—money owed to another individual, business, or tax collecting entity—includes such things as unpaid utility bills, mortgage and credit card payments, and real estate taxes. If you run into the situation where payments are due before you have an EIN and access to estate funds, call the business, utility billing, or real estate tax offices and explain the situation to them. Under these circumstances, they can suspend payment until you have access to the funds. You should not have to pay any late-fee penalties.

The billing office may require that you provide a certified death certificate and perhaps a letter of confirmation from the estate lawyer. If this sounds like it is more trouble than it is worth, pay the bills and any other debts with personal funds. Record these expenses as "gifts to the estate."

It's hard to remember all the services that a person once used or subscribed to. Going through the checkbook register and credit card bills, as well as finding the direct withdrawals on a bank statement, should reveal all those services you need to contact. Those services paid for in advance—newspaper and magazine subscriptions and house and car insurance, for example—will reimburse the estate for the amount of unused service. Record these refunds as estate income.

Legal Notice of Death

Although it is your responsibility to pay any outstanding bills, your lawyer will publish a legal notice in the newspaper. If you are not familiar with the legal notice page, it's the one with lots of classified ads in very small print.

The notice of the death and the estate invites the creditors to submit bills to an address listed in the notice. Usually there is a statute of limitations, for example, ninety days. The estate is not required to pay bills submitted after the statute of limitations has passed.

Credit Cards

Once you have paid a final credit card bill, notify the credit card company of the death. Call the toll-free number on the back of the card, give the recorded voice the information it needs—usually the last four digits of the credit card number and the zip code that corresponds to the one on the billing address. Once you have jumped that hurdle, ask to speak with a customer service representative. Tell the service representative that because of a death you are calling to close down the credit card account. From there, your call will be transferred to the Estates Department.

According to the service representative I spoke to, what happens next depends entirely on the circumstances and the type of account. Because I was only doing research and did not have an actual death to report, they would not transfer me to the Estates Department. But I bet they will want to know some of the information associated with the credit card, such as a date of birth and a maiden name. And as I recall from my real experience several years ago, they will ask that you send a certified death certificate and a cover letter.

To be on the safe side, record the names of the people you spoke with and ask about the best way to reach them should you need to speak with them again.

Communication Services

In addition to the telephone, you may also need to discontinue cell phone and internet service, movie subscriptions, and satellite or direct TV services. It's always a good idea to make these calls using the phone number or computer assigned to the bill.

Dorothy, like many other people of her generation, did not have a computer or any of the other accompanying internet services. She did, however, have a cell phone

Closing down the cell phone account was easy. I simply went to the cell phone store, waited in line, gave them documentation showing I was her PR, signed some papers, and that was it.

Closing down the house phone account was an entirely different story. First of all, I made the mistake of calling from my home phone. Even though Dorothy's phone bill was addressed to my house, calling from my phone, rather than hers, raised flags with the phone company. Even with my offer to send a certified death certificate and other documentation, the representative said he had no way of knowing if I was an abusive relative trying to isolate an elderly person from her family. So I said "thank-you" and ended the conversation.

Later, I called from Dorothy's home, and rather than telling them about a death, I said I (Dorothy) was moving to Peru and needed to close my account. The phone company was happy to oblige and hoped I would resume their services upon my return. I mumbled something about it being a permanent move.

HOUSE CLEANING

Cleaning the house is the time when we peel back the layers. In the process of sorting through belongings, we discover remnants of our childhood and our family's history. We may also find evidence that shows dementia was hovering in the background for much longer than anyone might have imagined.

The mismatched mittens I mentioned earlier instantly brought me back to the days of snowmen, sledding, and cold hands. There were other things, too: a dress I wore to a seventh-grade dance, paintings I made during my high school years, several pairs of outgrown ice skates, and a favorite winter hat, as well as a collection of preschool craft projects her grandchildren made twenty to thirty years ago.

I found boxes of photographs of people I do not know. One of the most interesting finds was the boat ticket showing that on November 22, 1913, my father and his parents sailed from Antwerp, Belgium, on the Red Star Line's SS *Zeeland* and arrived at Ellis Island eleven days later. How they traveled from Zambrow, Poland, to Belgium is a mystery.

No music box.

Other findings revealed more about Dorothy than she was willing to share with us. I found a large collection of still-boxed hair driers, drawers filled with unopened cosmetics, and jewelry hidden in the bottom of closet storage bags. Did she buy these things not remembering that she had already made a similar purchase? Perhaps she had forgotten the purpose of a hair drier or how to apply lipstick and face powder?

One can only assume that Dorothy, in the grips of dementia-related paranoia, hid her jewelry to protect her belongings from thieves. Finding jewelry in strange places both explained her insistence that people were stealing from her and made it mandatory that I sort through her belongings in a slow and methodical manner.

So Much Stuff!

At first, the amount of stuff in your family member's home is overwhelming. You wonder where to start. And no matter how much you put in the trash, it seems like the house looks just as it did before.

In an attempt to bring some kind of order, I made "trash," "donation," "estate sale," "family," and "take-home" piles. Sometimes it was hard to decide between the trash, the family, and take-home piles. Saying to myself, "now or later," meaning do I throw it out now or later, often solved the dilemma.

I donated Dorothy's clothing to an organization that helps homeless women dress for job interviews. Many charities that run thrift shops will come to the house at times outside of their normal neighborhood schedule. You can also deliver items to thrift shops at your own convenience. There are some items that charities like Goodwill, the Salvation Army, and Big Brothers and Big Sisters do not accept. Mattresses are one of them.

In many communities, you can call the waste management department and arrange for a "big trash" pickup. They do take mattresses and any other items too large to fit in the trash can. Other alternatives are renting a dumpster or taking things to the city dump.

As best you can, estimate the total value of everything you threw away, donated, kept, or gave to family and friends. The number you estimate becomes part of the overall value of the estate.

In most cases, you don't need to itemize. Putting a value of $750 on a used clothing donation is sufficient; however, do be more specific if you gave a valuable painting to your cousin or donated an item that other family members might have wanted.

For articles you believe may be of value, you can often find their worth online by keying in descriptive words and, if applicable, the name of the artist, the manufacturer, its location, and the year of manufacture. There are websites, such as "TinEye," that can identify flat works of art simply by uploading a photograph. Doing this sort of research is very time consuming, but in your role as archeological sleuth, it can be very interesting. Sometimes, online sales services can give you a sense of what people are willing to pay for such things as vintage Fiesta ware and Fire King mixing bowls or memorabilia like old election buttons and postcards.

Another alternative is taking items to an art or an antique appraiser. The appraisal fee is often a percentage of the item's value.

It Takes Sensitivity, Too

Distributing possessions often reveals big differences in feelings and emotional attachments. Some siblings want so much it almost seems as if they want to recreate their parent's home in their own house. Other siblings have a special attachment to one or a few objects or are happy to pick out a single memento.

In the process of cleaning and organizing, I did set aside items for specific family members—old cameras for the granddaughter who enjoys photography and tableware for my sibling who enjoys mid-century artifacts. I decided it was okay that I had first choice. I didn't want much; I asked permission and, as far as I know, no one complained.

Cleaning out the family home can be a time when smoldering family disharmony erupts into hostility and bitterness. Family members become concerned with who gets what and the relative value of what each receives. To make things seemingly equitable, siblings sometimes go as far as splitting china and silverware sets! It may be fair, but the end result is not particularly satisfying.

To minimize hurt feelings, some families develop rules for dividing belongings. They use the internet to research the monetary value of art and antiques and make efforts to see that each gets what they want of similarly valued items. "Heads or tails" is as good a way as any to distribute items that more than one person wants. And it's perfectly okay to ask your sister if she would be willing to trade her dining room set for your grandfather clock. Creating workable game rules encourages a more lighthearted approach to what is a difficult and painful job.

Here are some real-life scenarios that are guaranteed to create ill feelings: 1) inviting family members to come to the house to pick what they want and then informing them those items are already yours; 2) splitting sets of matching dessert dishes or wine glasses so no one has a useful number; 3) throwing out such things as recipe collections and family photographs before asking if others want them; and 4) refusing to respond to cousins, aunts, uncles, and partners who may want a small memento. These kinds of endings color the feelings immediate and extended families have for one another and become ingrained in the family lore.

Estate Sales

Estate sales, or tag sales, are great places to pick up tools, an extra folding chair, or some spare kitchen glasses. For the people who have the sale, it is an efficient way to clean out the house and increase the cash value of the estate.

People often hire an estate sale company to organize, run, and manage the sale for them. There are many advantages to taking this approach. First of all, the estate sale company often has a better idea of what things are worth. And because their charge is a percentage of the sales, anywhere from 30 to 50 percent, it is to everyone's advantage to get the highest possible price.

The estate sale company advertises, prices items, and organizes table displays. The sales table can accept cash, checks, or credit card payments. You do not have to be present. Afterward, the estate sales company clears away any remaining items. They may take remainders to another estate sale or donate them to charity.

It is easy to find local estate sale company listings on the internet. The keywords "estate sales" plus the location will bring up a list of resources.

I looked into using an estate sale company. I described the kinds of items available and how much stuff there was to sell. Several estate sale owners came to the house to look at specific items. Those businesses, plus the ones I spoke to by phone, all said there really wasn't enough in Dorothy's home to make a sale worth their time and my expense. A few offered to add Dorothy's belongings to another estate sale; however, the percentage they wanted to charge was too high.

In the end, I sold some of the furnishings to people who had just moved into a new house. I gave Dorothy's caregivers some things they wanted, and I spent a week or so pricing and organizing the remaining items for a home-grown estate sale.

Advertisement was nothing more than an ad in the classified section of the local newspaper and a few signs to direct people to the house. I asked a few friends to help. Many of them brought things from their house to sell. So in many respects, Dorothy's estate sale became a neighborhood event.

Be prepared! Customers show up early and are assertive about wanting to enter before opening time. Use signs, barricades, tape, or locked doors to close off private areas. Make sure there is a person in every room to keep an eye on things. Assign one person the task of money collector and another as the record keeper. Be willing to bargain, and prepare to be amazed at what people want to buy.

The estate sale didn't empty the house, but it did make cleaning out Dorothy's house considerably easier. Afterward, more stuff went to family and friends, was donated to charity, or put in the trash.

I recorded the money generated by the sale and deposited it in the estate bank account. I also recorded my expenses, such as the advertisement in the newspaper and the delivery pizza we had for lunch. Since I paid for these things, they were listed as "gifts to the estate."

CLOSING THE ESTATE

There isn't much more to do. The house is clean and is either for sale, rent, or belongs to the person named on the TODD. Without any more expenses or income, the estate account is quiet. Correspondences with Social Security and Medicare have ceased. Doctors and medical supply companies are no longer sending bills. It's time to work on the final accounting.

In total, the tabulations of expenses (i.e., the collection of sales slips and credit card bills) and income (i.e., the amount of money in the estate savings and checking accounts, as well as any other property once held in your family member's name) constitute the estate. Again, to be reimbursed, keep track of your out-of-pocket expenses. The lawyer will make a valuation based on the records they have and the information you have given them. Sometimes there is a difference between the value the lawyer determines and your estimate of the estate's value.

Discrepancies must be reconciled. In my case, it took many hours of going through records with the lawyer's legal assistant and then several more hours with the bank manager before the bank manager found the mistake—well, not really a mistake. The difference was finding a hidden CD in my name. Dorothy had left me a gift.

What you need to do next depends on the specifics of the estate, the stipulations of the will, and state laws. In my case, the lawyer sent the final reconciliation to probate court and to my sibling. Both the court and my sibling returned a signed copy to the lawyer, thus indicating we agreed with the value of the estate and its division among the heirs.

Now I could write checks to the heirs and divide any other property according to the stipulations of Dorothy's will. I have to admit I liked this step. It felt good to give Dorothy's grandchildren, all young adults, a little money toward their first house or some other special purchase.

DEATH AND TAXES

But wait! Before you can close the estate, you may still have to pay state and federal taxes. Some states have an estate tax, too.

Because Dorothy died on December 31, 2010, I only needed to pay her taxes for that year. Had she died the following day, the estate would have been responsible for any taxes due for 2011. On top of that, I wouldn't have been able to close the estate until January 1, 2012.

One day into the New Year is just an annoyance. But if your family member should die in July or September, then the estate must file taxes for the preceding seven or nine months of life. And don't forget estate tax if your family member lived in one of those states.

Although you can give heirs most of their inheritance, be sure to keep some funds in reserve in case the estate owes additional state or federal taxes. Your accountant should be able to estimate the amount the estate will owe or receive as a refund. Tell the heirs they will receive a final notification and payment sometime after the next taxable year. The other alternative is to hold off on distributing inheritances until the estate's tax issues have been resolved.

VERY LAST STEPS

There aren't too many "very last steps." You can close the estate bank accounts and cancel the associated EIN number once the government and heirs have made their deposits. To be on the safe side, be sure to check with your lawyer or accountant before you take those steps.

It is also a good idea to file and store the paperwork associated with your loved one's death and estate. Family members, interested in genealogy, may want to know some of the information contained in the death certificate. The state taxation bureau or the Internal Revenue Service may contact you if they find mistakes in the final tax filing. Medicare and Medicaid may discover similar reasons to contact you.

FREQUENTLY ASKED QUESTIONS

1. What is the difference between Social Security benefits and SSI?

Social Security without the "I" are benefits based on the amount of Social Security taxes you, or your spouse, paid while working. The purpose of the Social Security benefit is to increase economic security during the retirement years.

SSI, or Supplemental Security Income, is a federal program funded by general tax revenues. Its purpose is to help disabled people who are unable to work meet the basic needs of food, clothing, and shelter.

2. I'd like to get going on closing my mother's estate; however, the lawyer tells me it will take nearly two weeks before I become the personal representative of the estate and probably three weeks before I receive certified death certificates. Is there anything I can do now?

You can do things like collect and organize bills and other papers. If she was living at home, you can clean the kitchen and empty the refrigerator.

But until you become the personal representative of the estate, you should hold off doing anything that might get family members worried about your motivations. Use the time to recover from your mother's death and the years you spent as her caregiver. This is also a good time to talk to family members, explain the responsibilities of the personal representative, and tell them how they can help you.

3. What do I do about bills that come in after the estate is closed and money is already distributed to heirs?

If you or your lawyer posted a legal notice of death, and the statute of limitations has passed, then these creditors are out of luck; however, if you did not post a legal notice of death to creditors, then you or the heirs may be responsible for paying these bills. Should this be your situation, this would be a good time to consult with a lawyer. If cost is an issue, contact a local law school community clinic or a not-for-profit law practice.

4. My mother's estate consists of a small savings account and the contents of her assisted living apartment. It is really necessary that I go through all the steps and incur all the expenses described in this chapter?

As always, the rules, even for small estates, vary from state to state. You may find the information you need online. Use your internet search engine and the phrase "closing a small estate" plus the name of the state where the estate is located. Some states provide an online informational packet that a personal representative can use to close an estate that meets certain criteria. Another alternative is to get advice from a local law school community clinic or a not-for-profit law practice.

5. Between travel, legal fees, and time away from work, settling my father's estate is becoming more expensive than I can easily afford. What can I do to make this volunteer job more affordable?

The money you spend on travel, legal fees, and other expenditures like making photocopies are all gifts to the estate. Rather than a donation, the estate will reimburse the money you spend on these and other estate-related expenses.

You may also charge the estate for your time. Most states allow the PR to receive 3 to 5 percent of the estate value as their compensation. In particularly difficult situations, such as when the PR has to close or sell a business, the reimbursement rate may be higher; however, if you choose to be paid for your time, you will have to file forms and include the money earned as taxable income. Gifts to the estate are not taxable income.

WORKSHEET 15.1:
Dorothy's Blueberry Muffins

As promised, the following is the recipe for Dorothy's blueberry muffins. Unlike the sweet muffins we eat today, this recipe shows the frugality of World War II–era housewives. If you wish, add a teaspoon of vanilla extract or perhaps some finely chopped lemon peel.

Preheat oven to 400 degrees. Grease a muffin tin or line with paper muffin cups. This recipe makes approximately one dozen regular-sized muffins and six large muffins.

Dry Ingredients

Sift together the following:

> 2 cups flour
> ¾ teaspoon salt
> ⅓ cup sugar
> 2 teaspoons double-acting baking powder
> 1 cup blueberries

Wet Ingredients

In a separate bowl, beat 2 eggs and add the following:

> ¼ cup melted butter or oil
> ¾ cup milk

Add 1 cup blueberries to the flour mixture and stir to coat. Optional—add 1 teaspoon finely grated orange or lemon zest. Add egg mixture to the flour and berry mixture. Mix with a fork, just long enough to incorporate the liquid into the flour. Over-mixing will make tough, rubbery muffins!

Fill muffin tins about ⅔ full, bake for 20 to 25 minutes for small muffins and 25 to 30 minutes for large ones.

WORKSHEET 15.2:
The Family and the Relatives

The distribution of your loved one's possessions is one of the most emotionally charged aspects of closing your loved one's estate. Who gets what or, rather, who *doesn't* get what often leads to lifelong animosities. Basically, you have one chance to get it right. It's important that someone, not necessarily you, be in charge. The in-charge person, with the input with one or two impartial family members, should develop a plan that takes into consideration both monetary and sentimental value.

ACKNOWLEDGMENTS

I wish to thank the following individuals for their support, enthusiasm, encouragement, invaluable comments, and patience to answer what some would consider too many questions: Libby Golden Hopkins (RN), Edward Fancovic (MD), Elizabeth Roll (PhD), Sam Roll (PhD), Eric Roll, Susan Albright, Mae Green, Lauren Lockett, Dara Lockett, Rocky Stone, Barbara Shapiro, Carla Nichols, Hattie Johnson, Jeanne Johnson, Mary Ann Conley (PhD), and Susan Romano (PhD).

I also wish to thank the numerous families and the individuals in their care who allowed me to intrude into their lives. Their candor helped all of us learn about the difficulties caregivers face and the range of emotions family caregivers experience.

I would be remiss if I did not mention the efforts of doctors Edward Fancovic (MD) and Francesco Standoli (MD). Dr. Fancovic was Dorothy's primary caregiver for the last few years of her life. Despite the challenges, he was always patient, informative, and kind. Our family appreciates his efforts in helping to make things run as smoothly as possible.

Dr. Standoli provided Dorothy's care during her short stay in an assisted living facility. We will always remember him for his kindness, humor, and ability to gently guide Dorothy through the last stages of her life.

And to our caregivers—Carla Nichols, Hattie Johnson, and Jeannie Johnson—a thank-you hardly covers what you did for our family. Because of your patience, caring, and humor, too, Dorothy was able to spend all but a few weeks of her life in the home she loved.

And without question, extra special thanks go to Erin Conklin (RN, MSN). The combination of her keen editorial eye, medical experience, and generosity made a nearly overwhelming project doable. And a private joke: thank-you, Betty Crocker.

I would not have survived this unintended journey without the quiet support of my husband, Richard Shagam. He was always there to lend a hand, subdue my frustrations, and offer words of solace. Then, when the demands of dementia care and estate management were over, I spent the next eighteen months writing the first edition of this book. Now, my grateful thanks extend to the ten months it took to write the second edition. All I can say is, "What a good guy."

And to my granddaughters Camille and Pauline, both impressed by the pile of paper on my desk and floor, as of tomorrow you will have my full attention.

GLOSSARY

13-hour rule: Refers to the number of paid hours a home care worker can receive in a twenty-four-hour period. The 13-hour rule may exclude payment for five hours of uninterrupted sleep and three uninterrupted hours for meals.

911: In an emergency, dial 911 on your phone to contact local emergency services.

abuse: Harmful treatment of self or another person.

accountant: A professional who keeps track of and communicates financial information.

acetylcholine: A naturally occurring substance involved in the transmission of nervous system information to and from the brain.

acquiescence: A reluctant acceptance, submission.

active dying: A palliative care expression. Active dying refers to stepwise physical and mental changes that precede death.

ad litem (attorney): A court-appointed attorney who advocates for individuals unable to advocate for themselves. In cases involving competency and guardianship, the court assigns an ad litem attorney to advocate for the person who has dementia.

Adult Protective Services (APS): A required state-level case management program that arranges for services and support for at-risk or endangered physically and/or mentally impaired adults.

advance directive: A legal document to inform others of the kind of medical care you want if you are unable to speak for yourself. Examples: tube feeding and heroic measures (such as cardiopulmonary resuscitation and ventilation).

aggression/aggressive: A domineering, assaultive, or forceful action toward another person.

Alzheimer's Association: A nonprofit organization that focuses on Alzheimer's disease care, support, and research.

Alzheimer's disease: The most common type of dementia. Signs and symptoms include progressive memory loss and cognitive decline.

ambulate/ambulation: Refers to a person's ability to move or walk with or without a walker or wheelchair.

amyloid: A kind of naturally occurring, though abnormal, protein found in the brains of people who have Alzheimer's disease or other kinds of dementia.

anemia: A state of not having enough red blood cells. People who are anemic often feel weak and tired.

annuity: A kind of insurance that pays a person a fixed sum of money each year. Payments usually extend throughout the lifetime of the person named in the annuity.

antibiotic: A naturally occurring substance, such as penicillin or tetracycline, used to treat bacterial infections. Pharmaceutical chemists modify the chemical structure to improve antibiotic activity.

anticholinergic: A class of medications that *slow* the transmission of information between nerve cells. Anticholinergic medications can worsen dementia symptoms. Anticholinergic medications help manage bladder control problems, muscle spasms, and depression.

antidepressant(s): Medications used to treat depression. Some antidepressants act by slowing the transmission of information between nerve cells.

antipsychotic(s): Medications used to treat delusions and hallucinations that many people who have dementia experience.

antiseptic: Substances that reduce the growth of bacteria on skin.

antiviral: A medication that in various ways prevents the virus from either causing disease or reducing symptoms. For example, acyclovir (Zovirax®) both lessens and reduces the duration of symptoms that accompany genital herpes, cold sores, and shingles—a painful infection that many older people experience.

anxiety: The emotional and physiological response to anticipated dread and danger. People who are anxious may become restless or tense, have an increased pulse, or feel as though they cannot breathe.

art therapist: A health professional who uses art making as a therapeutic tool.

assets: Belongings, such as money, property, and stock, that comprise a person's estate.

assisted living facility: A place where people live and receive twenty-four-hour care and assistance.

atrophy: The wasting away or decrease in size of a body part or tissue. For example, a lack of exercise causes muscle weakening.

autopsy: An internal examination of a body after death that includes inspecting the organs to determine cause of death or to study the effects of disease or disease treatment (and the efficacy of experimental medications) on the body.

bacteria: Microscopic organisms that may cause disease.

bactericidal: A substance, such as a disinfectant or certain types of antibiotics, that kills bacteria.

barium: A naturally occurring element. When combined with a drinkable liquid, it improves contrast and the ability to see more detail in various X-ray imaging procedures.

belligerence: Aggressive, confrontational, and argumentative behavior.

beneficiary: The person who benefits or receives. With respect to estate law, the beneficiary is an heir.

biopsy: A small piece of tissue that receives assessment in a laboratory for signs of disease.

bipolar disease/disorder: A brain disease that causes big swings in mood—from mania to depression. Frontotemporal lobe dementia often mimics bipolar disease.

bisexual: A person who is sexually attracted to both men and women.

bladder infection: An infection that occurs when bacteria enter the bladder. In older people, a bladder infection can cause confusion and symptoms that mimic dementia.

bloating: Intestinal swelling caused by swallowed air or the gases that bacteria, living in the intestines, produce.

blog: Derived from the phrase "web log," a blog is a discussion or information site published on the internet.

blood: The fluid plus the cellular components that circulate through the body through veins and arteries. Among other functions, blood is responsible for transporting the oxygen we inhale to our body tissues.

blood pressure: The force of blood against the walls of arteries. The top number, the systolic pressure, is a measure of the force when the heart contracts. The bottom number, the diastolic pressure, is a measure of the force when the heart relaxes between beats. For most people, an ideal blood pressure ranges from 120/80 to 90/60.

blood transfusion: A common procedure in which a patient receives donated blood through an intravenous line.

blood–borne hepatitis: A liver infection caused by the hepatitis B and hepatitis C viruses. The route of entry into the body is through the circulatory system, often following use of dirty, virus-contaminated needles.

bone (mineral) density: An indicator of bone strength. Low bone density is a risk factor for bone fractures.

bowel: Another word for intestines.

brain bank: A facility that collects and stores donated normal and diseased brains for research purposes.

calorie: The energy contained within the molecules that compose food.

cancer: A group of diseases characterized by unregulated cell growth.

casket: A container where a body is placed prior to burial or cremation.

censor: With respect to dementia, the ability to withhold saying or doing impolite or inappropriate things.

Centers for Disease Control (CDC): A U.S. federal agency under the Department of Health and Human Services. Its scope of interest ranges from infectious diseases and environmental health to occupational safety and the promotion of healthful behaviors.

Centers for Medicare and Medicaid Services (CMS): The Centers for Medicare & Medicaid Services is a federal agency within the United States Department of Health and Human Services. The CMS administers the Medicare program and works in partnership with state governments to administer programs such as Medicaid.

certified death certificate: The original copy of a death certificate.

certified nursing assistant (CNA): Helps people with health care needs under the supervision of a registered nurse (RN) or a licensed practical nurse (LPN). Certified nursing assistants receive training at a school or on the job. Certification requires passing an exam.

chaplain: A clergyperson or layperson trained to provide pastoral care within an institution such as a hospital or hospice. Chaplains are often members of palliative care teams.

cholesterol: A naturally occurring substance found in animal tissues. Sources of dietary cholesterol include meat, dairy products, and eggs. High cholesterol blood levels are a risk factor for heart disease.

cholinesterase: An enzyme that breaks down acetylcholine and thereby terminates the transfer of information between nerve cells.

cognition: The ability to think, learn, and remember.

colonoscopy: A procedure that uses a small camera attached to a flexible tube to see the inner surface of the colon and large intestine. The purpose of the procedure is to find ulcers, colon polyps, tumors, and areas of inflammation or bleeding. During a colonoscopy, potentially abnormal growths can be removed for testing in the laboratory.

colorectal cancer: A cancer that originates in the lower part of the large intestine (the colon or the rectum).

commode: A portable toilet that looks like a chair. People who have difficulty walking may prefer to use a nearby commode.

competent: The ability to make well-founded decisions.

complementary medicine: Using a combination of conventional and alternative medical practices, such as a combination of physical therapy and acupuncture to reduce pain.

complicated grief: When feelings of loss become debilitating and do not resolve with time.

confabulation: When people fill in missing details with plausible information. For people who have dementia or other mental illnesses that distort memory, the fill-ins are often fanciful and usually contain detailed embellishments.

congestive heart failure (CHF): A condition where the heart can no longer efficiently pump blood through the body. Signs and symptoms include fatigue, coughing, difficulty breathing, and swollen legs.

conservator: A person appointed by the court to oversee the well-being and care of a person who cannot make well-founded decisions.

constipation: A condition where having a bowel movement is difficult or infrequent. Some medications used to manage dementia behaviors often cause constipation.

continuing medical education (CME): Course work that health professionals must take and pass to maintain their license to practice.

continuum of care facility/community: Provides a spectrum of care alternatives in one location. People may first live independently in an apartment and then, as need dictates, move into an assisted living facility or a nursing home.

contrast media: A liquid that contains substances, such as barium, that X-rays do not pass through. Using contrast media produces light and dark areas on the X-ray image and improves the ability to see anatomic details.

coronavirus: One of a large family of viruses that can cause disease in birds and animals including humans. In 2019, a newly identified coronavirus, which can spread from person to person, was responsible for the global outbreak of COVID-19, a severe respiratory disease.

Coronavirus Infectious Disease (20)19 (COVID-19): A new virus that is part of the larger coronavirus family. COVID-19 is contagious and spreads from person to person. Symptoms include fever, cough, and shortness of breath. According to the CDC, in the United States unvaccinated people between sixty-five and eighty-four years of age account for the majority of deaths.

coroner: A coroner is an official who investigates suspicious deaths. In some communities, the coroner is an elected official.

cremains: The substances that remain after a cremation. Rather than ashes, cremains are small bone fragments that look like small bits of gravel.

cremation: A funerary option.

Crisis Intervention Team (CIT): A community resource, often specially trained police officers, who intercede in emergency situations, such as when hallucinations cause unmanageable behaviors.

death certificate: A legal document that lists the location, time, and manner of death.

decedent: The person who died.

dehydration: Happens when a person doesn't drink enough water. Signs and symptoms include headaches, dry/sticky mouth, and the production of concentrated and smelly urine.

delusion: A false belief. People who have dementia may believe that people are stealing from them.

dementia: Progressive loss of cognitive skills often associated with observable changes in the brain.

demographic: Information, such as age distribution, occupation, or risk factors, used to describe the characteristics of specific groups of people.

Department of Health and Human Services (HHS): The federal government's principal agency for protecting the health of people living in the United States and providing essential human services, especially for those who are least able to help themselves.

depression: A mental disorder characterized by feelings of overwhelming sadness, loneliness, despair, and self-criticism.

diarrhea: Frequent and watery bowel movements.

digestion: The process of breaking down food into smaller pieces and finally into the molecules we need to nourish our bodies. The process, first beginning in the mouth, primarily involves the stomach and the small and large intestines.

disability: Lack of ability to perform normal or usual activities, such as walking or grasping objects.

disharmony: Conflict. Caring for a person who has dementia can make it difficult for family members to get along.

distraction and redirection: A behavior management strategy used to reduce anxiety.

do not resuscitate (DNR): Instructions not to perform heroic measures (such as CPR) to save or revive a patient who is not likely to recover and enjoy an acceptable quality of life.

durable power of attorney: A power of attorney that does not have a stated termination date.

dysphagia: Swallowing difficulties.

embalm: To use substances that slow or prevent decay.

embalming fluid: A substance, such as formalin, that slows or prevents decay.

embezzle: When a trusted person secretly steals money for their own use.

emotional blunting: Reduced ability to experience feelings like sadness or happiness. Not being able to show those emotions with words or facial expressions. Examples include frontotemporal dementia and dementia with Parkinson's disease.

Employer Identification Number (EIN): A unique nine-digit identification number assigned by the Internal Revenue Service (IRS) to business entities operating in the United States.

encephalopathy: A brain disease usually involving changes in brain structure.

endoscope: A medical instrument used to examine the interior of hollow organs such as the intestines or bladder.

enzyme: A specialized molecule that assists in the process of breaking down larger molecules or assembling large molecules from smaller ones. Many enzyme words end with the suffix *ase*.

epilepsy: A disorder characterized by seizures or other signs of altered consciousness.

esophagus: The tube-like structure that connects the back of the mouth to the stomach.

estate: Everything that a person owns in their name alone.

estate lawyer: A lawyer who specializes in the legal aspects of drafting documents like wills and trusts and eventually disburses the inheritances.

eulogy: A speech given at a memorial service or funeral intended to positively commemorate a person's life.

executive functions: The ability to apply past experiences to present activities, as well as the capability to plan, organize, strategize, and pay attention to details.

executor: A man who is designated to manage and close an estate.

executrix: A woman who is designated to manage and close an estate.

exhale: To let out a breath.

exploitation: To take advantage of a person or a situation.

faith-based not-for-profit: An organization founded by a religious group and whose income does not exceed expenses.

feces: The waste expelled from the digestive tract during a bowel movement.

Federal EIN: An official identification number the Internal Revenue Service (IRS) assigns to businesses in the United States. All businesses must have a Federal EIN to operate legally in the United States.

Federal Insurance Contributions Act (FICA): The tax employers and employees pay to fund Social Security and Medicare.

fiber: The indigestible material found in fruits and vegetables. Dietary fiber helps prevent constipation.

flatulence: The release of gas, a byproduct of digestion, through the rectum.

focus group: A group of people who report their perceptions, opinions, beliefs, and attitudes toward a product, service, concept, advertisement, or idea.

foodborne hepatitis: A contagious liver disease caused by eating food or drinking water contaminated with the hepatitis A virus. Food or water contaminated with fecal matter is the usual cause of foodborne hepatitis.

forensic psychiatry: A subspecialty of psychiatry. A forensic psychiatrist evaluates a person's behavior and capabilities to help the court reach an appropriate legal decision.

Freedom of Information Act: A law that gives the public access to government records.

frontal lobes: Located in the "forehead" part of the brain, these two lobes control short-term memory, appropriate behaviors, and the ability to plan ahead.

frontotemporal lobe dementia: A type of dementia. Symptoms include personality changes, loss of language, obsessive or inappropriate behaviors, and eventually memory loss.

funeral director: A person who has the education and licensure to embalm bodies, arrange burials and cremations, perform funeral rites, and counsel bereaved family members.

gag/cough reflex: The automatic response to having a foreign body stuck in the throat (gag) or a throat irritation (cough).

gay/homosexual: Sexual attraction between two men.

gender: The social attributes of being male or female. Male or female versus man or woman.

gene(s): A unit of inherited information that codes for a specific trait.

generic drug (name): A medication that in all ways, except for the name, works the same as the brand-name drug. For example, levothyroxine is the generic name for Levothyroxine®.

genetics: The study of inherited traits.

geriatric care manager: A person who helps find and coordinate the medical and social support services elderly people may need.

geriatrician: A doctor who specializes in treating older people.

gluten: A naturally occurring substance found in grains such as wheat and spelt. Sorghum rice, corn, quinoa, oats, and buckwheat do not contain gluten. Some normally gluten-free foods such as prepared sauces and soups contain added gluten as a thickener.

green burial: An environmentally sustainable burial. Burying the deceased in its natural state and in a biodegradable coffin or shroud allows natural decomposition to return the body to the earth. A simple wood casket, woven basket, or cotton or linen shrouds are examples of biodegradable caskets. Sometimes people add flower seeds to the burial container.

Green Card/Permanent Resident Card: An official legal document showing that a person can work and live permanently in the United States.

grief: (noun) A normal emotional response to loss.

grieve: (verb) The process of emotional response to loss, such as feelings of sadness and crying.

guardian: A person who protects another from harm.

guardianship: Describes the court-appointed responsibility of protecting another from harm.

hallucination: Sensations of sound, sight, touch, or taste without a source of sensory input. People who have dementia often see people or things that aren't present.

heart attack: Occurs when a blood clot blocks the flow of oxygen-rich blood to the heart and, if not restored, can cause permanent damage.

hepatitis: An inflammation of the liver, usually caused by a viral infection. Certain toxic chemicals, such as solvents and alcohol, are another cause for hepatitis.

hepatitis A: A foodborne virus that causes liver disease. People get hepatitis when they eat or drink virus-contaminated food or water. Hepatitis A is a vaccine-preventable infection.

hepatitis B: A virus found in blood and other body fluids that causes liver disease and some kinds of liver cancer. The virus gets passed from person to person when illegal drug users share needles. Tattoo needles and sexual contact are other modes of transmission. Hepatitis B is a vaccine-preventable infection.

HIV/AIDS: The abbreviations for "human immunodeficiency virus" and "acquired immunodeficiency syndrome." Some of the signs and symptoms of HIV include night sweats, weight loss, susceptibility to other infections, and increased risk for certain cancers.

home reverse mortgage: Converts home equity into monthly income.

hormone: A substance made in one organ that affects a distant organ. For example, the pituitary gland, located in the brain, produces hormones that affect the thyroid gland located at the base of the neck.

hospice: An organization that provides comfort care to those who are dying and emotional support to their families.

Housing and Urban Development (HUD): A federal department that provides adequate and safe rental housing for eligible low-income families, the elderly, and individuals with disabilities.

hygiene: The cleanliness that promotes health and well-being. People who have dementia often forget or refuse to bathe.

immune system: A multifaceted collection of molecular, cellular, and genetic components that helps the body fight off infections and other diseases.

immunization: A method that stimulates the immune system to protect people from various kinds of infections.

immunodeficiency: Occurs when the body is unable to respond to infection or injury with a strong enough response to fight infection or repair an injury. Cancer chemotherapy, medication to prevent tissue and organ transplants, and infections like HIV make people unable to fight off microbes and viruses that cause disease, as well as injuries like skin ulcers.

implicit memory: Learned skills we do without thinking (e.g., tying shoelaces).

incontinence: The inability to control the time or place when we urinate or have a bowel movement.

independent living: A facility that houses able-bodied older people who no longer want the work and responsibility of caring for their own home.

indwelling hardware: Metal implants that include pacemakers, joint replacements, and aneurysm clips.

infection: A condition when microbes cause symptoms.

infectious disease: A disease caused by bacteria, viruses, fungi, or parasites.

inflammation: The body's response to injury or infection. *PRISH* is the acronym health care providers use to remember the signs and symptoms that inflammation causes—*P*ain, *R*edness, *I*mmobility, *S*welling, and *H*eat.

influenza: A respiratory disease caused by the influenza virus that can put older people at increased risk for pneumonia and possibly death.

inhale: To take a breath.

inhibitor: A substance that slows or inhibits a biochemical reaction.

I-9 form: Verifies an employee's identity and eligibility to legally work in the United States.

insulin: A hormone produced in the pancreas that regulates the body's ability to use glucose.

ischemic: An area of reduced blood flow.

kidney: The bean-shaped organs located on either side of the lower back. The kidneys "filter" waste products from the blood and, in doing so, produce urine.

kosher: Food prepared according to traditional Jewish law, which includes humane slaughter and not eating dairy with meat or consuming shell fish.

lactose: A naturally occurring sugar found in milk and other unfermented dairy products. Lactose intolerance is a condition when a person cannot digest lactose and then experiences stomach cramps and bloating.

lesbian: A woman who is sexually attracted to other women.

Lewy bodies: Abnormal protein deposits in the brain associated with having dementia and Parkinson's disease.

life cycle event: Birth, certain religious ceremonies, marriage, and death are examples of events that occur at prescribed times over the course of a life.

life insurance: Purchased monetary protection that a beneficiary receives as one large payment upon the death of the individual who had the insurance.

life support: The technologies used to replace or supplement failed or failing organs, such as dialysis for kidney failure.

liver: A large organ located beneath the lungs. Some of its functions include the breakdown of the proteins and carbohydrates we eat and the production of bile that helps fatty substances mix with water.

living will: Another word for the term *advance directive* that informs others of your wishes concerning artificial life-sustaining measures.

lobe: Part of an organ, such as the thyroid gland, that, because of its shape, appears separate from the main structure.

long-term care facility: A residence providing care, such as an assisted living facility or a nursing home.

long-term care (LTC) insurance: An insurance policy that can help pay for some of the expenses associated with home care or living in an assisted living facility or nursing home.

malnourished: A diet lacking in key nutrients. A person who is malnourished may be of normal weight or heavier.

Medicaid: Funds that states use to help low-income individuals receive medical care.

medical alert device: A necklace or a bracelet that connects at-risk people to emergency help.

medical social worker: A person who has the education, experience, and licensure to provide counseling, practical advice, and services in clinical settings.

Medicare: A federal program that funds the medical care of people sixty-five years of age and older.

Medicare Conditions of Participation: Refers to the eligibility requirements one must have to receive Medicare coverage for hospice services.

melatonin: A substance made in the brain that helps regulate sleep cycles.

memory: The ability to retrieve information from specific areas of the brain; to remember.

metabolism: The biochemical reactions that harvest energy from the food we eat.

microscope: A laboratory tool, composed of many lenses and a light source, that makes it possible to see things too small to be seen by the unaided eye.

mild cognitive impairment (MCI): Having more than expected problems with remembering regularly scheduled events and appointments.

Many people who have mild cognitive impairment progress to having Alzheimer's disease.

Mini Mental Status Exam (MMSE): Also called the "mini mental," the MMSE evaluates such things as memory, cognition, and executive function.

mortuary: A place to prepare or store bodies before burial.

mucus: A clear, thick liquid secreted by the cells that line the respiratory and genital tracts and the intestines.

neglect: To purposefully ignore, often with detrimental outcomes to health and well-being.

neurofibrillary tangles: Aggregates of proteins found in the brain and associated with Alzheimer's disease and some other neurodegenerative conditions.

neuropsychologist: A clinical psychologist who specializes in the relationships between brain function and behavior. Neuropsychologists evaluate such things as cognition and executive function.

nondeclarative memory (implicit memory): Our collection of learned skills and procedures like riding a bicycle, typing, and tying shoelaces.

nonproprietary (drug) name: Uses the name of the main ingredients. The words *generic* and *nonproprietary* have the same meaning.

notary: A person licensed by the state to do such things as witness the signing of important documents.

not-for-profit/nonprofit: Organizations that use earned, donated, or foundation funds to provide information, support, and services to specific groups of people. The Alzheimer's Association is a nonprofit organization.

nurse case manager (CMCN): Oversees that patients receive the most efficient, effective, and cost-saving care.

nurse practitioner: A registered nurse who has completed a master of nursing or doctor of nursing practice degree. Nurse practitioners diagnose and treat physical and mental conditions. A nurse practitioner can be a primary care provider.

nursing home: A place for people who don't require hospitalization but are too ill or frail to stay in their own home or an assisted living facility. Nursing homes provide skilled nursing care. Unlike assisted living facilities, nursing homes are subject to federal health and safety regulations.

occupational therapy: Helps a person regain the dexterity to perform daily living skills like getting dressed or opening jars and cans.

Office of the Medical Investigator (OMI): A state-funded facility responsible for ruling out violence or malpractice as a cause of death.

off-label use: Using medication in ways not approved by the Food and Drug Administration (FDA). For example, some medications normally used to prevent seizures are sometimes used to modify behavior.

oncologist: A physician who specializes in diagnosing and treating cancer.

osteoporosis: A condition, especially for postmenopausal women and elderly men, where bones become thin, porous, and at high risk for fracture.

overactive bladder: Miscommunication between the brain and bladder that makes people continuously feel as though they have a full bladder and need to urinate.

palliative care: A philosophy of medical care that always takes into consideration patient comfort and dignity.

paranoia: A mental disorder characterized by delusions of harmful situations, such as being followed by strangers or poisoned by caregivers.

Parkinson's disease: A terminal neurological disease whose main signs and symptoms are shaking, slowed movements, impaired posture and balance, and rigid muscles.

pathologist: A medical practitioner who specializes in diagnosing disease and determining cause of death by looking at dissected organs, using a microscope to look at tissue specimens or medical imagery like an X-ray.

pelvic floor: A group of muscles that support and correctly position the pelvic organs like the bladder, rectum, and uterus (in females).

personal representative: The person identified in the will and/or appointed by the court to close an estate.

pH: Measurement units that describe the acidity or alkalinity of a substance.

physician assistant: A person educated, certified, and licensed to diagnose and treat commonly encountered medical problems. The physician assistant works under the supervision of a licensed physician.

pneumococcus: A microbe that can infect the lungs and cause pneumonia.

pneumonia: A lung inflammation that can be caused by chemical exposure or various bacterial, viral, or fungal infections.

pocketing: Collecting food between the teeth and cheek. People who cannot swallow may pocket their food.

power of attorney (POA): A competent adult assigned to oversee another's medical or financial needs.

probate: In a court of law, the process that determines if a will is valid.

probate court: A special court that deals with the administration of wills.

Programs of All-Inclusive Care for the Elderly (PACE): Available in some states to provide comprehensive long-term services and support to people enrolled in Medicaid or Medicare.

prostate: A gland (in males) that surrounds the upper part of the urethra. An enlarged prostate gland, a condition that affects older males, makes urination difficult.

protein: A biological molecule that is both an essential constituent of all living organisms and a required dietary nutrient.

pseudodementia: A condition where a psychiatric illness, for example, depression, makes it seem like a person has dementia. Treating the cause often treats the "not" dementia.

psychiatrist: A medical practitioner who specializes in the diagnosis and treatment of mental disorders.

psychologist: A licensed health care professional who helps people understand and cope with emotionally difficult situations.

psychosis: A mental disorder characterized by a gross distortion of reality.

quality of life: A state of personal satisfaction and general well-being.

radiologic technologist: A licensed health care professional who performs medical imaging procedures like X-ray, MR, and CT scans.

radiologist: A medical practitioner who evaluates X-ray, MR, and other medical imaging methods to detect and diagnose certain kinds of illness.

reflex: An involuntary or automatic response to a stimulus, such as a throat irritation making one cough.

registered nurse: A nurse who graduated from a nursing program at a college or university and has passed a national licensing exam.

rehabilitation hospital: A care facility that specializes in helping people regain physical functions, such as walking or using their hands. Many rehabilitation hospital patients have Parkinson's disease, have had a stroke, or have been in an accident.

Resources for Enhancing Alzheimer's Caregivers Health (REACH): A research program sponsored by the National Institute on Aging and the National Institute on Nursing Research. The Veterans Administration REACH program helps family caregivers manage challenging dementia behaviors and provides the skills needed to maintain their health and well-being.

respite: A short period of rest or relief from a stressful situation.

resuscitation: The action or process of reviving someone from unconsciousness or apparent death.

saliva: The liquid that keeps the mouth wet.

schizophrenia: A brain-based mental disorder characterized by delusions, hallucinations, and social isolation.

secretion: A substance produced and used in the body. The mucus that lubricates the intestinal tract is a secretion.

sedative/sedation: A quieting medicine that helps people feel less worried, anxious, or angry.

seizure: Usually referring to an epileptic seizure when changes in brain activity cause altered consciousness often leading to shaking and muscle contractions.

senile/senility: A word once used to describe mental disorders and physical condition associated with old age.

sign: A measurable feature of a disease, such as fever, a higher than normal amount of sugar in blood, or finding bacteria in urine.

skilled nursing: A type of nursing care that offers long- or short-term support for people who need rehabilitation or have serious health issues.

Social Security: A tax-funded program that provides a degree of economic security for retirees and their surviving spouse.

State Pharmaceutical Assistance Program (SPAP): A Medicare program that helps eligible people pay for drug premiums and other drug costs. Not all states have a State Pharmaceutical Assistance Program.

stress: A normal response to a mentally or emotionally disruptive situation.

stress hormone(s): Substances produced by the body during times of ongoing mental and emotional anxiety. Some stress hormones, such as cortisol and norepinephrine, cause—often temporary—high blood pressure and rapid heartbeat.

stroke: A "brain attack" caused by a blood clot or a broken vessel that blocks or prevents the flow of blood to or within the brain.

sundowner's syndrome: Describes the agitation, confusion, anxiety, disorientation, and depression that some people who have dementia experience toward the end of the day.

survivor: Someone who lives on after an event, such as a severe car accident.

swallow test: A type of X-ray examination used to determine the cause of swallowing difficulties.

symptom: A feeling experienced by the patient and not measurable by a lab test. A health care professional may ask the patient to rank pain or itchy skin from 1 to 10.

synagogue: A place where Jewish people attend religious services.

synchronize: To have or make events happen at the same or a certain time.

syndrome: A collection of signs and symptoms associated with a specific disease.

T-cells: A type of white blood cell that, as part of the immune system, protects us from getting infections.

terminal disease: A disease, such as advanced cancer, heart disease, and dementia, likely to eventually be the cause for death.

therapeutic deception: A harmless statement, though untrue, that calms the patient and deflects difficult-to-manage behavior.

trade name: Named by the pharmaceutical company that developed the medication. The ® indicates federal approval and registration. The words *proprietary* and *trade* mean the same thing.

tranquilizer(s): Drugs that make people feel calm.

transgender: A person whose anatomy is male or female but who feels they are in the wrong body. Some people opt to undergo hormone treatment and sex reassignment surgery.

transient ischemic attack (TIA): A very small stroke caused by a momentary interruption of blood flow to the brain. Symptoms are short-lived and sometimes go unnoticed.

tube feeding: A method of providing nutrition to people who cannot eat or swallow well enough to obtain sufficient calories.

tuberculosis (TB): Most often a lung infection caused by the bacterium *Mycobacterium tuberculosis.* This potentially fatal disease is highly contagious and spreads among people living in close quarters.

Twilight Zone: A phrase meaning an "other-worldly experience" where it is hard to tell the difference between what is real and what is fantasy. The phrase came into popular use with the original U.S. television show *The Twilight Zone*, which aired from 1959 to 1964.

type 1 diabetes: Usually occurring during childhood, it is a condition when the pancreas no longer produces insulin. People who have type 1 diabetes must take insulin shots for the rest of their lives.

type 2 diabetes: This most common type of diabetes happens when the pancreas makes insufficient insulin or the body does not respond to its presence. Obesity and lack of physical activity are two of the most common causes of type 2 diabetes.

unattended death: When the deceased has not been under a provider's care for the past thirty days, or one where a health care professional was not present to witness the death.

United States Census Bureau: The government office responsible for collecting, tabulating, and organizing data, such as the kinds of information recorded on death certificates.

urgency: Another word for the feeling of having to go to the bathroom right away.

urine: The water and dissolved substances produced by the kidneys and temporarily stored in the bladder.

U.S.-delivered work permit: A U.S. government document that eligible people receive to prove they can work legally in the United States. Also called the Employment Authorization Card (EAD).

vaccine/vaccination: A substance used to provide protection against infectious diseases like hepatitis, measles, mumps, pneumonia, and influenza.

vascular dementia: Stepwise, rather than steadily progressive, loss of cognition and other intellectual functions caused by many small strokes.

vegan: A type of diet that includes fruits, vegetables, beans, and nuts. This philosophy of eating excludes animal protein or any product derived from an animal including gelatin, eggs, honey, and dairy.

vegetarian: A type of diet that consists of fruits, vegetables, and plant-based proteins and avoids animal proteins like meat. Some vegetarians eat fish, shellfish, eggs, and dairy.

vertebrae: The thirty-three individual interlocking bones that make up the spinal column in humans. They surround and protect the spinal cord. Osteoporosis of the spine causes pain when the vertebrae compress on one another.

Veterans Administration (VA): A cabinet-level department of the U.S. government that provides patient care and federal benefits to veterans and their dependents.

virus: A small infectious "particle" that must enter the cells of a plant or animal (human) to replicate and make more virus particles.

vitamin(s): Substances found in small amounts in foods. Consuming insufficient amounts may cause such things as bone disease, blindness, and bleeding.

vomit: To eject food and water from the stomach through the mouth.

ward of the state: When a person is unable to care or make decisions for himself and has no family members to help do so, the state, through the court system, appoints a guardian to make decisions on the ward's behalf.

W-2 wage and tax statement form: A form that employers submit to the Internal Revenue Service (IRS) for each employee who receives payment or other types of compensation for services.

yogurt: A dairy protein-rich product that is easy to swallow and digest.

HELPFUL RESOURCES

U.S. Department of Health and Human Services
Website: Alzheimers.gov

This federal government portal is an entry way into the latest information for people whose lives have been touched by Alzheimer's disease and related dementias. You will find links to such topics as self-care, community support, and drug trial opportunities.

DEMENTIA ORGANIZATIONS

Alzheimer's Association
Website: https://www.alz.org/local_resources/find_your_local_chapter.

To find your local Alzheimer's Association chapter, search using your zip code or click on the state map to find contact information for your local Alzheimer's Association chapter.

Dementia Society of America
Website: https://www.dementiasociety.org.

This organization provides education, local resources and support to help enrich the lives of families and individuals impacted by dementia. Click on the "Resources" tab at the top of the website home page to access education-, program-, and awareness-raising information.

COGNITIVE AND GENETIC TESTING

Cognitive Assessment

Alzheimer's Association

Website: https://www.alz.org/professionals/health-systems-clinicians/cognitive-assessment.

Although this toolkit is designed for clinicians, it is full of information that can help you understand the different kinds of cognitive testing you can expect when your health care provider suggests assessing a loved one for dementia.

Genetic Testing

National Association of Genetic Counselors

Websites: http://www.nsgc.org/; https://www.aboutgeneticcounselors.org/About-Genetic-Counselors.

To learn more about what genetic counselors do click on the "Patient Resource Site," which can help you find a local genetic counselor and understand what genetic counselors do. You can also find information about the types of genetic testing available and what the results can tell you.

UNDERSTANDING THE TYPES OF DEMENTIA

AIDS Dementia Complex (ADC)

Website: http://hivinsite.ucsf.edu/InSite?page=id-01-08.

The University of California at San Francisco's website dedicated to HIV/AIDS treatment and prevention includes information about dementia related to HIV/AIDS. This information can be helpful in understanding cognitive changes your loved one with AIDS may be experiencing.

Alzheimer's Disease

Website: https://www.alz.org/alzheimers-dementia/what-is-alzheimers.

Learn about what makes Alzheimer's disease a distinct type of dementia with the Alzheimer's Association's "What Is Alzheimer's Disease?" home page, which also includes links to other topics, including symptoms, "plaques and tangles," and research related to Alzheimer's disease.

Creutzfeldt–Jakob Disease (CJD) Dementia

Website: https://www.alz.org/alzheimers-dementia/what-is-dementia/types-of-dementia/creutzfeldt-jakob-disease.

Learn more about this rare but extremely debilitating, rapidly progressing, and fatal dementia caused by infectious particles called prions.

Dementia with Lewy Bodies
Website: https://www.mayoclinic.org/diseases-conditions/lewy-body
-dementia/symptoms-causes/syc-20352025.
      The Mayo Clinic website includes details of symptoms, causes, risk factors, and complications of dementia with Lewy bodies. You will find a link at the bottom of the page regarding care offered at the Mayo Clinic for this type of dementia.

Frontotemporal Lobe Dementia (FTD)
Website: https://memory.ucsf.edu/dementia/ftd.
      The University of San Francisco's Memory and Aging Center website has a wealth of resources, including a video explaining frontotemporal lobe dementia, information on symptoms, types of FTD, and diagnosis. Scroll to the bottom of the page to locate links to numerous other resources for patients and providers, including support groups and key information about participating in research.

Huntington's Disease Dementia
Website: https://www.alz.org/alzheimers-dementia/what-is-dementia/types
-of-dementia/huntington-s-disease.
      This website offers links to information on symptoms, causes, diagnosis, and treatments focused on managing symptoms for Huntington's disease dementia as explained by the Alzheimer's Association.

Mild Cognitive Impairment (MCI)
Website: https://www.alz.org/alzheimers-dementia/what-is-dementia/
related_conditions/mild-cognitive-impairment.
      The Alzheimer's Association website contains an easy-to-understand overview of MCI and ways to manage the condition. The "Learn More" and "Read More" tabs direct readers to more detailed information.

Mixed Dementia
Website: https://www.alzheimercalgary.ca/learn/types-of-dementia/mixed
-dementia.
      The name says it all. The combination of Alzheimer's disease and vascular dementia is the most common form of mixed dementia. This website includes links to a Mixed Dementia factsheet and a brain diagram you can download. You can access them on the righthand side menu.

Multiple Sclerosis Dementia
Website: https://www.dementia.org/multiple-sclerosis-and-dementia.

While we think of Multiple Sclerosis (MS) as mainly impacting muscle movement, it attacks the entire nervous system including the brain. If your loved one has MS, learn more about cognitive changes that may occur and how they differ from other dementia diagnoses.

Parkinson's Disease Dementia
Website: https://www.alz.org/alzheimers-dementia/what-is-dementia/types -of-dementia/parkinson-s-disease-dementia.

The Alzheimer's Association website contains a wealth of information of other dementias, beyond Alzheimer's. Learn more about dementia related to Parkinson's disease, including prevalence, causes, risk factors, symptoms, outcomes, and treatment.

Traumatic Brain Injury (TBI)
Website: https://www.cdc.gov/traumaticbraininjury/index.html.

People who have a TBI, their family members, and health care professionals will find this well-designed Centers for Disease Control website useful. The "Basic Information" tab contains the practical information patients and their family members need.

Vascular Dementia
Website: https://www.mayoclinic.org/diseases-conditions/vascular -dementia/symptoms-causes/syc-20378793.

Learn about the second most common age-related dementia and what differentiates it from other dementias. You will find links to symptoms and causes, as well as diagnosis and treatment. Select a link from the menu bar under the title to find out more.

Wernicke–Korsakoff Syndrome (WKS)
Website: https://rarediseases.org/rare-diseases/wernicke-korsakoff-syndrome/.

WKS is considered a rare disease, and details about it can be found at this link to the Rare Disease Database. If you scroll to the end of the article, there are links and contact information related to investigational studies around WKS, as well as additional resources and supporting organizations.

RESEARCH AND CLINICAL TRIALS

Clinical Trials.gov
Website: https://clinicaltrials.gov.
This database gives details of privately and publicly funded clinical studies conducted around the world. The searchable database can help you find studies being conducted on dementia, including Alzheimer's disease. Use the "Find a Study" section to search for a condition or disease and related trials.

National Institute on Aging (NIA): Clinical Trials
Website: https://www.nia.nih.gov/health/clinical-trials.
This website provides information on the benefits and risks of participating in a clinical trial. The NIA also provides a direct link to help find a clinical trial related to Alzheimer's disease and other dementias: https://www.nia.nih .gov/alzheimers/clinical-trials.

Office for Human Research Protections (OHRP)
Website: https://www.hhs.gov/ohrp/.
This organization provides information about how the rights, welfare, and well-being of human subjects who take part in research studies are protected. The website also provides information on how you can participate in research. In the "I would like info on . . ." section of the website, you can find more information on participating in research.

BEING PREPARED:
ADVANCE DIRECTIVES AND LIVING WILLS

Advance Directives

Advance Directives: Information by State
Website: https://www.aarp.org/caregiving/financial-legal/free-printable-advance-directives/.
The American Association of Retired Persons (AARP) website has a map you can click on to access and download the advance directive forms used in your state. While state forms may differ somewhat, all include recommendations on what to do once you fill out the advance directive forms, including where to keep a copy and who to give copies to.

Advance Directive for Dementia
Website: www.dementia-directive.org.

You will learn how to define what type of care you would want if you were to develop worsening dementia. Starting with mild dementia and progressing to severe dementia, this form defines what can be expected at each stage and allows you to fill in what type of lifesaving care you would or wouldn't want.

Advance Directive Registries
Website: https://www.americanbar.org/groups/law_aging/publications/bifocal/vol_37/issue_6_august2016/tour-of-state-advance-directive-registries/.

Some states have registries where you can upload your advance directive with the idea that it would make it easier for health care providers to locate it. This American Bar Association website explains what a health care advance directive registry is and has links to registries for the dozen states that do have them.

Living Wills
Website: https://www.aarp.org/caregiving/financial-legal/info-2019/what-is-a-living-will.html?intcmp=AE-CAR-LEG-R2-C1.

Find out more about living wills and what to include, as well as how living wills and advance directives are related.

CREATIVITY

Alzheimer's Poetry Project (APP)
Website: http://www.alzpoetry.com/.

Founded by Gary Glazner, APP brings together individuals with dementia, their families, and their caregivers to improve quality of life by fostering creativity through poetry. APP hosts live and online events. Click on the "Events" tab in the top menu.

Dementia Arts: Celebrating Creativity in Eldercare
Website: http://www.dementiaarts.com.

Learn about the Institute of Dementia Arts and Education (IDEA), founded by poet and author Gary Glazner. IDEA uses innovative non-pharmacological creative art interventions to improve the quality of life for people with dementia, as well as their caregivers and families.

The Giving Voice Initiative
Website: https://givingvoicechorus.org.

This initiative creates choral communities to expand the possibilities for individuals living with dementia through music. For information on how to start your own chorus or join an existing chorus, click on the tabs in the top menu.

Meet Me at MoMA
Website: https://www.moma.org/visit/accessibility/meetme/.
The Museum of Modern Art (MoMA) was the trailblazer in bringing creativity and the arts to individuals with Alzheimer's disease and their caregivers. You can find resources on how to create similar programing in your community and learn more about Meet Me at MoMA events.
Follow these links to learn about planning an art outing for you and your family member or exploring art at home:

Outings: https://www.moma.org/visit/accessibility/meetme/practice/families.html#families_artoutings.
At home: https://www.moma.org/visit/accessibility/meetme/practice/families.html#families_artathome.

SENIORS AND DRIVING

Senior Driver Services Resources for Family and Friends
Website: https://seniordriving.aaa.com.
The American Automobile Association (AAA) offers a range of senior driver services and information including how to have conversations with seniors about driving. Click on the link at the top of the website titled "Resources for Family and Friends."

State-by-State Senior Driving Regulations
Website: https://seniordriving.aaa.com.
To find out senior driving regulations for your state, click on the "Know the Licensing Laws in Your State" box in the middle of the AAA website home page.

NOSTALGIA

Cook a Retro Recipe
Website: https://www.thedailymeal.com/cook/best-retro-recipes-gallery.
The website offers delicious and often simple recipes that can bring back good memories, including cinnamon toast, beef stroganoff, and scalloped

potatoes. If your family member had a favorite meal that they talked about you can easily recreate a modern version and bring back some tasty memories.

What Was for Dinner Way Back When?
Website: https://delishably.com/food-industry/A-1940s-Menu-Food-in-the-1940s.
   Put on an apron and whip up some nostalgia in the kitchen. While some foods may better be left in the past, you can create a fun menu based on old favorites and include family members of all ages.

Music and Dementia
Website: https://www.mayoclinic.org/diseases-conditions/alzheimers-disease/expert-answers/music-and-alzheimers/faq-20058173.
   Listening or singing along to music has been shown to provide emotional and behavioral benefits to individuals with dementia and to help relieve stress in their caregivers. Learn more about how to create a singalong that will benefit you and your loved one.

Radio Shows
Website: https://www.oldradioworld.com/.
   Despite the multitude of podcasts available today, the old radio programs still hold up. Maybe your loved one talked about a radio show they loved as a child. Check out this website to see if you can find it and spend time listening together. The old commercials are a hoot!

Vintage Jingles
Website: https://www.youtube.com/watch?v=mLRhsxJ8_GE.
   No matter when you were born, commercial TV and radio jingles stick in your head. To get started with an old-fashioned singalong, have a laugh remembering some old jingles from the 1950s and 1960s. An internet search for "jingles" will pull up more from across the decades.

DINNERTIME RESOURCES

Meals on Wheels America
Website: https://www.mealsonwheelsamerica.org.
   This organization provides nutritious meals to homebound seniors and to senior centers. Volunteers also provide companionship and keep watch over the health and safety of seniors in the community.

Click on the "Find Meals" tab in the website's menu bar to find a Meals on Wheels organization in your community that can assist you and your family members.

Ordering Groceries Online: Delivery and Pickup
Do an internet search for "grocery delivery near me" to find out which local stores will provide home grocery delivery. You can also order groceries online at many stores and then go pick them up without going into the store. Search for "grocery pickup near me" to find your nearest stores.

PLANNING AHEAD:
UNDERSTANDING PALLIATIVE CARE AND HOSPICE

National Hospice and Palliative Care Organization: Caring Information for Patients and Caregivers
Website: https://www.nhpco.org/patients-and-caregivers/.
This is a central website for information on palliative care and hospice. The main landing page is for patients and caregivers and provides direct links to help you and your loved one understand palliative care and hospice options. Some of the links are highlighted below.

What Is Palliative Care?
Website: https://www.nhpco.org/patients-and-caregivers/about-palliative-care/.
This link will lead you to direct responses to your questions about palliative care through a series of FAQs and an explanation of palliative care versus hospice.

Find Palliative Care in Your Area

Palliative Care Provider Directory
Website: https://getpalliativecare.org/provider-directory/.
To help locate a palliative care team in your area, follow this link to a provider directory that you can search by zip code, city, and state.

What Is Hospice?
Website: https://www.nhpco.org/patients-and-caregivers/about-hospice-care/.
This helpful link connects you to information on what hospice is, how to choose a hospice, and how and when hospice starts. A question-and-answer section provides clear responses to frequently asked questions about hospice.

Hospice Knowledge Quiz
Website: https://hospicefoundation.org/hfa/media/Files/8-5x11_booklet_
Hospice_Cagle_Sept1.pdf.

Take the "Hospice Knowledge Quiz" to find out when it may be time for you and your loved one to discuss/consider hospice care. This comprehensive booklet answers a multitude of questions about hospice through "true and false" questions.

FINANCIAL MATTERS MATTER

Guardianship and Conservatorship
Website: https://files.consumerfinance.gov/f/documents/cfpb_msem_court
-appointed-guardians_guide.pdf.

This link provides help for court-appointed guardians of property and conservators. Get expert advice and guidance on how to manage someone else's money with this useful guide.

Elder Law

National Academy of Elder Law Attorneys
Website: www.naela.org.

Need help finding an expert in elder law? Click on "Find a Lawyer" to access a state-by-state directory to get help with estate planning and completing decision-making documents, as well as planning for long-term care.

Reverse Mortgages

Ten Things You Should Know about Reverse Mortgages
Website: https://www.aarp.org/money/credit-loans-debt/info-02-2011/
10-questions-answered-about-reverse-mortgages.html.

This introductory guide to reverse mortgages includes pros and cons to consider before signing any paperwork.

Five Signs a Reverse Mortgage Is a Bad Idea
Website: https://www.investopedia.com/mortgage/reverse-mortgage/
5-signs-reverse-mortgage-bad-idea/.

This is a quick, clear reference guide to assess whether a reverse mortgage is the best choice for you or your loved one.

COSTS OF CARE

Genworth Cost of Care Survey (2019)
Website: https://pro.genworth.com/riiproweb/productinfo/pdf/282102.pdf.
    This report offers information by state comparing the cost of care for in-home caregiving, community and assisted living, and nursing homes. Breakdowns are provided for annual, monthly, and daily costs, as well as hourly costs for in-home care.

Alzheimer's/Dementia Care Costs: Home Care, Adult Day Care, Assisted Living, and Nursing Homes
Website: https://www.dementiacarecentral.com/assisted-living-home-care -costs/.
    This useful cost breakdown by type of care can help you in your decision-making process about care for your loved one. The website includes links to programs that compensate you or another family member who provides care for your loved one with Alzheimer's/dementia.

Search for Assisted Living and Alzheimer's Care by Price
Website: https://www.assistedlivingcosts.org.
    This interactive map allows you to search by state and county to identify different levels of cost for assisted living and Alzheimer's care residences that you can match to you or your loved one's budget.

Payment Options and Financial Assistance for Alzheimer's/Dementia Care
Website: https://www.payingforseniorcare.com/memory-care.
    This comprehensive website has links to all the various payment options including Medicare, Medicaid, and state-based financial assistance, as well as links to finding affordable assisted living and Alzheimer's care and identifying other types of financial assistance. Follow the links under "Table of Contents" and on the righthand sidebar.

HOME CARE AND CAREGIVERS

State-by-State Eldercare Locator
Website: https://eldercare.acl.gov.
    Use this website created by the U.S. Administration on Aging to search by zip code or city/state to find eldercare options and services in your family

member's community. You can also reach the Eldercare Locator by calling 1-800-677-1116 (Monday through Friday, 9 a.m. to 8 p.m. ET).

Caregiving Resources from the American Association of Retired Persons (AARP)
Website: www.aarp.org/home-family/caregiving/.
    This very comprehensive website from AARP is the gateway to a multitude of links related to caregiving, focused on how to find help and support. Follow the link to "AARP Local Caregiver Resource Guides" to find caregivers in your area. There are also links to "Finding LGBT-Friendly Care" and to support groups (click on "Find Support"), as well as information on financial aspects of caregiving and many other topics.

Small Business Ownership Requirements

Guide to Small Business Ownership
Website: http://financesonline.org/small-business-ownership/.
    There's a lot of information here, but click on some key topics like "Getting a Tax Identification Number" and "Filing and Paying Taxes" to get the information you need to keep yourself and your employees legal.

Get Your Employer Identification Number (EIN) / Federal Employer Identification Number (FEIN) Online
Website: https://www.irs.gov/businesses/small-businesses-self-employed/apply-for-an-employer-identification-number-ein-online.
    This step-by-step online guide from the Internal Revenue Service (IRS) provides all the details on how to obtain your EIN/FEIN, including what documentation you need and links to the online application.

Employer's Tax Guide from the Internal Revenue Service (IRS)
Website: https://www.irs.gov/forms-pubs/about-publication-15.
    This comprehensive website explains what forms and information you must obtain from your employees as a small business owner, as well as what you need to report to the IRS each year to avoid penalties.

Form W-4: Employee's Withholding Certificate
Website: https://www.irs.gov/pub/irs-pdf/fw4.pdf.
    This free copy of the W-4 is available from the Internal Revenue Service (IRS). You must ask any employees to fill out this form upon engaging them in employment. It is their opportunity to indicate their current tax situation

to you as their employer. It helps determine how much tax will be withheld from their paychecks.

Form I-9: Employment Eligibility Verification
Website: https://www.uscis.gov/i-9.

Find information about the I-9 and free downloads of the form provided by the U.S. Citizenship and Immigration Services. Employers must verify that their employees have the legal right to work in the United States. You must have all your employees fill out an I-9. They also must provide you with a copy of (and you should ask to see the originals upon hire) of supporting documentation for legal employment. You will find a list of acceptable documents on the last page of the I-9 form, which you can download here: https://www.uscis.gov/i-9-central/form-i-9-acceptable-documents.

Form W-2: Wage and Tax Statement
Website: https://www.irs.gov/forms-pubs/about-form-w-2.

As a small business owner, if you pay an employee more than $600 in any tax year, you must file a W-2 for that employee with the Internal Revenue Service (IRS). For details of what must be reported on the W-2, follow the link above. You can download a copy of a blank W-2 at https://www.irs.gov/pub/irs-pdf/fw2.pdf.

Consequences of Paying Employees under the Table
Website: https://www.irs.gov/compliance/criminal-investigation/employer-and-employee-responsibilities-employment-tax-enforcement.

Paying employees under the table is illegal and punishable by civil and criminal penalties, including fines that would far exceed any savings you think you might make by not paying taxes.

Paying under the table is not the same as paying an employee in cash. You can pay in cash as long as you also pay the required employment taxes. The Internal Revenue Service (IRS) has a step-by-step guide here: https://www.irs.gov/taxtopics/tc756.

ADULT DAY CARE

Medicaid's Adult Day Care / Adult Day Health Care Benefits and Eligibility
Website: https://www.payingforseniorcare.com/medicaid-waivers/adult-day-care.

You will find a state-by-state guide to locating adult day care and a description of Medicaid's benefit for adult day care, as well as other adult day care benefits.

The Older Americans Act
Website: https://www.aarp.org/content/dam/aarp/research/public_policy_
institute/health/2014/the-older-americans-act-AARP-ppi-health.pdf.
Published by the AARP's Public Policy Institute, this document explains what the Older Americans Act provides and offers a history of the act itself.

GERIATRIC CARE MANAGEMENT

What Is a Geriatric Care Manager?
Website: https://www.nia.nih.gov/health/what-geriatric-care-manager.
Find out more about what a geriatric care manager does and how they can help you on your caregiving journey.

Aging Life Care Association (ALCA)
Website: https://www.aginglifecare.org//.
The Aging Life Care Association provides resources for families including how to locate an aging life care professional (another name for geriatric care manager) in your area. Click on the "Find an Aging Life Care Expert" box to search for help in your area.

National Academy of Certified Care Managers (NACCM)
Website: https://www.naccm.net/.
As the certifying body for care managers in the United States, NACCM provides guidelines for qualification as a care manager. It is a good starting point for verifying if the care manager you are thinking of working with has the proper training and credentials.

MEDICARE

Medicare: General Information
Website: https://www.medicare.gov/what-medicare-covers/your-medicare
-coverage-choices/whats-medicare.
It can be daunting to understand just what Medicare is, as the details seem endless. A good starting point can be found at the bottom of this "What's Medicare?" web page. Scroll down to "Not sure what kind of coverage you

have?" to get started figuring out where your loved one stands in relationship to Medicare coverage.

Medicare Hospice Benefit
Website: https://www.medicare.gov/Pubs/pdf/02154-medicare-hospice -benefits.pdf.

This comprehensive downloadable booklet explains Medicare hospice benefits in detail, including who is eligible, what is covered, how to find a hospice provider, and where to get more information.

Aging Services Division: Resources Near You
Website: https://www.hhs.gov/aging/state-resources/index.html.

Click on the link for your state to find out what resources are available to support older adults and their caregivers, including Area Agencies on Aging and State Health Insurance Assistance Programs (SHIPs) that provide counseling and assistance to people with Medicare and their families.

All-Inclusive Eldercare

Programs of All-Inclusive Care for the Elderly (PACE) and Living Independence for the Elderly (LIFE)
Website: https://www.payingforseniorcare.com/medicare/pace_medicare.

Both PACE and LIFE are government programs that can help you find options for caring for your loved one at home. Click on the "Table of Contents" entries to learn more about pros and cons of PACE versus skilled nursing, who can apply, and how to apply, as well as what benefits and services are included in PACE.

PACE/LIFE Program Provider List 2019
Website: https://www.payingforseniorcare.com/medicare/pace_medicare/ provider_list.

Find PACE/LIFE providers in your loved one's community using this provider list updated in June 2019. More up-to-date information may also be found at http://www.pace4you.org.

MEDICAID

Medicaid Eligibility
Website: https://www.hhs.gov/answers/medicare-and-medicaid/who-is -eligible-for-medicaid/index.html.

Understanding Medicaid can be a draconian task; however, this is a good starting point. Under "Who Is Eligible for Medicaid?" you can find out whether the state where your loved one lives has expanded Medicaid and, if so, what you or your loved one may qualify for based on income and family size.

Payment for Family Caregivers

How to Receive Financial Compensation via Medicaid to Provide Care for a Loved One
Website: https://www.medicaidplanningassistance.org/getting-paid-as-caregiver/.

The American Council on Aging site provides a free service to help you understand how to get compensation for caring for your loved one at home. Follow the links to read about Medicaid programs that may apply to your situation and then click on "How to Apply / Getting Started."

VETERANS

Services for Veterans

There are no services offered by the U.S. Department of Veterans Affairs that are specifically for individuals with dementia or Alzheimer's disease. See below for some programs and benefits for veterans that are available and may be helpful, including aid and attendance, respite care, caregiver support, and geriatrics services for veterans.

VA Aid and Attendance: https://www.payingforseniorcare.com/veterans/veterans-pension.

VA Respite Care: https://www.va.gov/GERIATRICS/docs/Respite_Care.pdf.

Veteran's Directed Care Program (VDC): https://www.payingforseniorcare.com/veterans/veterans-directed-hcbs.

Other Geriatric Services for Veterans

VA Community Living Centers: https://www.va.gov/GERIATRICS/docs/Community_Living_Center.pdf.

Community Residential Care Facility: https://www.va.gov/GERIATRICS/pages/community_residential_care.asp.

Adult Day Health Care Center: https://www.va.gov/GERIATRICS/ pages/Adult_Day_Health_Care.asp.

VA Caregiver Support
Website: https://www.caregiver.va.gov/.

This comprehensive website includes everything from how to tell if you are a "caregiver" to what services and resources are available for you if you answer "yes." Self-care for caregivers is vital, and the VA offers information here on a variety of support programs for you and your veteran loved one, as well as information on support groups and other self-care activities for caregivers. Just check the left-hand menu for helpful links.

VA Caregiver Support: Resources for Enhancing All Caregivers Health (REACH)
Website: https://www.caregiver.va.gov/REACH_VA_Program.asp.

The REACH VA Caregiver Program provides assistance to caregivers of veterans on topics that range from self-care and peer support to managing finances and problem solving.

SAFETY AWAY FROM HOME

The Complete Guide to Financial Elder Abuse
Website: https://www.medicareadvantage.com/complete-guide-to-elder -financial-abuse.

In addition to valuable information about what elder abuse is and how to protect yourself or your loved one, you can easily access links to your state and national resources for assistance if you suspect elder abuse.

Adult Protective Services and Elder Abuse Hotline
If you suspect elder abuse of your loved one in any setting, the first thing to do is assure safety and call 911 to request immediate emergency care. If you suspect abuse and you or your loved one are not in immediate danger, you can also call the National Domestic Abuse hotline at 1-800-799-7233.

The following link will provide you with contact information for the Elder Abuse hotline in the state where your loved one lives, as well as contact information for local Adult Protective Services agencies: https://www.care giver.org/adult-protective-services-and-elder-abuse-hotline-1.

National Center on Elder Abuse (NCEA)
Website: https://ncea.acl.gov/Suspect-Abuse.aspx.

This site offers a quick guide to what to do if you suspect abuse of your loved one, including a description of what constitutes elder abuse. Other links are "Get Help" and "Reporting Abuse." You can find a map with direct links to state resources here: https://ncea.acl.gov/Resources/State.aspx. You can also contact the Eldercare Locator at 1-800-677-1116 weekdays. Remember, if it is an immediate safety emergency, call 911.

FUNERAL PLANNING

Funeral Planning Checklist
Website: https://www.agingcare.com/articles/funeral-planning-checklist-145646.htm.
This necessary checklist will help you make decisions with your loved one, or after their death, as to what components of a funeral are wished for and affordable. There is also a breakdown of funeral costs to help make planning for cost easier to understand.

Funeral Consumer Alliance (FCA)
Website: www.funerals.org.
The FCA provides a free complete four-step online guide to funeral planning. Click on "Consumers" and "Learn More" to get started.

Green Burials
Website: https://www.greenburialcouncil.org/.
This website is a one-stop shop for all things "green burial," including how to locate certified cemetery stewards, funeral professionals, and funerary product sellers in your area. An "Interactive Provider Map" allows you to click on your state to locate green burial–certified cemeteries and products. Access the map by clicking on "Find Providers" in the top menu bar.

Urns and Art
Website: http://www.funeria.com.
Funeria's slogan is "Art honors life." Options of how to display ashes after cremation can include beautiful urns that are original works of art. Use this website to help your loved one choose an urn or choose one for them, or why not choose one for yourself while you are at it!

Employment Leave Handbook
Website: https://www.employmentlawhandbook.com/leave-laws/bereavement-leave-laws/.

What are the laws for your state regarding leave from work following the death of a loved one? This helpful site provides a list by state of bereavement leave and the applicable laws.

DEATH, GRIEF, AND EMOTIONAL HEALTH

What to Do When a Loved One Dies Checklist
Website: https://www.aarp.org/home-family/friends-family/info-06-2012/when-loved-one-dies-checklist.html.

This very comprehensive checklist from the American Association of Retired Persons (AARP) can help you keep practical things organized when a loved one dies, starting with what to do immediately and continuing with what to do in the days and weeks to come.

Diversity in Dying: Death across Cultures
Website: https://courses.lumenlearning.com/suny-nursing-care-at-the-end-of-life/chapter/diversity-in-dying-death-across-cultures/.

Sometimes your loved one may be from a different cultural or religious background than yours. This helpful article, written for nurses, is great at explaining common funeral traditions, as well as beliefs about death and dying, across a range of cultures and religious traditions.

Grief: Hospice Foundation of America
Website: https://hospicefoundation.org/Grief-(1).

This site offers useful resources about the grief journey, including how to find a support group, answers to commonly asked questions about grief, and links to helpful articles about grief.

Other Helpful Websites for Grieving
Website: https://griefcounselor.org/resources/helpful-websites/.

The grieving process is unique for each of us. No one can tell you how you should be grieving, but this list of grief programs, resources, and helpful information about the grief process can be a starting point for healing whatever step you may be at on your journey.

Ten Tips to Help You Stop Ruminating
Website: https://www.healthline.com/health/how-to-stop-ruminating#bottom-line.

Once your loved one is gone, you may keep going over in your head things you wish you had said or done. This helpful website provides tips on how to help calm racing thoughts and offers positive advice on taking control back over your thought cycle.

FINANCIAL CHECKLIST AND BENEFIT INFORMATION

Surviving Spouse Financial Checklist
Website: https://www.balancepro.net/education/pdf/survivingspouse.pdf.
    This clear and practical checklist helps you focus on what needs to get done after your spouse or partner dies.

Federal Benefits for Veterans, Dependents, and Survivors
Website: https://www.va.gov/opa/publications/benefits_book/benefits_chap13.asp.
    Information provided here by the Office of Public and Intergovernmental Affairs explains in detail the various benefits for surviving family members of a veteran who dies.

VA Survivors Pension
Website: https://www.va.gov/pension/survivors-pension/.
    Find out if you or your unmarried dependent children qualify for a survivors pension after your veteran spouse dies.

BIBLIOGRAPHY

CHAPTER 1

Schultz, Richard, and Scott R. Beach. "Caregiving as a Risk Factor for Mortality: The Caregiver Health Effects Study." *Journal of the American Medical Association* 282, no. 23 (1999): 2,215. Accessed October 31, 2012. http://jama.jamanetwork.com/article.aspx?articleid=192209.

CHAPTER 2

Schultz, Richard, and Scott R. Beach. "Caregiving as a Risk Factor for Mortality: The Caregiver Health Effects Study." *Journal of the American Medical Association* 282, no. 23 (1999): 2,215. Accessed October 31, 2012. http://jama.jamanetwork.com/article.aspx?articleid=192209.

CHAPTER 3

Alzheimer's Association. "Lewy Body Dementia." Accessed May 21, 2020. https://www.alz.org/alzheimers-dementia/what-is-dementia/types-of-dementia/lewy-body-dementia.
———. "Parkinson's Disease Dementia." Accessed May 21, 2020. https://www.alz.org/alzheimers-dementia/what-is-dementia/types-of-dementia/parkinson-s-disease-dementia.
———. "Stages of Alzheimer's." Accessed May 21, 2020. https://www.alz.org/alzheimers-dementia/stages.
———. "10 Early Signs and Symptoms of Alzheimer's." Accessed May 20, 2020. https://www.alz.org/alzheimers-dementia/10_signs.

———. "2018 Alzheimer's Facts and Figures." Accessed May 21, 2020. https://www .alz.org/media/documents/facts-and-figures-2018-r.pdf.

———. "2019 Alzheimer's Facts and Figures." Accessed May 21, 2020. https://www .alz.org/media/documents/alzheimers-facts-and-figures-2019-r.pdf.

Centers for Disease Control and Prevention. "Creutzfeldt–Jakob Disease, Classic (CJD)." Accessed May 21, 2020. https://www.cdc.gov/prions/cjd/occurrence -transmission.html.

———. "U.S. Burden of Alzheimer's Disease, Related Dementias to Double by 2060." Press release, September 20, 2018. Accessed March 22, 2021. https://www.cdc .gov/media/releases/2018/p0920-alzheimers-burden-double-2060.html.

Geda, Yonas. "Mild Cognitive Impairment in Older Adults." *Current Psychiatry Report* 14, no. 4 (2012): 320–27. Accessed May 20, 2020. https://www.ncbi.nlm.nih.gov/ pmc/articles/PMC3963488/.

Janssen. "Causes of Dementia." Accessed March 15, 2021. https://www.dementia. com/causes.html.

Mayo Clinic. "Huntington's Disease." Accessed May 21, 2020. https://www.mayo clinic.org/diseases-conditions/huntingtons-disease/symptoms-causes/syc-20356117.

National Organization for Rare Disorders. "Wernicke–Korsakoff Syndrome." Accessed May 21, 2020. https://rarediseases.org/rare-diseases/wernicke-korsakoff-syndrome/.

Price, Richard W. "AIDS Dementia Complex." *HIV InSite.* Accessed May 21, 2020. http://hivinsite.ucsf.edu/InSite?page=kb-04-01-03.

Rahn, Kristen, Barbara Slusher, and Adam Kaplin. "Cognitive Impairment in Multiple Sclerosis: A Forgotten Disability Remembered." *Cerebrum* (November–December 2012). Accessed May 21, 2020. https://www.ncbi.nlm.nih.gov/pmc/articles/ PMC3574761/.

U.S. Department of Veterans Affairs. "PTSD: National Center for PTSD." Accessed May 21, 2020. https://www.ptsd.va.gov/understand/related/tbi_ptsd.asp.

Weill Institute for Neurosciences. "Behavioral Variant Frontotemporal Dementia." Accessed May 21, 2020. https://memory.ucsf.edu/dementia/ftd/behavioral-vari ant-frontotemporal-dementia.

———. "Familial FTD." Accessed May 21, 2020. https://memory.ucsf.edu/genetics/ familial-ftd.

CHAPTER 4

Death, John, Adam Douglas, and Rose Anne Kenny. "Comparison of Clock Draw- ing with Mini Mental State Examination as a Screening Test in Elderly Acute Hos- pital Admissions." *Postgraduate Medical Journal* 69, no. 815 (1993): 696. Accessed May 7, 2020. http://europepmc.org/backend/ptpmcrender.fcgi?accid=PMC2399 767&blobtype=pdf.

Internet Stroke Center. "Blessed–Roth Assessment Scale." Accessed March 23, 2021. http://www.strokecenter.org/wp-content/uploads/2011/08/blessed_dementia .pdf.

Medical Xpress. "Blood Test May Accurately Predict Alzheimer's: Study." November 30, 2020. Accessed March 18, 2021. https://medicalxpress.com/news/2020 -11-blood-accurately-alzheimer.html#:~:text=Scientists%20said%20Monday%20 they%20had,fight%20against%20the%20debilitating%20condition.

National Institute on Aging, U.S. Department of Health and Human Services. "Scam Susceptibility May Signal Risk for Cognitive Decline." Published June 6, 2019. Accessed March 25, 2020. https://www.nia.nih.gov/news/scam-susceptibility-may -signal-risk-cognitive-decline.

Office of Civil Rights (OCR), U.S. Department of Health and Human Services. "Summary of the HIPAA Privacy Rule." Last reviewed 2013. Accessed May 6, 2020. https://www.hhs.gov/hipaa/for-professionals/privacy/laws-regulations/index.html.

U.S. Census Bureau. "Population 60 Years and over in the United States." Accessed April 6, 2021. https://data.census.gov/cedsci/table?q=S0102&tid=ACSST1Y2018 .S0102.

CHAPTER 5

American Association of Retired Persons (AARP). "Caregiving in the U.S.: 2020 Report." Accessed March 15, 2021. https://www.aarp.org/content/dam/ aarp/ppi/2020/05/full-report-caregiving-in-the-united-states.doi.10.26419 -2Fppi.00103.001.pdf.

Area Agency on Aging of Pasco-Pinellas (AAAPP). "Are You a Caregiver?" Accessed May 21, 2020. https://agingcarefl.org/wp-content/uploads/2013/04/Intro duction_-_page_1-_12.pdf.

Kreider, Rose M., and Renee Ellis. "Living Arrangements of Children: 2009." *U.S. Census Bureau*, June 2011. Accessed June 2, 2020. https://www.census.gov/ prod/2011pubs/p70-126.pdf.

Stepfamily Foundation. "Stepfamily Statistics." Accessed May 8, 2020. http://www .stepfamily.org/stepfamily-statistics.html.

CHAPTER 6

Alzheimer's Association. "2020 Facts and Figures: Alzheimer's Disease Facts and Figures." Accessed June 1, 2020. https://www.alz.org/media/Documents/alzheimers -facts-and figures_1.pdf.

Bailey, Regan L. "Current Regulatory Guidelines and Resources to Support Research of Dietary Supplements in the United States." *Critical Reviews in Food Science and Nutrition* 60, no. 2 (2020): 298. Accessed June 1, 2020. https://www.ncbi.nlm.nih .gov/pmc/articles/PMC6513729/.

Douglas, David. "Bladder and Dementia Therapy May Be Incompatible." *Reuters*, June 4, 2008. Accessed June 1, 2020. https://www.reuters.com/article/us-bladder-dementia/ bladder-and-dementia-therapy-may-be-incompatible-idUSTON47359520080604.

Jameson, Kevin W. (founder and CEO of the Dementia Society of America). Personal communication with author, May 27, 2020.

Khachiyants, Nina, David Trinkle, Sang Joon Son, and Kye Y. Kim. "Sundown Syndrome in Persons with Dementia: An Update." *Psychiatry Investigation* 8, no. 4 (2011): 275. Accessed June 1, 2020. https://www.ncbi.nlm.nih.gov/pmc/articles/PMC3246134/.

Kosberg, Jordan I. "Preventing Elder Abuse: Identification of High Risk Factors Prior to Placement Decisions." *Gerontologist* 28, no. 1 (1988): 43. Accessed June 1, 2020. https://academic.oup.com/gerontologist/article-abstract/28/1/43/552632.

Maust, Donovan T., Hyungjin Myra Kim, Lisa S. Seyfried, Claire Chiang, Janet Kavanagh, Lon S. Schneider, and Helen C. Kales. "Antipsychotics, Other Psychotropics, and the Risk of Death in Patients with Dementia." *JAMA Psychiatry* 72, no. 5 (May 2015): 438–45. Accessed March 18, 2021. https://doi.org/10.1001/jamapsychiatry.2014.3018.

Mayo Clinic Staff. "Alzheimer's: Managing Sleep Problems." *Mayo Clinic.* Accessed June 1, 2020. https://www.mayoclinic.org/healthy-lifestyle/caregivers/in-depth/alzheimers/art-20047832.

Medicare Advantage. "A Complete Guide to Elder Financial Abuse." Accessed June 1, 2020. https://www.medicareadvantage.com/complete-guide-to-elder-financial-abuse.

National Center on Elder Abuse. "Statistics and Data." Accessed March 18, 2021. https://ncea.acl.gov/About-Us/What-We-Do/Research/Statistics-and-Data.aspx.

National Council on Aging. "Elder Abuse Facts." Accessed June 1, 2020. https://www.ncoa.org/public-policy-action/elder-justice/elder-abuse-facts/.

National Institute on Aging. "Caring for a Person with Alzheimer's Disease: Your Easy-to-Use Guide." Accessed March 17, 2021. https://order.nia.nih.gov/publication/caring-for-a-person-with-alzheimers-disease-your-easy-to-use-guide?_gl=1*ay8x90*_ga*MTI1NDc1ODU4NS4xNjA3NDYxNTkw*_ga_TK3CE80DBZ*MTYxNjUyNjExMy4xMi4xLjE2MTY1MjYzNDEuNjA.

———. "Helping Family and Friends Understand Alzheimer's Disease." Updated May 17, 2017. Accessed June 1, 2020. https://www.nia.nih.gov/health/helping-family-and-friends-understand-alzheimers-disease.

Rosengren, John. "7 Ways to Prevent Financial Elder Abuse." AARP, August 29, 2018. Accessed March 13, 2020. https://www.aarp.org/money/scams-fraud/info-2018/financial-elder-abuse.html.

Stranger, Tobie. "Financial Elder Abuse Costs $3 Billion a Year: Or Is It $36 Billion?" *Consumer Reports,* September 29, 2015. Accessed June 1, 2020. https://www.consumerreports.org/cro/consumer-protection/financial-elder-abuse-costs--3-billion-----or-is-it--30-billion-.

CHAPTER 7

Alzheimer's Association. "Alzheimer's Disease Caregivers Factsheet." Updated March 2020. Accessed May 21, 2020. https://act.alz.org/site/DocServer/caregivers_fact_sheet.pdf?docID=3022.

Associated Counselors and Therapists. "Evaluating Competency." Accessed May 21, 2020. http://www.beachpsych.com/pages/cc97.html.

Centers for Disease Control and Prevention (CDC). "Deaths from Falls among Persons Aged ≥65 Years—United States, 2007–2016." *Morbidity and Mortality Weekly Report (MMWR)*. Accessed April 7, 2021. https://www.cdc.gov/mmwr/volumes/67/wr/mm6718a1.htm.

Centers for Disease Control and Prevention (CDC), National Center for Health Statistics. "Leading Causes of Death." Last reviewed March 17, 2017. Accessed May 21, 2020. https://www.cdc.gov/nchs/fastats/leading-causes-of-death.htm.

Family Caregiving Alliance. "Caregiving." Accessed June 5, 2020. https://www.caregiver.org/caregiving.

Glynn, Sarah Jane. "Breadwinning Mothers Continue to Be the U.S. Norm." *Center for American Progress*, May 10, 2019. Accessed May 21, 2020. https://www.americanprogress.org/issues/women/reports/2019/05/10/469739/breadwinning-mothers-continue-u-s-norm/.

Hausman, Ken. "Competency Evaluations Start with the Five Senses." *Psychiatric News*, May 16, 2003. Accessed June 5, 2020. https://psychnews.psychiatryonline.org/doi/full/10.1176/pn.38.10.0034.

Lund, Dale A., Rebecca L. Utz, Michael S. Caserta, Scott D. Wright, Sarah M. Llanque, Chris Lindfelt, Herb Shon, Carol J. Whitlatch, and Julian Montoro-Rodriquez. "Time for Living and Caring: An Intervention to Make Respite More Effective for Caregivers." *International Journal of Aging and Human Development* 79, no. 2 (2014): 157. Accessed May 22, 2020. https://www.ncbi.nlm.nih.gov/pmc/articles/PMC4388419/.

Medicare Advantage. "A Complete Guide to Elder Financial Abuse." Accessed June 1, 2020. https://www.medicareadvantage.com/complete-guide-to-elder-financial-abuse.

Nolo. "Conservatorships and Adult Guardianships." Accessed May 22, 2020. https://www.nolo.com/legal-encyclopedia/conservatorships-adult-guardianships-30063.html.

Seniorliving. "1900–2000: Changes in Life Expectancy in the United States." Updated July 25, 2019. Accessed May 21, 2020. https://www.seniorliving.org/history/1900-2000-changes-life-expectancy-united-states/.

Vandergriendt, Carla. "What to Know about Palliative Care." *Healthline.* Reviewed January 9, 2020. Accessed May 22, 2020. https://www.healthline.com/health/palliative-care#what-is-it.

CHAPTER 8

Alzheimer's Association New Mexico. "Thursday Art Project." Accessed May 23, 2020. https://docplayer.net/52735647-Thursday-art-project-page-13-summer-2014.html.

Glazner, Gary. *Dementia Arts: Celebrating Creativity in Elder Care.* Baltimore, MD: Health Professions Press, 2014.

Miller, Bruce L. "Dementia and Creativity." Vimeo video, 50:43. Recorded November 30, 2009. https://vimeo.com/14395155.

Together in This. "Alive with Alzheimer's: A Skydiving Adventure." Accessed April 5, 2021. https://togetherinthis.com/alive-alzheimers-skydiving-adventure/.

U.S. Senate Special Committee on Aging. "Fighting Fraud: Senate Aging Committee Identifies Top 10 Scams Targeting Our Nation's Seniors." Accessed April 5, 2021. https://www.aging.senate.gov/imo/media/doc/Fraud%20Book%202017.pdf.

Online Resources

Alzheimer Poetry Project: http://www.alzpoetry.com/.

CHAPTER 9

Internal Revenue Service. "About Form W-2, Wage and Tax Statement." Accessed May 14, 2020. https://www.irs.gov/forms-pubs/about-form-w-2.

———. "Topic No. 751: Social Security and Medicare Withholding Rates." Accessed May 14, 2020. https://www.irs.gov/taxtopics/tc751.

Online Resources

I-9 form and acceptable documents: https://www.uscis.gov/i-9-central/acceptable -documents; https://www.medicare.gov/what-medicare-covers/your-medicare -coverage-choices/whats-medicare.

Small business ownership: http://www.irs.gov/businesses/small/article/0,,id=99021,00 .html; https://www.dol.gov/agencies/oasam/orientation/forms/new-employee (Office of the Assistant Secretary for Administration and Management, forms for new employees; this link will take you to the I-9 Employee Eligibility Verification and the W-4 Federal Withholding forms); https://www.irs.gov/pub/irs-pdf/fss4.pdf (application for an Employer Identification Number; you can apply for your EIN/ FEIN Tax ID [SS-4] here).

W-4 forms: https://www.irs.gov/pub/irs-pdf/fw4.pdf (what they are and where to find them free online).

CHAPTER 10

Betty Crocker's Cooky Book. New York: General Mills, 1963.

Merriam-Webster, s.v. "Umami." Accessed May 9, 2020. https://www.merriam-web ster.com/dictionary/umami.

Raman, Ryan. "How Your Nutritional Needs Change as You Age." *Healthline*, September 5, 2017. Accessed May 9, 2020. https://www.healthline.com/nutrition/nutritional-needs-and-aging.

Sollitto, Marlo. "Why Seniors' Tastes Change with Age." *Aging Care*. Accessed May 9, 2020. https://www.agingcare.com/articles/loss-of-taste-in-the-elderly-135240.htm.

Weiss, Toby. "Caring for Holocaust Survivors and Survivors of Other Traumatic Events at the End of Life." *National Hospice and Palliative Care Organization*. Palliative Care Resource Series, 2016. Accessed May 9, 2020. https://www.nhpco.org/wp-content/uploads/2019/04/PALLIATIVECARE_Holocaust_Survivors.pdf.

Online Resources

Alzheimer's Disease Education and Referral (ADEAR) Center: https://www.nia.nih.gov/health/about-adear-center.

Meals on Wheels America: https://www.mealsonwheelsamerica.org. (Provides nutritious meals to homebound seniors and to senior centers. Volunteers also provide companionship and keep watch over the health and safety of seniors in the community. Click on the "Find Meals" tab in the website's menu bar to find a Meals on Wheels organization in your community that can assist you and your family members.)

CHAPTER 11

American Association of Retired Persons (AARP). "New State Law to Help Family Caregivers." Accessed May 19, 2020. https://www.aarp.org/politics-society/advocacy/caregiving-advocacy/info-2014/aarp-creates-model-state-bill.html.

Centers for Disease Control and Prevention (CDC). "Preparing for COVID-19 in Nursing Homes." Accessed March 30, 2020. https://www.cdc.gov/coronavirus/2019-ncov/healthcare-facilities/prevent-spread-in-long-term-care-facilities.html.

Dementia Care Central. "The Role of Antipsychotics to Control Disruptive Behavior with Dementia." Last updated August 2, 2019. Accessed May 19, 2020. https://www.dementiacarecentral.com/aboutdementia/treating/antipsychotics.

Fredriksen-Goldsen, Karen I., Hyun-Jun Kim, Charles A. Emlet, Anna Muraco, Elena A. Erosheva, Charles P. Hoy-Ellis, Jayn Goldsen, and Heidi Petry. "The Aging and Health Report: Disparities and Resilience among Lesbian, Gay, Bisexual, and Transgender Older Adults." *Seattle: Institute for Multigenerational Health*, 2011. Accessed May 19, 2020. https://depts.washington.edu/agepride/wordpress/wp-content/uploads/2012/10/Executive_Summary10-25-12.pdf.

Medicare. "PACE." Accessed May 18, 2020. https://www.medicare.gov/your-medicare-costs/get-help-paying-costs/pace.

National Center for Assisted Living (NCAL). "Assisted Living." Accessed May 18, 2020. https://www.ahcancal.org/ncal/Pages/index.aspx.

National LGBTQ Task Force. "LGBT Elders Raise Serious Fears about Long-Term Care Facilities." Accessed May 19, 2020. https://www.thetaskforce.org/lgbt-elders-raise-serious-fears-about-long-term-care-facilities/.

National Senior Citizens Law Center (NSCLC), National Gay and Lesbian Task Force (NGLTF), SAGE (Services and Advocacy for LGBT Elders), Lambda Legal, National Center for Lesbian Rights (NCLR), and National Center for Transgender Equality. "LGBT Older Adults in Long-Term Care Facilities." Accessed May 19, 2020. https://www.lgbtagingcenter.org/resources/pdfs/NSCLC_LGBT_report.pdf.

U.S. Department of Veterans Affairs. "VA Nursing Homes, Assisted Living, and Home Health Care." Accessed May 18, 2020. https://www.va.gov/health-care/about-va-health-benefits/long-term-care/.

CHAPTER 12

Centers for Disease Control and Prevention (CDC). "Viral Hepatitis Statistics: Health-care-Associated Hepatitis B and C Outbreaks (≥ 2 Cases) Reported to the Centers for Disease Control and Prevention (CDC) 2008–2016." Accessed April 22, 2020. https://www.cdc.gov/hepatitis/statistics/healthcareoutbreaktable.htm.

Hawes, Catherine. "Elder Abuse in Residential Long-Term Care Settings: What Is Known and What Information Is Needed?" In *Elder Mistreatment: Abuse, Neglect, and Exploitation in an Aging America*, edited by Richard J. Bonnie and Robert B. Wallace, 14. Washington, DC: National Academies Press, 2003. Accessed May 20, 2020. https://www.ncbi.nlm.nih.gov/books/NBK98786/.

National Center on Elder Abuse (NCEA). "Nursing Home Abuse Risk Prevention Profile and Checklist." 2005. Accessed May 20, 2020. http://www.aaaceus.com/courses/NL1008/Article6.pdf.

Nursing Home Abuse Center. "Understanding Nursing Home Abuse." Accessed May 20, 2020. https://www.nursinghomeabusecenter.com/nursing-home-abuse/.

"*The Twilight Zone* Intro." YouTube video, 0:34. Posted July 31, 2008. Accessed May 20, 2020. https://www.youtube.com/watch?v=cxf_Dvy0VLs.

CHAPTER 13

Alzheimer's Association. "Feeding Issues in Advanced Dementia" (2015). Accessed May 11, 2020. https://www.alz.org/media/Documents/feeding-issues-statement.pdf.

Compassus. "Hospice Eligibility for Adult Failure to Thrive." Accessed May 11, 2020. https://www.compassus.com/healthcare-professionals/determining-eligibility/adult-failure-to-thrive.

Crisis Prevention Institute. "The Adapted FAST: Introduction and Application." Accessed May 11, 2020. https://www.crisisprevention.com/Blog/The-Adapted-FAST-Introduction-and-Application.

Crossroads Hospice and Palliative Care. "Renal Disease Hospice Eligibility Criteria." Accessed May 11, 2020. https://www.crossroadshospice.com/hospice-care/hospice-eligibility-criteria/renal-disease/.

Lynch, Matthew C. "Is Tube Feeding Futile in Advanced Dementia?" *Linacre Quarterly* 83, no. 3 (August 2016): 283. Accessed May 11, 2020. https://www.ncbi.nlm.nih.gov/pmc/articles/PMC5102197/.

National Hospice and Palliative Care Organization. "Hospice Volunteering Worth over $469 Million Annually Reports NHPCO." Published April 5, 2019. Accessed May 11, 2020. https://www.globenewswire.com/news-release/2019/04/05/1797674/0/en/Hospice-Volunteering-Worth-Over-469-Million-Annually-Reports-NHPCO.html.

———. "NHPCO Releases Updated Edition of Hospice Facts and Figures Report." Accessed May 11, 2020. https://www.nhpco.org/nhpco-releases-updated-edition-of-hospice-facts-and-figures-report/.

Reisberg, B., E. Franssen, S. Hasan, et al. "Retrogenesis: Clinical, Physiologic, and Pathologic Mechanisms in Brain Aging, Alzheimer's, and other Dementing Processes." *European Archives of Psychiatry and Clinical Neurosciences* 249, no. S28–S36 (1999). Accessed April 5, 2021. https://doi.org/10.1007/PL00014170.

CHAPTER 14

Axelrod, Julie. "The 5 Stages of Grief and Loss." *PsychCentral.* Last updated November 20, 2019. Accessed May 17, 2020. https://psychcentral.com/lib/the-5-stages-of-loss-and-grief/.

Burgess, Lana. "What Are the Signs That Someone Is Close to Death?" *Medical News Today.* Reviewed January 31, 2020. Accessed May 16, 2020. https://www.medicalnewstoday.com/articles/320794#is-death-near.

Caba, Justin. "Can Coma Patients Hear You? Families Should Tell Stories to Loved Ones in a Coma." *Medical Daily*, January 23, 2015. Accessed May 16, 2020. https://www.medicaldaily.com/can-coma-patients-hear-you-families-should-tell-stories-loved-ones-coma-319148.

CBC News. "Beyond the Scalpel: Why 'Virtual' Autopsies May Be the Way of the Future." Last updated October 4, 2018. Accessed May 17, 2020. https://www.cbc.ca/news/health/minimally-invasive-autopsy-ct-mri-1.4850464.

Karnes, Barbara. *Gone from My Sight.* RN End of Life Educational Materials, 2005. Accessed May 16, 2020. https://bkbooks.com/products/gone-from-my-sight-the-dying-experience.

Potts, Leanne. "Smart Ways to Cover the Cost of a Funeral." *AARP*, November 27, 2017. Accessed May 17, 2020. https://www.aarp.org/home-family/friends-family/info-2017/funeral-payment-options-fd.html.

Schulz, Richard, Randy Hebert, and Kathrin Boerner. "Bereavement after Caregiving." *Geriatrics* 63, no. 1 (2008): 20. Accessed May 17, 2020. https://www.ncbi.nlm.nih.gov/pmc/articles/PMC2790185/.

Steinhauser, Karen E., Elizabeth C. Clipp, and Maya McNeilly. "In Search of a Good Death: Observations of Patients, Families, and Providers." *Annals of Internal Medicine*

132, no. 10 (2000): 825. Accessed May 17, 2020. https://www.acpjournals.org/doi/10.7326/0003-4819-132-10-200005160-00011.

U.S. Department of Veterans Affairs. "Eligibility for Burial in a VA National Cemetery." Accessed May 17, 2020. https://www.va.gov/burials-memorials/eligibility/.

CHAPTER 15

U.S. Department of Veterans Affairs. "Eligibility for Veterans Pension." Accessed May 15, 2020. https://www.va.gov/pension/eligibility/.

INDEX

Page references for tables and worksheets are italicized; t = table; w = worksheet.

345

CPSIA information can be obtained
at www.ICGtesting.com
Printed in the USA
BVHW031044300821
615079BV00012B/5

9 781633 886940